Indian Army
MER NURSING ASSISTANT
Recruitment EXAM

Indian Army MER NURSING ASSISTANT Recruitment EXAM

Author
Major RD Ahluwalia

arihant
Arihant Publications (India) Ltd.

arihant

ARIHANT PUBLICATIONS (INDIA) LIMITED

Administrative & Production Offices

Regd. Office

'Ramchhaya' 4577/15, Agarwal Road, Darya Ganj, New Delhi -110002
Tele: 011- 47630600, 43518550

Head Office

Kalindi, TP Nagar, Meerut (UP) - 250002
Tel: 0121-7156203, 7156204

Sales & Support Offices

Agra, Ahmedabad, Bengaluru, Bareilly, Chennai, Delhi, Guwahati, Hyderabad, Jaipur, Jhansi, Kolkata, Lucknow, Nagpur & Pune.

ISBN 978-93-24193-91-9

PRICE ₹195.00

Published by Arihant Publications (India) Ltd.

For further information about the books published by Arihant, log on to www.arihantbooks.com or e-mail at info@arihantbooks.com

Follow us on

CONTENTS

ALL ABOUT

Indian Army MER Nursing Assistant

ELIGIBILITY CRITERIA *(only for Females)*

Age	Height	Educational Qualification
17.5 to 23	152 cm	10 + 2/ Intermediate Examination passed in Science with Physics, Chemistry, Maths and English with 50% marks in aggregate and 40% marks in each subject.

SELECTION PROCESS

During recruitment rally, first of all documents will be verified. After verification, the following tests will be conducted:

1. Written Exam (Computer Based)
2. Interview & Document Check
3. Medical Test

The tests mentioned below are mandatory for all :

1. PAPER PATTERN

S.N.	Subject	Questions	Marks	Passing Marks
1	GK & Reasoning	10	40	80
2	Maths	5	20	
3	Physics	5	20	
4	Biology	15	60	
5	Chemistry	15	60	

2. INTERVIEW

Candidates selected in Online Examination will be called for interview and document verification

3. MEDICAL TEST

(i) As per laid down medical standards at the Rally Site.

(ii) Unfit candidates will be referred to MH/CH/BH for specialist review. Candidates referred for specialist review should present themselves to the nominated MH/CH/BH within 14 days of the referral and report back to ARO for issue of Admit Cards for CEE, in case declared FIT.

SYLLABUS

GENERAL KNOWLEDGE

The test will include questions related to India and its neighbouring countries especially pertaining to History, Culture, Geography and who's who. In addition Abbreviations, Sports, Awards and Prizes, Terminology, Indian Armed Forces, Continents and Sub-continents, Inventions and Discoveries, The Constitution of India, International Organisations, Books and Authors, Knowledge of Important events that have happened in India and at world level in the recent years, Current important world events, Prominent personalities etc.

MATHEMATICS

According to class 10 syllabus.

PHYSICS

Physical Properties and States of Matter, Mass, Weight, Volume, Density and Specific Gravity, Principle of Archimedes, Pressure Barometer, Motion of objects, Velocity and Acceleration, Newton's Laws of Motion, Force and Momentum, Parallelogram of Forces, Stability and Equilibrium of bodies, Gravitation, Elementary ideas of work, Power and Energy, Heat and its Effects, Sound waves and their properties, Reflection and refraction, Spherical mirrors and Lenses, Type and properties of magnet, Static and Current Electricity, Conductors and Non-conductors, Ohm's Law, Simple Electrical Circuits, Heating.

BIOLOGY

Basic Biology, Life Process, Study of Birds, Human Beings, Uniqueness of human body, Food and Health, Necessity of balanced diet, Wasteful Food Practices, Food Yield, Essentials for good health, Cycles of materials, Ecological balance, Living resources, Habitat and Organisms, Adaptation.

CHEMISTRY

Physical and Chemical changes, Elements, Mixtures and Compounds, Symbols, Formulae and simple Chemical Equations, Law of Chemical Combination, Properties of Air and Water, Preparation and Properties of Hydrogen, Oxygen, Nitrogen and Carbondioxide, Oxidation and Reduction, Acids, Bases and Salts, Carbon and its forms, Natural and Artificial Fertilizers, Elementary ideas about the Structure of Atom, Atomic, Equivalent and Molecular Weights, Valency.

Types of Questions

Asked in Exam and Sample Questions*

General Knowledge

Though as per syllabus, this section is in examination, 10 questions will be asked from this section including reasoning.

- After analysing previous papers, it has been concluded that rare questions are asked from History, Geography and Constitution till now.
- Majority of questions are asked from Sports, Culture, Static GK like Books and Author, Country and Capital etc.
- Sometimes 1-2 Question are also asked from current affairs.

Sample Questions

1. Who elects the Deputy Chairman of the Rajya Sabha?
   (a) Loksabha and Rajya Sabha
   (b) Vice President
   (c) Lok Sabha
   (d) Rajya Sabha
2. Which religion was started by Akbar ?
   (a) Deen-e-elahi (b) Buddhism
   (c) Muslim (d) Sufi
3. Where is the location of HQ 'SAARC' ?
   (a) Kabul
   (b) Dhaka
   (c) Islamabad
   (d) Kaathmandu

Note Though only 1-2 questions are be asked from this section but candidate must be required of proper knowledge and practice of basic reasoning chapters.

Mathematics

- Questions asked from this section are easy to moderate, means, out of 5 questions, questions are easy and some questions are moderate in level.

Sample Questions

4. The print price of an article is Rs 125, if 8% discount is given on it then selling price is ....
   (a) 110 (b) 118
   (c) 115 (d) 120
5. Area of a Trapezium is ....
   (a) $b \times h$
   (b) $1/2(b \times h)$
   (c) $1/2(a+b) \times h$
   (d) $1/2\ (d_1 \times d_2)$
6. The sum of the ages of Rinku and Gopal is 40 yr. 5 yr hence, the ratio of their ages will be 3 : 7. The age of Rinku is ?
   (a) 10 yr (b) 25 yr
   (c) 30 yr (d) 15 yr

Physics

- This section is most important from examination point of view as 5 questions are asked from this section.
- Questions asked from this section generally covers entire syllabus.
- As type of question is concerned, questions are asked either directly from theory, formulae or numericals.
- Sometimes 2-3 questions of applied type also has been asked.
- Mostly questions have been asked from various topics viz; Mass, Weight, Volume, Motion, Laws of Motion, Archimede's Principal, Force, Work, Power and Energy, Heat, Waves, Ohm's Law, Magnet and Current Electricity etc.

Sample Questions

7. Sound of frequency below 20 Hz is called ....?
   (a) Infrasonic sound
   (b) Audio sounds
   (c) Ultrasonic sound
   (d) Supersonic sound

8. Dyne is a unit of ....
   (a) Momentum (b) Power
   (c) Work (d) Force

9. If a car travels a distance of 100 km & it takes 25 minutes to reach its destination, the speed of the car is ....
   (a) 4 km/min
   (b) 400 m/min
   (c) 4 m/min
   (d) None of these

Biology

- This section is most important from examination point of view as 15 questions are asked from this section.

Sample Questions (Official)

10. Synagamy is fusion of two ....
    (a) Gametic nuclei (b) Nuclei
    (c) Gametes (d) Cells

11. The essential organs for reproduction in a flower are ....
    (a) Stamens and Pistils
    (b) Petals and pistils
    (c) Sepal and stamens
    (d) Sepals and Petals

12. Vascular Cambium is a type of ....
    (a) Lateral meristem
    (b) Intercalary meristem
    (c) Apical meristem
    (d) Permanent or mature meristem

Chemistry

- 15 questions will be asked from this section.
- Type of question from this section till now has been asked either based on direct chemical formulae, symbol or direct theory.
- Sometimes 2-3 questions also has been asked based on chemical equations, applied questions, and numerical problems.
- Most of the topics of syllabus like Physical and Chemical Changes, Mixture and Compound, Symbols and Formulae, Carbon and its Compound, Atom, Molecular Weight, have been asked in the examination on regular basis.

Sample Questions (Official)

13. Thomson model of atom is also known as
    (a) Raisin pudding model
    (b) Plum pudding model
    (c) All
    (d) Watermelon model

14. Galvanised iron sheets have a coating of :
    (a) Zinc (b) Tin
    (c) Lead (d) Chromium

15. Nessler's reagent is given by ....
    (a) Hg_2I_2 (b) K_2HgI_4
    (c) KI_3 (d) $Au(CN)_2$

Promotion & Other Areas for Entry in Indian Army

Subedar Major

Subedar

Naib Subedar

Havaldar

Naik

Sepoy

Catering JCO (ASC)

Age - 21 - 27 Years

Qualifications - 10+2 with Diploma in Hotel Management & Catering Technology

Havaldar (Education)

Age - 21 - 25 Years

Qualifications - For Group X- MA/MSc/MCA or BA/BSc/BCA with BEd BSc(IT) for Group Y - BSc/BA/BCA (IT) without BEd

Surveyor Auto Carto (Engineers)

Age - 20 - 25 Years

Qualifications - BA/BSc with Maths 10+2 (Math & Science)

Religious Teacher (JCO)

Age - 27-34 Years

Qualifications - Graduate + He is qualified in his religion

Soldier General Duty

Age - 17½ - 21 Years

Qualifications - 10th pass with 45% & each subject must contain 33%

Soldier Clerk/Store Keeper

Age - 17½ - 23 Years

Qualifications - 10+2 pass (60% marks) (Each subject must have 50% marks) with Maths & English

Soldier Tech

Age - 17½ - 23 Years

Qualifications - 10+2 pass (50% Marks) (Each subject must have 40% marks) with Physics, Chemistry, Maths

Soldier Nursing Assistant/ Tech (RVC)

Age - 17½ - 23 Years

Qualifications - 10+2 pass (50% Marks) (Each subject must have 40% marks) with Physics, Chemistry, Biology

Soldier Tradesman

Age - 17½ - 23 Years

Qualifications - 10th / ITI and 8th pass (for some trades)

For Officer Entry

General

Lt General

Major General

Brigadier

Colonel

Lt Colonel

Major

Captain

Lieutenant

TGC (Education)
Age - 23 - 27 Years
Qualifications - MA/MSc in 1st or 2nd division

UES
Age - 18-24 Years
Qualifications - Pre Final Student of Engineering Degree Course

TGC
Age - 21-27 Years
Qualifications - BE / B.Tech streams of Engineering / B.Arch MSc computer

JAG (Men & Women)
Age - 21-27 Years
Qualifications - Law Graduate LLB with 55% marks Registered with Bar Council of India / State

National Defence Academy
Age - 16½-19½ Years
Qualifications - 10+2

10+2 Tech
Age - 16½-19½ Years
Qualifications - 10+2 (70% marks with PCM)

Indian Military Academy
(Non Tech)
Age - 19-24 Years
Qualifications - Graduate

Short Sevice Commission
(Non Tech)
Age - 19-25 Years
Qualifications - Graduate

Short Sevice Commission
(Tech Men & Women)
Age - 19-27 Years
Qualifications - BE/BTech stream of Engineering/B.Arch, MSC Computer

NCC Special (Men & Women)
Age - 19-25 Years
Qualifications - Graduate 50% aggregate "A" or "B" grade in NCC "C" certificate

GENERAL KNOWLEDGE

Chapter 01

History of India

Ancient India

Indus Valley Civilisation (2500 BC – 1750 BC)

- Harappan civilisation named by John Marshall after the first discovered site Harappa in 1921 by Dayaram Sahni. It was an urban civilisation.
- In this civilisation people were familiar with gold, silver, bronze, lead and copper, but iron was not know to them.
- Indus people first produced cotton which the Greeks termed as **Sindon.**

Major Indus Valley Sites

Name of Sites	Years	Excavators	Location
Harappa	1921	Dayaram Sahni	Pakistan
Mohenjodaro (Mound of Dead)	1922	RD Bannerjee	Pakistan
Chanhudaro	1931	N Gopal Majumdar	Pakistan
Kalibangan	1955	A Ghosh	India (Rajasthan)
Lothal	1955-1960	SR Rao	India (Gujarat)
Banawali	1974	RS Bisht	India (Haryana)
Dholavira	1990	RS Bisht	India (Gujarat)

Vedic Period (1500 BC – 600 BC)

- It was a rural civilisation and started with the arrival of Aryans in Indian subcontinent from Central Asia.
- They settled in Afghanistan, Pakistan and India. This region is known as the land of seven rivers or *Sapta Sindhu.*

Four Vedas

Veda	Important Facts
Rig Veda (oldest Veda)	▪ Collection of Hymns ▪ Contains 10 Mandals and Gayatri Mantra
Sama Veda	▪ Book of Mantra related to music
Yajur Veda	▪ Book of sacrificial prayers
Atharva Veda	▪ Book of magical formulae

- 'Satyameva Jayate' (Truth alone triumps) is taken from **Mundkopanishad**.

Buddhism

- Gautam Buddha founded Buddhism. He established eight fold path-'Ashtangika Marg'. Alara Kalama was his first teacher.
- 'Tripitakas' i.e. are the most important Buddhist texts-Sutta Pitaka, Vinaya Pitaka and Abhidhama Pitaka.

Gautam Buddha : At a glance

▪ Birth	In 563 BC at Lumbini (Nepal)
▪ Family Members	Father-Suddhodhana, Mother-Mahamaya (Kosala dynasty), Wife-Yashodhara, Son-Rahul
▪ Renunciation/Mahabhi nish-kramana	At the age of 29 years
▪ Enlightment/Nirvana	At the age of 35 years at Uruvella (Bodh Gaya) under pipal tree on the bank of Niranjana river.
▪ Dharmachakra Pravartana (Symbol-Wheel)	At Sarnath to his five disciples
▪ Death/Mahaparinirvana	In 483 BC at Kushinagar

Jainism

There were 24 tirthankaras, Rishabhdev being the 1st and Mahavira being the last.

Mahavira : At a glance

Birth	In 540 BC in a village Kundalgram near Vaishali in Bihar
Family Members	Father-Siddharth a Mother-Trishala (Lichchhavi Princess and sister of Chetak) Wife-Yashoda, Daughter-Priyadarshana
Renunciation	At the age of 30
Kaivalya (Supreme knowledge)	At the age of 42, under a sal tree at Jambhikagram on the bank of river Rijupalika
First Sermon	At Pavapuri to his 11 disciples known as Gandharas
Death	In 436 BC at Pavapuri

Mahajanapadas

The Anguttara Nikaya (Buddhist Literature) and Bhagavi Sutta (Jain Literature) mention the list of 16 Mahajanapadas.

Magadha Empire

- Magadha was one of the most powerful Mahajanapadas.
- **Bimbisara** was the founder of **Haryanka dynasty**. Magadha came into prominent under the leadership of Bimbisara.
- **Ajatashatru** was the son of Bimbisara and occupied the throne by killing his father.
- **Udayin**, son of Ajatashatru, founded the city of Pataliputra and shifted the capital of Magadha from Rajagriha to Pataliputra.
- **Naga Dasak** was the last ruler of Haryanka dynasty.
- **Shishunaga** was the founder of Shishunaga dynasty. He was succeeded by Kalashoka and Nandivarman.
- **Mahapadmananda** was the founder of the Nanda dynasty.
- The last Nanda king **Dhanananda** ruled Magadha during the Alexander's invasion of India.

Alexander's Invasion (326 BC)

- Alexander of Macedonia fought the 'Battle of Vitasta' or 'Battle of Hydaspes' with Porus (ruler of India) to conquer Indian territory.
- This battle was fought on the bank of river Jhelum.
- He failed to conquer India and died in 323 BC at Babylon.

Mauryan Empire (322-185 BC)

- **Chandragupta Maurya**, assisted by Chanakya overthrew Dhanananda to lay the foundation of Maurayan dynasty.
- During his region Megasthenese wrote **Indica** and Kautilya (Vishnugupta, Chanakya) wrote **Arthashastra**.
- **Bindusara** son and successor of Chandragupta Maurya was famous as Amitroghata.
- **Ashoka** was a great ruler, he succeeded Bindusara. He fought Kalinga war in 261 BC.
  It was the last war fought by Ashoka.
- His Rock Edict XIII talked about Kalinga war. Ashoka is also called Devanampriya and Piyadasi.
- Sanchi stupa was built by Ashoka.
- **Brihadratha** was the last Mauryan ruler.

The Gupta Age (AD 319-AD 540)

- **Sri Gupta** was the founder of this dynasty who was succeeded by **Ghatotkachh.**
- **Chandra Gupta-I** was first Gupta ruler to assume the title of Maharajadhiraj.He started Gupta Era in AD 319-20.
- **Samudragupta** is also called 'Napoleon of India' by VA Smith. His court poet Harisena composed Prayag Prashasti (Allahabad Pillar Inscription).
- **Chandragupta-II** (Vikramaditya) was a great ruler of Gupta dynasty. Mehrauli Iron Pillar (near Qutub Minar, Delhi) is dedicated to him. The famous poet Kalidasa (also known Shakespeare of India) lived in his court.
  Fa-hien, a chinese pilgrim, visited his court.
- **Kumaragupta-I** founded Nalanda Mahavihara.
- **Skandagupta** repaired Sudarshan lake. Gupta empire was attacked by Huns during his reign.
- After Guptas, the most powerful ruler was Harshavardhana of **Pushyabhuti dynasty.**
- His capital was Kannauj and Hieun Tsang visited during his reign.

Medieval India

Muslim Invasions in India

- **Mohammad Bin Qasim** was the first Muslim invader. He invaded India in AD 712.
- **Mahmud Ghaznavi** was the first Turkish invader. He invaded India in AD 998. He led 17 expeditions to India and destroyed Somnath temple in AD 1025.
- **Mohammad Ghori** was defeated by Prithviraj Chauhan III in first Battle of Tarain (1191).
- He was defeated him in second Battle of Tarain (1192). After his death, his slave Qutubuddin Aibak established Delhi Sultanate.

Delhi Sultanate

Slave Dynasty (AD 1206-90)

- **Qutubuddin Aibak** founded Slave dynasty. He started the construction of Qutub Minar (Delhi). He died while playing Chaugan or Polo in AD 1206 at Lahore.
- **Iltutmish** was the slave of Aibak. He introduced silver coin (tanka) and copper coin (jittal), and completed the construction of Qutub Minar.
- **Razia Sultan** was the daughter of Iltutmish and the first woman emperor of India.
- **Ghiyasuddin Balban** took the title of Zil-i-Ilahi. He introduced Sijda and Pabos (forms of salutation).
- **Kaiqubad** was the last ruler of Slave dynasty.

Khilji Dynasty (AD 1290-1320)

- **Jalaluddin Khilji** was the founder of Khilji dynasty.
- **Alauddin Khilji** proclaimed 'Kingship knows to kinship'. He introduced Dagh (branding of horse) and Chehra (descriptive role of soldiers). He also introduced market reforms. He built Alai Darwaja (Delhi).
- **Malik Kafur** was the chief of Military under Alauddin Khilji and was given the title 'Hazar Dinari'.

Tughlaq Dynasty (AD 1320-1414)

- **Ghiyasuddin Tughlaq** was the founder of the Tughlaq dynasty.
- **Mohammad Bin Tughlaq** transferred capital from Delhi to Devagiri (later named Daulatabad). He also introduced tocken currency.
- **Firoz Shah Tughlaq** made Jaziya as a separate tax. He also imposed water tax (Hasil-i-Sharb). He built many canals and established a hospital (Dar-ul-Shifa) at Delhi.
- Timur, the lame, was a Turkish chief. He invaded India in AD 1398 during the reign of **Muhammad Shah Tughlaq.**

Lodhi Dynasty (AD 1451-1526)

- **Bahlol Lodhi** founded this dynasty. It was the first Afghan dynasty.
- **Sikandar Lodhi** introduced Gaz-i-Sikandari. He also shifted his capital from Delhi to Agra.
- **Ibrahim Lodhi** was the last king of Lodhi dynasty and also last Sultan of Delhi.

Mughal Dynasty

- **Babur** laid the foundation of Mughal empire in India in AD 1526. His autobiography is Tuzuk-i-Baburi. He died at Agra and his tomb is at Kabul.
- **Humayun** was the son of Babur, he built Din Panah at Delhi as his second capital. His biography 'Humayunama' was written by his sister Gulbadan Begum. He was burried in Delhi after his death in AD 1556. His Tomb (Delhi) built by his wife Haji Begum.

Sher Shah Suri

- Sher Shah Suri was the founder of Sur dynasty.
- He issued coin called Rupia.
- He built the Grand Trunk Road (G.T. Road).

- **Akbar** ascended the throne under the title of Jalaluddin Muhammad Akbar Badshah Ghazi. He founded Fatehpur Sikri and proclaimed a new religion called, Din-i-Ilahi, and Birbal was the only hindu who joined it.

- He abolished Jaziya and built Agra Fort, Lahore Fort, Buland Darwaja, Allahabad Fort. His court had nine jewels (navaratnas). He was buried at Sikandra near Agra.
- **Jahangir** son of Akbar, established Zanzir-i-Adal (chain of justice). He wrote his memoirs Tuzuk-i-Jahangiri. He was buried in Lahore.
- **Shah Jahan** was the son of Jodhabai and Akbar. He built Moti Masjid (Agra), Taj Mahal (Agra), Jama Masjid (Delhi). He was buried at Taj Mahal (Agra).
- **Aurangzeb** adopted the title of Alamgir. He executed Guru Tegh Bahadur (9th Sikh Guru). He built Moti Masjid in Red Fort, Delhi. He was called Zinda Pir and was buried at Daulatabad.

Marathas and Peshwas

- **Shivaji** was born at Shivneri fort in AD 1627. He was helped by Ashtapradhan (8 ministers). He introduced Chauth and Sardesh Mukhi taxes.
- **Balaji Viswanath** was the first Peshwa.
- **Baji Rao I** was greatest exponent of Guerrilla tactics.
- **Balaji Baji Rao** was popularly known as Nana Saheb.

Important Battles of Medieval India

Battles	Details
First Battle of Panipat (AD 1526)	Babur defeated Ibrahim Lodhi.
Battle of Khanwa (AD 1527)	Babur defeated Rana Sanga.
Battle of Chanderi (AD 1528)	Babur defeated Medini Rai.
Battle of Ghagra (AD 1529)	Babur defeated Muhammad Lodhi.
Battle of Chausa (AD 1539)	Humayun defeated by Sher Shah.
Battle of Kannauj (AD 1540)	Delhi was captured by Sher Shah Suri and Humayun escaped from India.
Second Battle of Panipat (AD 1556)	Hemu was defeated by Bairam Khan (regent of Akbar).
Battle of Haldighati (AD 1576)	Rana Pratap defeated by Akbar.
Third Battle of Panipat (AD 1761)	Fought between Ahmad Shah Abdali and Marathas. Ahmad Shah Abdali emerged victorious.

Sikh Gurus

Sikh Gurus	Details
Guru Nanak	Founded Sikh religion
Guru Angad	Invented Gurumukhi Script
Guru Amardas	Established 22 Gadiyans.
Guru Ramdas	Founded Amritsar
Guru Arjan	Founded Golden Temple and composed Adi Granth.
Guru Hargobind	Established Akal Takht.
Guru Har Rai	Supported Dara Shikoh
Guru Har Kishan	Died in early age
Guru Tegh Bahadur	Executed by Aurangzeb
Guru Gobind Singh	Last Sikh Guru and founded the Khalsa Pant

Modern India

Advent of European

- **Portugese East India Company** (AD 1498) Vasco-da-gama was the first European to reach India (at Calicut) in 1498. Francisco de Almeida was the first Portugese Governor in India.
- **English East India Company** (AD 1600) First factory was opened at Surat in 1613 and established Fort William of Calcutta in 1700.
- **Dutch East India Company** (AD 1602) Pulicat was their main centre till 1690. Defeated by British troops in Battle of Bedera (1759).
- **Danish East India Company** (AD 1616) established first factory at Tranquebar in Tamil Nadu (1620). Serampur in Bengal was their headquarters in India.
- **French East India Company** (AD 1664) It was founded by Colbert. First factory was established at Surat in 1668.

Important Wars in Modern History

War	Details
Bengal Battle of Plassey (1757)	Fought between Siraj-ud-Duala and Robert Clive
Battle of Buxar (1764)	Fought between Mir Qasim, Shuja-ud-Duala, Shah Alam and Robert Clive
First Anglo-Mysore War (1766-69)	Haider Ali defeated the British Army
Fourth Anglo-Mysore War (1799)	Tipu Sultan was killed and territories divided among British and Nizam of Hyderabad
Third Anglo-Maratha War (1817-18)	Fought between Lord Hastings and Peshwa Baji Rao II.

Revolt of 1857

- The revolt of 1857 consists of series of revolts that took place in different parts of the country. It is considered as the **first war of Indian independence.**
- It began on 10th May, 1857, when the sepoys of 3rd native Regiment of Meerut raised the cry of 'Delhi Chalo'.
- They moved to Delhi, where Bahadur Shah Zafar (the last Mughal emperor) was declared as the leader of the revolt. He was given the title of 'Shahenshahi-e-Hindustan'.

List of Important Centres Revolt

Centre of Revolt	Leader
Delhi	Bahadur Shah Zafar and Bakht Khan
Kanpur	Nana Sahib and Tantiya Tope, Azimullah
Lucknow	Begum Hazarat Mahal
Jhansi	Rani Laxmi Bai
Allahabad	Liyaqat Ali
Faizabad	Maulvi Ahmadullah

Socio-Religious Reform Movements

Religious Institutions	Founder	Ideas
Brahmo Samaj (1828)	Raja Rammohan Roy	Propagated monotheism, opposed sacrifices, idolatory, superstition and sati.
Young Bengal Movement (1826-31)	Henry Louis Vivian Derozio	Opposed the vices in society and believed in truth, freedom and right.
Wahabi Movement (1820)	Syed Ahmed of Rai Bareilly	Popularised the teachings of Waliullah, stressed the role of individual conscience in religion.
Prarthana Samaj (1867)	Atmaram Pandurang	Monotheism, upliftment of women, abolition of caste discrimination.
Arya Samaj (1875)	Dayanand Saraswati (original name Mulshankar)	Gave the slogan Go Back to the Vedas
The Theosophical Society (1875)	Madam HP Blavatsky and Col. HS Olcott	Drew inspiration from Upanishads, philosophy of the Vedanta and a spiritual belief.

Indian National Movement

Indian National Congress

- Indian National Congress (INC) was formed in 1885 by A.O. Hume.
- First session was held at Gokuldas Tejpal Sanskrit college, Bombay and presided over by W.C. Banerjee.

Swadeshi and Boycott Movement

- Partition of Bengal came into effect on 16th October, 1905. It was announced by Lord Curzon.
- The Congress leaders and nationalists of Bengal firmly opposed the partition of Bengal.
- INC took Swadeshi call in 1905 at Benaras session.
- Rabindranath Tagore composed 'Amar Sonar Bangla' song.

Muslim League and Surat Split

- Muslim League was established in 1906 by Nawab Salimullah at Dhaka (Bangladesh). In Surat splits (1907), Congress got divided into two wings : **Moderates** and **extremists.**
- Moderates were led by **Gopal Krishna Gokhale**.
- Extremists were led by **Lala Lajpat Rai** (Lal), Bal Gangadhar Tilak (Bal) and Bipin Chandra Pal (Pal). Also famous for frio Lal, Bal, Pal.

Home Rule Movement

- It was started by Tilak on 28th April, 1916 and Annie Besant in September, 1916. The main objective of this movement was 'Swaraj'.

Gandhi's Arrival in India

- In 1915, Gandhiji arrived in Bombay from South Africa.
- In 1916, he founded Sabarmati Ashram on the banks of river Sabarmati in Gujarat. He led the three major struggles.
  1. **Champaran Satyagrah** (1917) was the first Civil Disobedience Movement in India by Gandhiji. He redressed the grievances of the Indigo cultivators of Champaran (Bihar) and fought against teen-kathia system.
  2. **Ahmedabad Satyagraha** (1918) Mahatma Gandhi supported the workers against mill owners, as workers demanded increase in wages. It was Gandhiji's first hunger strike and resulted in increase in wages.
  3. **Kheda Satyagraha** (1918) He supported the cause of peasants for remission of revenue demand, due to crop failure. It was first Non-cooperation movement led by Gandhiji.

Jallianwala Bagh Massacre

- The massacre took place on 13th April 1919, in Jallianwala Bagh, at Amritsar (Punjab) where people gathered to protest against the arrest of Satyapal and Dr. Kitchlu.
- General O'Dyer opened fire on the peaceful protesters. Sardar Udham Singh murdered General Dyer in London in 1940.

Non-cooperation Movement

- INC at its Calcutta Session (1920) passed Non-cooperation resolution.
- Non-cooperation movement launched by Gandhiji in August 1920. There was boycott of schools, colleges, courts, surrender of titles etc.
- Local police station was put on fire by a group of angry peasants it is known as Chauri-Chaura Incident (1922).
- Gandhiji called off the Non-cooperation movement after this.

Swaraj Party and Kakori Conspiracy

- Swaraj Party founded by Motilal Nehru, C.R. Das and N.C. Kelkar in 1923.
- A train robbery was took place at Kakori station on 9th August, 1925.
- The robbery conspiracy was executed by Ram Prasad Bismil, Ashfaqula Khan and others of Hindustan Republican Association (HRA).

Simon Commission

- It was constituted in Chairmanship of John Simon to review the political situation in India and suggest constitutional reforms. It came India in 1928.
- Indian leaders opposed the commission as all the members were white and they raised the slogan of 'Go Back Simon'.

Lahore Session (1929)

- In this session, Jawaharlal Nehru became the President of INC and Poorna Swaraj was declared as ultimate goal of INC.
- 26th January, 1930 was adopted as the first independence day and tri-colour flag was unfurled.

Dandi March (1930)

- It was also called the Salt Satyagraha.
- Gandhiji started march from Sabarmati Ashram to Dandi on 12th March, 1930.
- The aims of the movement included non-payment of land revenue, boycott of courts of law, school, colleges, civil services etc.

Round Table Conferences

- **First Round Table Conference** (1930) held in London between the British and Indians to discuss Simon Commission report, but failed due to the absence of INC.
- **Second Round Table Conference** (1931) held in London during Viceroyalty of Lord Willingdon.
- First time Indian National Congress participate in Round Table Conference.
- **Third Round Table Conference** (1932) This conference failed in achieving its target because all national leaders were in jail.

Gandhi-Irwin Pact (1931)

- It was signed between Lord Irwin and Gandhiji (representing INC).
- In this pact, INC agreed to called off Civil Disobedience Movement and join the Second Round Table Conference.

Poona Pact (1932)

- It was signed between Gandhiji and BR Ambedkar.
- In this joint electorate was accepted, but seats reserved for depressed class in provincial legislature were increased.

Cripps Mission (1942)

- This Mission was sent to get Indian cooperation in World War II.
- It was headed by Stafford Cripps and offered 'Dominion Status' for India.

Quit India Movement (1942)

- INC passed the Quit India Resolution at Gwoliya Tank, Bombay. In this movement Gandhiji gave the slogan of 'Do or Die'.
- Parallel governments were established like : Balia (UP) led by Chittu Pandey, Tamluk (Bengal) led by Satish Samanta, Satara (Maharashtra) led by YB Chavan and Talcher (Odisha).
- The slogan of 'Quit India' was given by Yusuf Meher Ali.

Indian National Army

- INA was founded by General Mohan Singh in 1942.
- In 1943, Rashbehari Bose handed over the leadership of INA to Subhash Chandra Bose.Subhash Chandra Bose set-up Indian League at Berlin around 1941.

Cabinet Mission Plan (1946)

- Members in Cabinet mission were Lord Pethick Lawrence, Stafford Cripps and AV Alexander.
- It provided that the Constituent Assembly would be elected by the members of Provincial Legislative Assembly.
- This was followed by 'Direct Action Day' on 16th August, 1946.

Attlee's Announcement and Mountbatten Plan

- British PM Attlee announced that the British would withdraw from India by 30th June, 1948.
- The Mountbatten plan was announced on 3rd June, 1947 which decided to India to be divided into two independent dominions of India and Pakistan.

Indian Independence Act (1947)

- It abolished the sovereignty of British Parliament and established dominions of India and Pakistan.
- Sardar Vallabhbhai Patel integrated all princely states by 15th August, 1947.

Governor Generals/Viceroys

Governor-Generals/Viceroys	Important Details
Warren Hastings (1772-1785)	▪ First Governor-General of Bengal. ▪ Introduced 'Dual Government' by Regulation Act, 1773. ▪ Sir William Jones founded Asiatic society during this time in 1784.
Lord Cornwallis (1786-1793)	▪ Introduced permanent settlement in Bengal, Bihar (1793) ▪ Also called Father of Civil Services in India.
Lord Wellesley (1798-1805)	▪ Introduced Subsidiary Alliance (1798), Hyderabad was the first state to sign Subsidiary Alliance.
Lord Minto I (1807-1813)	▪ Signed Treaty of Amritsar with Maharaja Ranjit Singh.
Lord Hastings (1813-1823)	▪ Established Ryotwari system (suggested by Thomas Munro) in 1820.
Lord William Bentinck (1828-1835)	▪ First Governor-General of India ▪ Prohibition of Sati (1929)
Lord Hardinge I (1844-1848)	▪ Signed the Treaty of Lahore with Sikhs, after first Anglo-Sikh war.
Lord Dalhousie (1848-1856)	▪ Passed Widow Remarriage Act (1856); introduced Doctrine of Lapse in 1848 (Satara was first state to be captured) ▪ First railway line (1853) and Postal system (1854).
Lord Canning (1856-1862)	▪ Last Governor-General of India and first Viceroy. ▪ Revolt of 1857 took place during his period.
Lord Lytton (1876-1880)	▪ Passed Vernacular Press Act, (1878) and reduced the minimum age of civil services from 21 to 18.
Lord Ripon (1880-1884)	▪ Father of local self-government in India.
Lord Curzon (1899-1905)	▪ Partition of Bengal (1905).
Lord Hardinge (1910-1916)	▪ Delhi Durbar of 1911, annulment of Partition of Bengal.
Lord lrwin (1926-1931)	▪ Gandhi-Irwin Pact was signed (1931); First Round Table Conference and Dandi March took place.
Lord Linlithgow (1936-1943)	▪ Congress ministries resigned (1939); Quit India movement took place.
Lord Wavell (1943-1947)	▪ Shimla Conference of 1945; Cabinet Mission Plan.
Lord Mountbatten (March-August 1947)	▪ First Governor-General of free India; appointed 2 boundary commissions under Sir Cryil Radcliffe

Books, Journals and Newspapers

Book/Journal/Newspaper	Author/Writer/Editors	Book/Journal/Newspaper	Author/Writer/Editors
Ghulam Giri	Jyotiba Phule	Young India, Harijan, Indian Opinion, Hind Swaraj	MK Gandhi
Satyarth Prakash	Swami Dayanand	Bengal Gazette	JA Hicky
Anand Math	Bankim Chandra Chatterji	Kesari, Maratha	BG Tilak
Unhappy India	Lala Lajpat Rai	Vande Mataram	Aurobindo Ghosh
India Divided	Rajendra Prasad	Yugantar	Bhupendranath Datta and Barindra Kumar Ghosh
Neel Darpan	Dinbandhu Mitra	Indian Mirror	Devendranath Tagore

Important Sayings

Saying	Said by	Saying	Said by
'Dilli Chalo'	Subhash Chandra Bose	'Vande Matram'	Bankim Chandra Chatterjee
'Do or Die'	MK Gandhi	'Jai Hind'	Subhash Chandra Bose
'Give Me Blood and I will give you freedom'	Subhash Chandra Bose	'Purna Swaraj'	Jawaharlal Nehru
'Swaraj is my birthright and I will have it'	Bal Gangadhar Tilak	'Jai Jawan Jai Kisan'	Lal Bahadur Shastri

Exam Pattern Questions

Ancient History

1. The evidences of Indus valley civilisation were first discovered at
(a) Lothal (b) Harappa
(c) Mohenjodaro (d) Chanhudaro

2. The Indus valley civilisation has been asigned the period 2500-1750 BC on the basis of
(a) Radio carbon dating
(b) Accounts written by travellers
(c) Markings on seal
(d) Harappan seals

3. Which among the following civilisation belongs to bronze age?
(a) Indus valley (b) Rig Vedic
(c) Sumerian (d) Mesopotamian

4. Dholavira is situated on the bank of which river?
(a) Luni (b) Narmada
(c) Ravi (d) Beas

5. Which of the following is the largest Indus valley site of India?
(a) Mohenjodaro (b) Lothal
(c) Harappa (d) Rakhigarhi

6. The Great Granary of Indus valley civilisation has been discovered at which place?
(a) Harappa (b) Kalibangan
(c) Mohenjodaro (d) Ropar

7. Who excavated the Indus site of Harappa in year 1921?
(a) Daya Ram Sahani (b) Rakhaldas Banerjee
(c) SR Rao (d) RS Bisht

8. Which metal was not known to Indus valley people?
(a) Gold (b) Silver (c) Bronze (d) Iron

9. Which of the following was the main port to the Indus people?
(a) Harappa (b) Kalibangan
(c) Lothal (d) Mohenjodaro

10. Which among the following Indus valley site is situated in India?
(a) Harappa (b) Mohenjodaro
(c) Kalibangan (d) Chanhudaro

11. Which is the Southern most extent of the Indus valley civilisation?
(a) Alamgirpur (b) Daimabad
(c) Mandu (d) Sutkagender

12. Which is the earliest civilisation of the world to cultivate cotton?
(a) Sumerian (b) Mesopotamia
(c) Indus valley (d) Crete

13. Which among the following is the oldest Veda?
(a) Sam Veda (b) Yajur Veda
(c) Rig Veda (d) Atharva Veda

14. Identify the Veda which is called 'The Book of Chants'.
(a) Atharva Veda (b) Sam Veda
(c) Yajur Veda (d) Rig Veda

15. Atharva Veda deals with which among the following?
(a) Hymns (b) Charms and spells
(c) Songs (d) Rituals

16. Rig Veda contains how many mandals?
(a) Eleven (b) Twelve
(c) Nine (d) Ten

17. 'Upnishads' are books on
(a) Religion (b) Yoga
(c) Philosphy (d) Law

18. The words ' Satyameva Jayate' inscribed below the base plate of the emblem of India are taken from
(a) Rigveda (b) Satpath Brahmana
(c) Mundaka Upanishada (d) Ramayana

19. Purusha Sukta hymn of Rigveda deals with which of the following?
(a) Varna system (b) Trimurti
(c) Gods (d) Nature

20. 'Gayatri Mantra' is contained in which among the following Vedas?
(a) Rig Veda (b) Atharva Veda
(c) Sam Veda (d) Yajur Veda

21. The Purushasukta hymn is contained in which mandala?
(a) 10th mandala (b) 3rd mandala
(c) 1st mandala (d) 2nd mandala

22. Gautam Buddha was born at which place in year 563 BC?
(a) Lumbini (b) Kapilavastu
(c) Sarnath (d) Gaya

23. Buddha attained enlightenment (Nirvana) on the bank of which river?
(a) Sabarmati (b) Niranjana
(c) Penner (d) Ganga

24. 'Dharmachakrapravartan' is associated with which event of Buddha's life?
(a) Birth (b) Death
(c) First Sermon (d) Nirvana

25. Who was the first teacher of Buddha?
(a) Jamali (b) Alara Kalama
(c) Channa (d) Makkhali Gosala

26. The first Buddhist Council was held at which place?
(a) Rajagriha (b) Vaishali
(c) Pataliputra (d) Kundalvana

27. Who was the patron of third Buddhist Council?
(a) Ajatashatru (b) Ashoka
(c) Kanishka (d) Kalashoka

28. The second Buddhist council was held at which place?
(a) Pataliputra (b) Vaishali
(c) Rajagriha (d) Kundalvana

29. Who was the chairman of the last (fourth) Buddhist council?
(a) Sabakami (b) Vasumitra
(c) Mahakashyapa (d) Mogaliputta Tissa

30. Which Buddhist council was held during the reign of Ashoka?
(a) First (b) Second (c) Third (d) Fourth

31. Which among the following is a Buddhist text?
(a) Tripitaka (b) Mahakavya
(c) Shad Darshan (d) Brahmanas

32. Abhidhama pitaka deals with which among the following?
(a) Buddha's Teachings (b) Rules of Monks
(c) Buddha's Sermon (d) Buddhist Philosophy

33. The language of the discourses of Gautam Buddha was
(a) Bhojpuri (b) Magadhi
(c) Pali (d) Sanskrit

34. How many tirthankaras are there in Jainism?
(a) 24 (b) 25 (c) 20 (d) 30

35. Who was the founder of Jainism?
(a) Mahavira (b) Rishabhadeva
(c) Ajitnatha (d) Naminatha

36. At which place Mahavira attained Kaivalya?
(a) Pavapuri (b) Vaishali
(c) Jimbhikagrama (d) Rajgriha

37. Which among the following is not one of the five teachings of Jainism?
(a) Ahimsa (b) Asteya (c) Satya (d) Karma

38. The first Jain Council was held at which place?
(a) Rajagriha (b) Vaishali
(c) Pataliputra (d) Lumbini

39. What is the name of the Jain sect that was formed under the leadership of Bhadrabahu?
(a) Swetambars (b) Hinayana
(c) Digambaras (d) Yogachara

40. Which was the most powerful Mahajanapada?
(a) Kashi (b) Kosala
(c) Avanti (d) Magadh

41. What was the capital of Gandhara Mahajanapada?
(a) Ujjain (b) Raipur
(c) Kaushambi (d) Taxila

42. Which of the following dynasty was the first to rule over Magadha?
(a) Haryanka (b) Nandas
(c) Shishunagas (d) Mauryas

43. Who was the first ruler of Magadha empire?
(a) Bimbisara (b) Udayin
(c) Ajatashatru (d) Nanda

44. The city of Rajgriha was built by whom?
(a) Ajatshatru (b) Bimbisara
(c) Mahapadmananda (d) Ashoka

45. Who was the first Indian ruler to have a regular standing army of his own?
(a) Udayin (b) Ajatshatru
(c) Kalashoka (d) Bimbisara

46. Who was the contemporary of Pushyamitra Sunga?
(a) Patanjali (b) Kalidas
(c) Helidorus (d) Vasudeva

47. 'Jaladurga' at a village named Patali and the fort of Rajgriha was built by whom?
(a) Anuruddha (b) Somdeva
(c) Munda (d) Ajatshatru

48. Udayin founded the new capital at the confluence of two rivers namely Son and Ganga, what was its name?
(a) Pataliputra (b) Vaishali
(c) Rajagriha (d) Kampilya

49. Who was the last ruler of Nanda Dynasty?
(a) Ajatashatru (b) Dhananand
(c) Bimbisara (d) Udayin

50. Ajatashatru was the son of
(a) Udayin (b) Dhananand
(c) Alexander (d) Bimbisara

51. Who shifted the capital of Magadha from Rajagriha to Pataliputra?
(a) Ajatashatru (b) Dhananand
(c) Bimbisara (d) Udayin

52. Alexander fought the 'Battle of Vitasta' with which ruler?
(a) Ambhi (b) Porus
(c) Ashoka (d) Chandragupta

53. Who was known as 'Amitraghat'?
(a) Bindusara
(b) Bimbisara
(c) Ajat shatru
(d) Chandra Gupta Maurya

54. Who wrote the book 'Indica'?
(a) Kautilya (b) Charak
(c) Panini (d) Megasthenese

55. Who sent Megasthenes as an ambassador to the court of Chandragupta Maurya?
(a) Darius (b) Seleucus Nicator
(c) Alexander (d) Ptolemy-II

56. Which ruler fought the Kalinga war in year 261 BC?
(a) Chandragupta Maurya
(b) Ashoka
(c) Bindusara
(d) Brihadratha

57. Which rock edict of king Ashoka contains information about the Kalinga war?
(a) X (b)XIII (c) IX (d)IV

58. Most of the Ashoka's edicts are written in the script of
(a) Brahmi (b) Kharoshthi
(c) Devanagri (d) Prakrit

59. Who were the founders of the first great united Empire in India?
(a) The Mauryans (b) The Nanda
(c) Kushanas (d) The Shakas

60. Who was the last Maurya ruler?
(a) Chandragupta II (b) Kalashoka
(c) Bimbisara (d) Brihadratha

61. Who was the first Gupta ruler to assume the title of 'Maharajadhiraja'?
(a) Chandragupta I (b) Samudragupta
(c) Chandragupta II (d) Kumaragupta

62. Which Gupta ruler is popularly known as 'Napolean of India'?
(a) Kumaragupta (b) Samudragupta
(c) Chandragupta (d) Skandagupta

63. Prayag Prashasti in praise of Samudragupta was composed by whom?
(a) Kalidas (b) Amarsimha
(c) Harisena (d) Tulsidas

64. Mehrauli Iron Pillar is dedicated to which ruler?
(a) Chandragupta II (b) Chandragupta I
(c) Samudragupta (d) Skandagupta

65. Which Mahavihara was founded by Kumaragupta I ?
(a) Vikramashila (b) Nalanda
(c) Taxila (d) All of these

66. Huns invaded India during the reign of which ruler?
(a) Kumargupta I (b) Skandagupta
(c) Chandragupta (d) Ashoka

67. Sanchi Stupa was built by which ruler?
(a) Chandragupta (b) Ashoka
(c) Kumargupta (d) Bindusara

68. Ellora caves are dedicated to which religion?
(a) Hinduism (b) Jainism
(c) Buddhism (d) All of these

69. The most ornate temple belonging to Gupta age is ....
(a) Dasavatara Temple
(b) Teli Ka Mandir
(c) Sun Temple
(d) Brihadeshvara Temple

70. Who is known as the 'Shakespeare of India'?
(a) Aryabhatta (b) Kalidasa
(c) Amarsimha (d) Galibh

71. Suryasindhanta was composed by which Indian Mathematician?
(a) Bhaskara (b) Varahamihira
(c) Aryabhatta (d) Brahmagupta

72. Vikram Samvat was started during which period?
(a) AD 78 (b)BC 58 (c) AD 28 (d)AD 17

73. Which Kushan ruler started the Saka era in AD 78?
(a) Kanishka (b) Rudradaman
(c) Vima Kadphises (d) Vasudeva I

74. Hiuen-Tsang, a Chinese pilgrim, visited India during the reign of which ruler?
(a) Harshavardhana (b) Kanishka
(c) Samudragupta (d) Jayasimha

75. Harshavardhana was defeated by which Chalukyan ruler on the banks of river Narmada?
(a) Pulakeshin II (b) Yasovarman
(c) Narsimvarman (d) Mahipala

Medieval History

76. Who was the first Muslim to invade India in AD 712?
(a) Mahmud Ghaznavi
(b) Qutubuddin Aibak
(c) Mohammad Bin Qasim
(d) Kaiqubad

77. Who was the King of Sindh at the time of Muslim Invasion?
(a) Dahir (b) Iraq
(c) Afganistan (d) Iran

78. Name the Turkish invader, who invaded India 17 times and destroyed Somnath temple.
(a) Iltutmish (b) Alauddin Khilji
(c) Malik Kafur (d) Mahmud Ghaznavi

79. Qutubuddin Aibak constructed a mosque named Quwat-ul-Islam at which place?
(a) Delhi (b) Agra
(c) Ajmer (d) Lahore

80. Which ruler of Slave dynasty started the construction of Qutub Minar?
(a) Qutubuddin Aibak (b) Iltutmish
(c) Razia Sultan (d) Balban

81. Which ruler of the Slave dynasty was given the title of 'Lakh Baksh' (giver of lakhs)?
(a) Qutubuddin Aibak (b) Razia Sultan
(c) Iltutmish (d) Rukunuddin Firoz

82. What was the name of the copper coin introduced by Iltutmish?
(a) Rupiya (b) Tanka
(c) Jittal (d) None of these

83. Which ruler of Slave dynasty set up Chalisa?
(a) Razia Sultan (b) Kaiqubad
(c) Iltutmish (d) Qutubuddin Aibak

84. Who was the first woman ruler of India?
(a) Gulbadan Begum
(b) Razia Sultan
(c) Rani Lakshmi Bai
(d) Begum Hazarat Mehal

85. The power of Chalisa was broken by which Sultan of Delhi?
(a) Jalaluddin Khilji (b) Ghiyasuddin Balban
(c) Kaiqubad (d) Iltutmish

86. Which Muslim ruler of Delhi introduced token currency?
(a) Khizr Khan
(b) Kaiqubad
(c) Mohammad Bin Tughlaq
(d) Firoz Shah Tughlaq

87. What was 'Dar-ul-Shifa' established by Firoz Shah Tughlaq?
(a) Water tax (b) Hospital
(c) Market (d) Granary

88. Who was the founder of Lodhi dynasty?
(a) Bahlol Lodhi (b) Sikandar Lodhi
(c) Ibrahim Lodhi (d) Daulat Khan Lodhi

89. 'Gaz-i-Sikandari' was introduced by which ruler?
(a) Sikandar Lodhi (b) Bahlol Lodhi
(c) Ghiyasuddin Tughlaq (d) Ibrahim Lodhi

90. Which Mughal emperor wrote Tuzuk-i-Baburi?
(a) Humayun
(b) Babur
(c) Abul Fazal
(d) Abdul Rahim Khan-i-Khana

91. Which of the following battle took place between Babur and Rana Sangha?
(a) Battle of Khanwa (b) Battle of Ghagra
(c) Battle of Chanderi (d) Battle of Plassey

92. In the first Battle of Panipat, Ibrahim Lodhi was defeated by whom?
(a) Babur (b) Rana Sanga
(c) Muhammad Lodhi (d) Akbar

93. Babur defeated Muhammad Lodhi at which battle?
(a) Battle of Khanwa (b) Battle of Chanderi
(c) Battle of Ghaghra (d) Battle of Panipat

94. Who defeated Humayun in the battle of Chausa and Kannauj?
(a) Sher Shah Suri (b) Muhammad Lodhi
(c) Medini Rai (d) Alam Khan

95. Humayun founded his second capital 'Din Panah' at which place?
(a) Ajmer (b) Agra
(c) Delhi (d) Fatehpur Sikri

96. Biography of Humayun named 'Humayunama' was written by whom?
(a) Gulbadan Begum (b) Faizi
(c) Abul Fazal (d) Akbar

97. Which among the following rulers conferred the title of 'Sher Khan' to 'Sher Shah Suri'?
(a) Sikandar Lodhi (b) Humayun
(c) Babur (d) Bahar Khan Lohani

98. Sher Shah's real name was
(a) Hemu (b) Faizi (c) Bahadur (d) Farid

99. Which among the following is not related to Sher Shah Suri?
(a) Rupiah (b) Grand Trunk Road
(c) Patta (d) Tanka

100. Which ruler of Mughal dynasty shifted his capital from Agra to Fatehpur Sikri?
(a) Akbar (b) Babur
(c) Humayun (d) Sher Shah

101. Which of the following was the court language during the regime of Akbar?
(a) Hindi (b) Urdu (c) Persian (d) Arabic

102. Which among the following was not the part of Akbar's Navaratna?
(a) Tansen (b) Abul Fazal
(c) Todarmal (d) Amarsimha

103. When did the second battle of Panipat fought?
(a) 1556 (b)1576 (c) 1520 (d)1528

104. Who among the following established the system of Justice called 'Zanzir-i-adal'?
(a) Shah Jahan (b) Tansen
(c) Jahangir (d) Abul Fazal

105. During the reign of which Mughal emperor, the French travellers like Bernier, Travernier visited India?
(a) Humayun (b) Jahangir
(c) Babur (d) Shah Jahan

106. Name the architecture built by Shah Jahan?
(a) Qutub Minar (b) Alai Darwaza
(c) Agra Fort (d) Taj Mahal

107. What title was given to Mughal emperor Aurangzeb?
(a) Zil-i-Ilahi (b)Hazar Dinari
(c) Alamgir (d) Badshah Salamat

108. 'Chauth' and 'Sardeshmukhi' were introduced by which ruler?
(a) Shivaji (b) Sambhaji
(c) Baji Rao I (d) Baji Rao II

109. Who got the title of 'Sena Karte'?
(a) Balaji Vishwanath (b) Baji Rao I
(c) Balaji Baji Rao (d) Shivaji

110. Who emerged victorious in the third battle of Panipat?
(a) Aurangzeb (b) Ahmad Shah Abdali
(c) Rana Pratap (d) Babur

111. Who was the founder of the Sikh religion?
(a) Guru Gobind Singh (b) Guru Angad
(c) Guru Nanak (d) Guru Ramdas

112. Which among the following can be contributed to Guru Arjan?
(a) Gurumukhi Script (b) Akal Takht
(c) Golden Temple (d) Amritsar

113. Khalsa Pant was discovered by which Sikh Guru?
(a) Guru Nanak (b) Guru Angad
(c) Guru Har Rai (d) Guru Gobind Singh

114. Which Mughal ruler executed Guru Tegh Bahadur?
(a) Babur (b) Humayun
(c) Akbar (d) Aurangzeb

Modern India

115. Which of the Europeans came to India first?
(a) The Portuguese (b) The British
(c) The French (d) The Germans

116. Which Hindu ruler received Vasco da Gama, when he reached Calicut?
(a) Zamorin (b) Kanishka
(c) Chandragupta (d) Dharmapala

117. In which year, Vascoda Game visited India?
(a) 1512 (b) 1498 (c) 1478 (d) 1598

118. The first trading centre of Dutch East India Company was established at which place?
(a) Goa (b) Surat
(c) Daman and Diu (d) Masulipatanam

119. The English East India Company opened their first factory in 1613 at which place?
(a) Surat (b) Bombay
(c) Calcutta (d) Madras

120. Captain William Hawkins obtained farman from which Mughal ruler?
(a) Akbar (b) Jahangir
(c) Aurangzeb (d) Babur

121. English East India Company established fort William at which place?
(a) Madras (b) Calcutta
(c) Bengal (d) Bombay

122. Dutch East India Company was defeated at which battle?
(a) Khanwa (b) Waterloo
(c) Bedera (d) Chanderi

123. During India's freedom struggle, the Sepoy Mutiny started from which one of the following places?
(a) Agra (b) Gwalior (c) Jhansi (d) Meerut

124. Mangal Pandey fired the first shot of the Revolt of 1857 at
(a) Barrackpore (b) Meerut
(c) Kanpur (d) Jhansi

125. Kunwar Singh led the revolt of 1857 in
(a) Punjab (b) Bengal
(c) Bihar (d) Maharashtra

126. Rani Jhansi was related to
(a) Congress
(b) Revolt of 1857
(c) Champaran
(d) Civil disobedience Movement

127. The first session of Indian National Congress was held at which place?
(a) Lucknow (b) Calcutta
(c) Bombay (d) Madras

128. Which Governor-General of British India announced the partition of Bengal in 1905?
(a) Lord Curzon
(b) William Bentinck
(c) Lord Ripon
(d) Lord Canning

129. Who was the leader of the Swadeshi and Boycott movement in Punjab?
(a) Ajit Singh
(b) Lala Lajpat Rai
(c) Dada Bhai Naoroji
(d) Madan Mohan Malviya

130. Who was the founder of Muslim League?
(a) Nawab Salimullah
(b) Mohammad Ali Jinnah
(c) Maulana Abul Kalam Azad
(d) Shaukat Ali

131. Who was the founder of Brahmo Samaj?
(a) Raja Ram Mohan Roy
(b) Ishwar Chandra Vidyasagar
(c) Keshab Chandra Sen
(d) Swami Dayananda

132. Which socio-religious organisation emerged to counter Brahmo Samaj?
(a) Tattvabodhini Sabha
(b) Dharma Sabha
(c) Arya Samaj
(d) Seva Sadan

133. Who gave the slogan of 'Go back to the Vedas'?
(a) Swami Dayananda
(b) Annie Basant
(c) Atmaram Pandurang
(d) Raja Ram Mohan Roy

134. In India, the headquarters of Theosophical Society was set up at which place?
(a) Adyar (b) Pune
(c) Belur (d) Bombay

135. The Surat session of INC took place in which year?
(a) 1907 (b) 1921
(c) 1905 (d) 1916

136. The Congress got divided into two wings during which session?
(a) Haripur (b) Calcutta
(c) Bombay (d) Surat

137. In which year, Gandhiji established Sabarmati Ashram?
(a) 1915 (b) 1914
(c) 1916 (d) 1917

138. During Champaran Satyagraha, Gandhiji fought for the cause of which among the following groups?
(a) Indigo Cultivators (b) Tea Planters
(c) Trade Union (d) Peasants

139. Which was the first non-cooperation movement led by Gandhiji?
(a) Kheda Satyagraha
(b) Ahmedabad Satyagraha
(c) Champaran Satyagraha
(d) Bardoli Satyagraha

140. Who among the following started the Home Rule Movement first?
(a) Annie Besant
(b) BG Tilak
(c) Firoz Shah Mehta
(d) Subramaniyam Swami

141. The Lucknow Session of the Congress was presided over by which among the following?
(a) Ambika Charan Mazumdar
(b) Maulana Abul Kalam Azad
(c) Shaukat Usmani
(d) Dadabhai Naoroji

142. 'Dyarchy' was introduced in 1919 through which initiative of the British Government?
(a) Morley Minto Reform
(b) Montague Chelmsford Reforms
(c) Government of India Act, 1935
(d) Government of India Act, 1858

143. Rowlatt Act of 1919 was passed during the viceroyalty of which Governor-General?
(a) Lord Chelmsford (b) Lord Canning
(c) Lord Dalhousie (d) William Bentinck

144. The Jallianwala Bagh Massacre took place at Amritsar in which year?
(a) 1919 (b) 1920
(c) 1921 (d) 1930

145. Which British official opens fired at a peaceful crowd gathered at Jallianwala Bagh?
(a) Lord Ripon (b) Lord Lytton
(c) General O' Dyer (d) Lord Curzon

146. Ali brothers organised which movement in 1920?
(a) Non-cooperation (b) Khilafat
(c) Civil Disobedience (d) Swadeshi

147. The Chauri-Chaura incidence of 1922 was held at which place?
(a) Kolkata (b) Madras
(c) Gaurakhpur (d) Bombay

148. Which movement was called off by Gandhiji as a result of Chauri-Chaura incidence?
(a) Civil Disobedience Movement
(b) Non-cooperation Movement
(c) Swadeshi and Boycott Movement
(d) Quit India Movement

149. Swaraj Party was formed by Motilal Nehru, NC Kelkar and which other leader?
(a) CR Das
(b) Jawaharlal Nehru
(c) Dadabhai Naoroji
(d) Bal Gangadhar Tilak

150. Name the leaders who designed the Nehru Report.
(a) Tej Bahadur Sapru (b) Motilal Nehru
(c) Jawaharlal Nehru (d) Both (a) and (b)

151. At which INC session, 'Swaraj' was adopted as the ultimate goal?
(a) Lahore (b) Calcutta
(c) Bombay (d) Madras

152. Which leader died as a result of the brutal lathi charge?
(a) Bal Gangadhar Tilak
(b) Bipin Chandra Pal
(c) Lala Lajpat Rai
(d) Motilal Nehru

153. First independence day was celebrated on which date?
(a) 26th November, 1930
(b) 26th January, 1930
(c) 15th August, 1947
(d) 26th January, 1950

154. Gandhiji started 'Dandi March' to launch which movement?
(a) Civil Disobedience Movement
(b) Non-cooperation Movement
(c) Swadeshi Movement
(d) Quit India Movement

155. Who was the first nationalist to gave the idea of Pakistan?
(a) Shaukat Usmani
(b) Mohammad Ali Jinnah
(c) Chaudhary Rehmat Ali
(d) CR Das

156. Who among the following did not participate in First Round Table Conference?
(a) Muslim League (b) INC
(c) BR Ambedkar (d) Hindu Mahasabha

157. The demand for Pakistan was put forward during which session of Muslim League?
(a) Surat (b) Lahore
(c) Bombay (d) Calcutta

158. The objective of Cripps Mission; headed by Sir Stafford Cripps was
(a) to prevent Quit India Movement
(b) to secure the Indian Cooperation in World War II
(c) to set up a Constitution making body
(d) to convince the INC to attend to second Round Table Conference

159. Who was the congress President when India became free?
(a) Mahatma Gandhi (b) Jawaharlal Nehru
(c) JB Kriplani (d) Sardar Patel

160. Which session of Indian National Congress witnessed Bose and Sitaramaya conflict in 1939?
(a) Tripuri Session (b) Haripur Session
(c) Banaras Session (d) Calcutta Session

161. Congress failed to form ministries in which of the following provinces during 1937 provincial elections?
(a) Bengal (b) Bombay
(c) Madras (d) Bihar

162. Who laid the foundation of Indian National Army?
(a) Subhash Chandra Bose
(b) Rash Bihari Bose
(c) Mohan Singh
(d) Sohan Singh Bakhna

163. Name the female fighting brigade of INA?
(a) Rani of Jhansi (b) Sarojini Naidu
(c) Aruna (d) Indira Gandhi

164. Who was the first individual Satyagrahi?
(a) Sarojini Naidu (b) Jawaharlal Nehru
(c) Vallabhbhai Patel (d) Vinoba Bhave

165. Which plan is also known as 3rd June Plan?
(a) Shimla Plan (b) Wavell Plan
(c) Mountbatten Plan (d) All of these

166. Who was the head of interim Government of India?
(a) CR Das (b) Jawaharlal Nehru
(c) BR Ambedkar (d) Gandhiji

167. Who was the first Muslim President of INC?
(a) Badrudin Tyabji
(b) Maulana Abul Kalam Azad
(c) Jinnah
(d) Muhammad Ali

168. Mahatma Gandhi presided which session of Congress?
(a) Calcutta (b) Belgaum
(c) Surat (d) Haripur

169. The plan to transfer of power to the Indians and Partition of the country was laid down in the
(a) Cabinet Mission Plan
(b) Cripps Mission
(c) Simon Commission
(d) Mountbatten Plan

170. Which among the following state was the last one to be the part of India?
(a) Goa
(b) Hyderabad
(c) Puducherry
(d) Junagarh

171. Which slogan was raised by Mahatma Gandhi during the Quit India Movement of 1942?
(a) Do or Die (b) Dilli Chalo
(c) Inqalab Zindabad (d) Jai Hind

172. Who is the author of the 'Anandamath'?
(a) Aurobindo Ghosh
(b) Bankim Chandra Chatterjee
(c) MK Gandhi
(d) Rabindranath Tagore

173. Name the first newspaper of British India.
(a) Al-Hilal (b) National Herald
(c) Bengal Gazette (d) Rast Goftar

174. The famous slogan 'Delhi Chalo' was given by
(a) Subhash Chandra Bose
(b) Bal Gangadhar Tilak
(c) Mahatma Gandhi (d) Jawaharlal Nehru

Answers

1 (b)	2 (a)	3 (a)	4 (a)	5 (d)	6 (c)	7 (a)	8 (d)	9 (c)	10 (c)
11 (b)	12 (c)	13 (c)	14 (b)	15 (b)	16 (d)	17 (c)	18 (c)	19 (a)	20 (a)
21 (a)	22 (a)	23 (b)	24 (c)	25 (b)	26 (a)	27 (b)	28 (b)	29 (b)	30 (c)
31 (a)	32 (d)	33 (c)	34 (a)	35 (b)	36 (c)	37 (d)	38 (c)	39 (c)	40 (d)
41 (d)	42 (a)	43 (a)	44 (b)	45 (d)	46 (c)	47 (d)	48 (a)	49 (b)	50 (d)
51 (d)	52 (b)	53 (a)	54 (d)	55 (b)	56 (b)	57 (b)	58 (a)	59 (a)	60 (d)
61 (a)	62 (b)	63 (c)	64 (a)	65 (b)	66 (b)	67 (b)	68 (d)	69 (a)	70 (b)
71 (c)	72 (b)	73 (a)	74 (a)	75 (a)	76 (c)	77 (a)	78 (d)	79 (a)	80 (a)
81 (a)	82 (c)	83 (c)	84 (b)	85 (b)	86 (c)	87 (b)	88 (a)	89 (a)	90 (b)
91 (a)	92 (a)	93 (c)	94 (a)	95 (c)	96 (a)	97 (d)	98 (d)	99 (d)	100 (a)
101 (c)	102 (d)	103 (a)	104 (c)	105 (d)	106 (d)	107 (c)	108 (a)	109 (a)	110 (b)
111 (c)	112 (c)	113 (d)	114 (d)	115 (a)	116 (a)	117 (b)	118 (d)	119 (a)	120 (b)
121 (b)	122 (c)	123 (d)	124 (a)	125 (c)	126 (b)	127 (c)	128 (a)	129 (b)	130 (a)
131 (a)	132 (b)	133 (a)	134 (a)	135 (a)	136 (d)	137 (c)	138 (a)	139 (c)	140 (b)
141 (a)	142 (b)	143 (a)	144 (a)	145 (c)	146 (b)	147 (c)	148 (b)	149 (a)	150 (d)
151 (a)	152 (c)	153 (a)	154 (a)	155 (c)	156 (b)	157 (b)	158 (b)	159 (c)	160 (a)
161 (a)	162 (c)	163 (a)	164 (d)	165 (c)	166 (b)	167 (a)	168 (b)	169 (d)	170 (a)
171 (a)	172 (b)	173 (c)	174 (a)						

Chapter 02 Art and Culture

Classical Dances

The Sangeet Natak Academy has recognised 8 dances as the Classical dances of India.

Dance	Famous Dancers
Bharatanatyam (Tamil Nadu)	Rukmini Devi Arundale, T Balasaraswati, Sonal Mansingh, Yamini Krishnamurthy, Leela Samson
Kuchipudi (Andhra Pradesh)	Vempati Chenna Satyam, Radha Reddy, Yamini Krishnamurthy, Vijaya Prasad
Kathakali (Kerala)	Kalamondalan Gopi, Kalamondalam Nair,, Narayan Menon, Mrinalini Sarabhai, Shanta Rao.
Odissi (Odisha)	Guru Pankaj Charan Das, Keluchara, Mohapatra, Sonal Mansingh, Sanjukta Panigrahi
Manipuri (Manipur)	Jhaveri sisters, Guru Bipin Singh, Sohini Roy, Charu Mathur, Ponshali Chatterjee
Kathak (Uttar Pradesh)	Birju Maharaj, Sitara Devi, Damyanti Joshi, Gopi Krishna
Sattriya (Asom)	Jatin Goswami, Maniram Muktiyar, Bapu Ram Muktiyar
Mohiniattam (Kerala)	Kalyani Amma, Bharati Shivaji, Hema Malini

State and their Folk Dances

Andhra Pradesh	Ghantamardala, Ottam Thedal, Veedhi Natakam
Asom	Bihu, Bichhua, Natpuja, Maharas, Kaligopal, Bagurumba, Khel Gopal
Bihar	Jata-Jatin, Panwariya, Sama-Chakwa, Bidesia
Gujarat	Garba, Dandiya Ras, Tippani
Haryana	Jhumar, Phag, Daph, Dhamal, Loor, Gugga, Khor, Gagor
Himachal Pradesh	Jhora, Jhali, Chharhi, Dhaman, Chhapeli, Mahasu, Nati, Dangi
J & K	Rauf, Hikat, Mandjas
Karnataka	Yakshagan, Huttari, Suggi, Kunitha, Karga, Lambi
Kerala	Ottam Thulal, Kaikottikali
Maharashtra	Lavani, Nakata, Koli, Lezim, Gafa, Dahikala Dasavtar or Powada
Odisha	Savari, Ghumara, Painka, Munari
West Bengal	Kathi, Gambhira, Dhali, Jatra, Baul, Marasia, Mahal, Keertan
Punjab	Bhangra, Giddha, Daff, Dhaman, Bhand, Naqual
Rajasthan	Ghumar, Ganagor, Jhuma, Suisini, Ghapal, Kalbeliya
Tamil Nadu	Kumi, Kolattam, Kavadi
Uttar Pradesh	Nautanki, Raslila, Kajri, Jhora, Chappeli, Jaita
Uttarakhand	Garhwali, Kumayuni, Kajari, Jhora, Raslila, Chappeli

Musical Instruments and Instrumentalists

Instrument	Instrumentalists
Sarod	Ustad Alauddin Khan, Ali Akbar Khan, Amjad Ali Khan
Tabla	Ustad Allah Rakha, Mian Kader Baksh, Ustad Zakir Hussain, Lal Ahmad
Sitar	Pandit Ravi Shankar, Akshay Kumar Ghosh, Ustad Vilayat Khan
Violin	Dr Balamurali Krishna, V.G. Jog, Lal Gudie Jay Araman, Karaikudi Sambasiva Iyer
Shehnai	Bismillah Khan, Ali Bor 'Vilayati'
Flute	Hariprasad Chaurasia, Pannalal Ghosh, Pandit Bholanath
Sarangi	Pandit Ram Narayan, Sabri Khan, Bundu Khan, Pandit Udayalal
Santoor	Shiv Kumar Sharma

Folk Painting in India

Style/Painting	Area
Madhubani	Bihar
Phad	Rajasthan
Warli	Maharashtra
Kalamkari	Andhra Pradesh
Kalighat	Bengal
Patachitra	Odisha and West Bengal

Important Festivals and their State

Festival	State
Bihu	Asom
Onam	Kerala
Pongal	Tamil Nadu
Lusar	Arunachal Pradesh
Hornbill	Nagaland
Ganesh Chaturthi	Maharashtra
Lohri	Punjab
Navratri	West-Bengal
Saga Dawa	Sikkim
Dree Festival	Arunachal Pradesh
Gangaur	Rajasthan
Losoong	Sikkim

Famous Fairs in India

Name of Fair	Held at
Kumbh Mela	Haridwar, Prayagaraj, Nashik and Ujjain
Pushkar Mela	Pushkar (Rajasthan)
Surajkund Crafts Mela	Faridabad (Haryana)
Sonepur Cattle Fair	Sonepur (Bihar)
Hemis Gompa Fair	Ladakh (Jammu and Kashmir)
Gangasagar Mela	Sagardwip (West Bengal)
Goa Carnival	Goa
Cattle Fair of Nagaur	Nagaur (Rajasthan)

Exam Pattern Questions

1. Kathakali asssociated with the state
(a) Tamil Nadu
(b) Andhra Pradesh
(c) Karnataka
(d) Kerala

2. Which of the following pair about dance and associated states is wrong ?
(a) Kuchipudi – Andhra Pradesh
(b) Garba – Gujarat
(c) Bhangra – Punjab
(d) Bihu – Bihar

3. Which among the following is not a classical dance form of India?
(a) Kalaripayattu
(b) Mohiniattam
(c) Bharatanatyam
(d) Kathakali

4. Padma Subramaniam is an exponent of which of the following classical dance form?
(a) Kuchipudi (b) Odissi
(c) Bharatanatyam
(d) Manipuri

5. Which among the following dance form incorporates an important elements namely 'Tribhanga'?
(a) Odissi (b) Manipuri
(c) Sattriya (d) Mohiniattam

6. Which of the following pairs is wrongly matched?
(a) Mrinali Sarabhai : Bharatanatyam
(b) Kalamandalam Gopi : Kathakali
(c) Sonal Mansingh : Odissi
(d) Singhajit Singh : Kathak

7. Lavani is one of the most popular forms of dance and music that is practised in which state?
(a) Maharashtra (b) Bihar
(c) Gujarat (d) Andhra Pradesh

8. Dance forms like Chodiya, Jagaus, Jhora, Pandav Nritya deals with which of the following state?
(a) Mizoram (b) Uttarakhand
(c) Meghalaya (d) Bihar

9. Match the following.

List I		List II	
A.	Maharashtra	1.	Hultari
B.	Karnataka	2.	Garba
C.	Gujarat	3.	Tamasha
D.	Assam	4.	Tahal Chongli

Codes

	A	B	C	D		A	B	C	D
(a)	3	1	2	4	(b)	4	3	1	2
(c)	1	2	3	4	(d)	3	4	2	1

10. Birju Maharaj is well known for
(a) Manipuri dance (b) Odissi dance
(c) Kathak dance (d) Bhangra

11. Pandit Shivkumar Sharma is associated with which musical instrument?
(a) Tabla (b) Sitar
(c) Sarod (d) Santoor

12. Which of the following pair of the person and their musical instrument is wrong?
(a) Flute – Hariprasad Chaurasia
(b) Violin – Dr Rajan
(c) Santoor – Bhajan Chaudhari
(d) Sitar – Kishan Maharaj

13. Which among the following pairs is correctly matched?
(a) Asad Ali Khan : Rudra Veena
(b) Shiv Kumar Sharma : Santoor
(c) Sajjad Hussain : Surb Ahar
(d) TN Krishnan : Violin

14. Which among the following pairs are incorrectly matched?
(a) Kalighat Paintings : Kolkata
(b) Madhubani Paintings : Rajasthan
(c) Kalamkari Paintings : Andhra Pradesh
(d) Wauli Paintings : Maharashtra

15. Name the paintings that are known for the use of bright colours, animals and bird representations.
(a) Apabhramsa paintings
(b) Pahari paintings
(c) Rajput paintings
(d) Mughal paintings

16. Which festival of Karnataka is celebrated in veneration of the statue of Siddha Bahubali?
(a) Mahamastakabhisheka
(b) Brahmotsav
(c) Ugadi
(d) Onam

17. Which fair takes place twice a year during the Navaratri of Chaitra and Assiy?
(a) Christian Mela (b) Pushkar Fair
(c) Jwalamukhi Mela (d) All of these

18. Name the fair which is also known as the 'Livestock Fair' and is held in the state of Rajasthan.
(a) Nagaur Fair
(b) Pushkar Fair
(c) Baneshwar Fair
(d) Kolayat Fair

19. Pongal festival is related to
(a) Tamil Nadu (b) North India
(c) Assam (d) None of these

20. Onam is the festival of
(a) Kerala (b) Assam
(c) Tamil Nadu (d) Punjab

Answers

1 (d)	2 (d)	3 (a)	4 (c)	5 (a)	6 (d)	7 (a)	8 (b)	9 (a)	10 (c)
11 (d)	12 (d)	13 (b)	14 (b)	15 (b)	16 (a)	17 (c)	18 (b)	19 (a)	20 (a)

Chapter 03

Geography

World Geography

Universe

- The study of universe is known as **Cosmology**.
- The universe is commonly defined as the totality of everything that exists including all physical matter and energy, the planets, stars, galaxies and the contents of intergalactic space.
- A **galaxy** is a vast system of billions of stars, dust and gases bound by their own gravity.
- There are 100 billion galaxies in the universe and each galaxy has on average 100 billion stars.
- Our galaxy is **Milky Way Galaxy** (or the **Akash Ganga**) formed after the Big Bang.
- **Stars** are the heavenly bodies made up of hot burning gases and they shine by emitting their own light.
- **Satellites** are the heavenly bodies that revolve around the planets. Moon is the natural satellite of the Earth.

Solar System

- The solar system consists of the Sun, the eight planets and their satellites (or Moons) and thousands of other smaller heavenly bodies such as asteroids, comets and meteors.
- The **Sun** is at the centre of the solar system and all these bodies revolve around it. It is the nearest star to the Earth.
- Eight planets according to their distance from the Sun are **Mercury, Venus, Earth, Mars, Jupiter, Saturn, Uranus** and **Neptune**.
- The ninth planet 'Pluto' has just been removed from the family of the solar system in 2006.

Planets and their Characteristics

Planets	Characteristics
Mercury	Nearest planet to Sun and Smallest planet.
Venus	Known as evening star. It is brightest planet, nearest planet to Earth, Hottest planet.
Earth	It is known as 'Blue planet' due to presence of water. Life is possible only on Earth.
Mars	It is also known as 'Red planet'.
Jupiter	It is Biggest Planet. Fastest revolution in solar system (9.8 hr only).
Saturn	Second biggest planet.
Uranus	It is Green planet.
Naptune	Slowest revolution in solar system. Farthest planet farm Sun.

Earth

- The Earth is an **oblate spheroid**. It is almost spherical, flattened a little at the poles with a slight bulge at the centre (equator).
- Earth rotates on its axis from West to East once in every 24 hours. This rotation causes day and night on Earth.
- Earth revolves arround the Sun in a orbit once in every $365\frac{1}{4}$ days. The revolution is the cause of different seasons on Earth.
- **Perihelion** is the nearest position of the Earth to the Sun. It occures on 3rd January.

- **Aphelion** is the farthest position of the Earth from Sun. It occures on 4th July.
- The Earth's interior is composed of three major layers -the **crust** (SiAl), the **mantle** (SiMa) and the **core** (NiFe).

Equinox and Solstice

- Equinox is when day and night are equal.
- Solstice is when either day or night is longest or shortest.

Date	Feature
21st March	Equal day and night (Vernal Equinox)
21st June	Longest day in Northern hemisphere (Summer Solstice)
23rd September	Equal day and night (Autumnal Equinox)
22nd December	Longest night in Northern hemisphere (Winter Solstice)

Eclipses

Generally, there are two types of eclipses i.e. Solar eclipse and Lunar eclipse.

1. **Solar Eclipse** It is a situation when the Moon comes between Sun and Earth. It occurs only on a new Moon day.
2. **Lunar Eclipse** It occurs when the Earth comes between Sun and Moon. It only occurs on a full Moon day.

Rocks

- The solid part of the Earth's crust is called 'Rock'.
- Rocks are made up of two or more minerals.
- *Rocks are classified into three main types*
  1. **Igneous Rocks** (Granite, Basalt, Gabbro)
  2. **Sedimentary Rocks** (Sandstone, Gypsum, Limestone, Dolomite)
  3. **Metamorphic Rocks** (Marble, Quartzite, Gneiss, Slate)

Volcano

A volcano is a vent or opening through which Lava comes out. Types of volcanoes on the basis of periodicity of eruption

1. **Active Volcano** A volcano is said to be active if it shows signs of unrest and have erupted in recent past. e.g. Mount Etna, Mount Stromboli etc.
2. **Dormant Volcano** A volcano which has not erupted in near past but it is capable of erupting in future. e.g. Fujiyama.
3. **Extinct Volcano** A volcano which shows no signs of eruption in future. e.g. Hawaiian Emperor, Kohala etc.

Major Mountain Ranges

Range	Location	Highest Peak
Andes	South-America	Mount Aconeagna (Argentina, 3962 m)
Himalayas	Asia	Mount-Everest (Nepal, 8848 m)
Rockies	North-America	Mount Elbert (Canada, 4401 m)
Atlas	North West Africa	Mount-Toubkal (Morocco, 4167 m)
Great- Dividing Range	Australia	Mount-Kosciuszko (South Wales, 2228 m)
Alaska	USA	Mount Denali (USA, 6190 m)
Alps	Europe	Mount Blanc (France, 4804 m)
Western Ghat	India	Anamudi (Kerala, 2695 m)

Important Deserts of the World

Desert	Country/Region
Sahara (Libyan, Nubian)	North Africa
Gibson, Simpson, Victorian, Great Sandy	Australia
Arabian	Saudi Arabia
Dasht-e-Lut	Iran
Atacama	North Chile
Patagonia	Argentina
Kalahari	Botswana
Thar	India
Gobi	Central Asia
Namib	Southern Africa (Angola and Namibia)

Cyclones

Cyclones are known by different names in different parts of the world.

Name	Region
Hurricane	Atlantic Ocean and Caribbean Sea
Typhoon	Western North Pacific and Philippines
Cyclone	Indian and South Pacific Ocean
Tornado	USA and Eastern Pacific
Willy Willy	Northern Australia

List of Local Winds

Wind	Nature of Wind
Chinook	Hot, dry wind in Rockies, also called 'Snow Eater'.
Fohn	Hot, dry wind in the Alps.
Khamsin	Hot, dry wind in Egypt.
Sirocco	Hot, moist wind from Sahara to Mediterranean Sea. It is also known as 'Blood rain'.
Harmattan	Hot, dry wind blowing in Western Africa. Also called 'Guinea Doctor'.
Bora	Cold, dry wind blowing outwards from Hungary to the North of Italy (near Adriatic Sea).
Mistral	Very cold wind, which blows from the Alps over France.
Blizzard	Very cold winds in Tundra region.
Purga	Cold wind in Russian Tundra.
Levanter	Cold wind in Spain.
Norwester	Hot wind in New Zealand.

Major Rivers of the World

River	Origin	Important facts
Nile	Victoria Lake	Longest river of the world (6670 km)
Amazon	Andes (Peru)	Largest river of the world.
Yangtze	Tibetan Kiang Plateau	Deepest river in the world and Longest river in Asia.
Mississippi Missouri	Itaska Lake (USA)	Longest river of North America.
Huang Ho	Kurlun mountains	Also called 'Yellow river'.
Mekong	Tibetan Highlands	Connects six countries in South-East Asia. Contributes immensely to the biodiversity.
Niger	Guinea	The country Niger has been named after this river.

Important Canals of the World

Canal	Region
Panama	Pacific Ocean to Caribbean Sea
Suez	Mediterranean Sea to Red Sea
Erie	Atlantic Ocean to Great Lakes
Kiel	North Sea to Baltic Sea

Important Lakes

Lakes	Location
Caspian Sea (Largest lake)	Kazakistan, Iran, Russia, Turkmenistan
Superior	Canada, USA
Victoria	Uganda, Kenya, Tanzania
Huron	Canada, USA
Michigan	USA
Tanganyika	Tanzania, Burundi
Baikal	Russia
Erie	Canada, USA
Winnipeg	Canada
Ontario	Canada, USA
Titicaca	Bolivia, Peru
Great Salt lake	USA

Important Waterfalls

Falls	Location
Angel Falls (Highest in the world)	Venezuela
Tugela Falls	South Africa
Victoria Falls	Zambia
Hannoki	Japan
Niagara Falls	Canada
Yosemite Catarata	United States
Yumbilla	Peru

Continents of the World

Features	Asia	Africa	North America	South America	Europe	Australia	Antarctica
Area	29.5%	20.2%	16.5%	11.8%	6.5%	5.3%	9.6%
Largest country	China	Algeria	Canada	Brazil	Russia	Australia	—
Smallest country	Maldives	Mayotte	Centre Pierre	Falkland Island	Vatican city	Nauru	—
Longest river	Yangtze	Nile	Mississippi Missouri	Amazon	Volga	Murray Darling	—
Highest Mountain peak	Mt. Everest (8848 m)	Mt. Kilimanjaro (5895 m)	Mt. Mckinley (6194 m)	Aconcagua (6960 m)	Mt. Elbrus	Mt. Kosciuszko	Vinson Massif
Deepest point	Dead sea	Asia Lake	Death Valley	Valdes Island	—	Eyre lake	Bentley Trench

Continents and their Sub-continent

Continent	Sub-continent
Africa	Central Africa, Eastern Africa, Northern Africa, Southern Africa, Western Africa
Americas	Central America, West Indies
Asia	Central Asia, East Asia, Northern Asia, South Asia, South-East Asia, South-West Asia
Europe	Central Europe, Eastern Europe, Northern Europe, South-East Europe, South-West Europe, Southern Europe, Western Europe

Indian Geography

- India is the 7th largest country in the world, with an area of 32, 87, 263 sq.km it covers 2.42% of world area.
- It ranks second in the world in terms of population after China.
- India is located in Northern and Eastern hemisphere.
- The Latitudinal extent of India is 8°4′ North to 37°6′ North and Longitudinal extent of India is 68°7′ East to 97°25′ East.
- Its Southernmost point is Indira Point (Pygmalion Point) and Indira Col is Northernmost point whereas, Ghuar Mota is the Westernmost point and Kibithu is Easternmost point.
- The 82°30′E longitude is taken as the Standard Time Meridian of India.
- Rajasthan is the largest state in India (in terms of area) and Uttar Pradesh is the most populous state in India.
- Tropic of Cancer (23½ ° N) divides the country into almost two equal halves.
  It passes through 8 states.
- Andaman & Nicobar and Lakshadweep Islands are parts of Indian Territory.

Indian States Situated on the Border

Country	Indian States on Border
Pakistan	Gujarat, Rajasthan, Punjab, Jammu and Kashmir
Afghanistan	Jammu and Kashmir
China	J & K, Uttarakhand, Himachal Pradesh, Sikkim, Arunachal Pradesh
Nepal	Uttar Pradesh, Uttarakhand, Bihar, West Bengal, Sikkim
Bhutan	Sikkim, West Bengal, Assam, Arunachal Pradesh
Bangladesh	West Bengal, Assam, Meghalaya, Tripura, Mizoram

Highest Peaks of India

Highest Peak	Height (m)	State
Mt K-2	8611	Kashmir (Pok)
Kanchenjunga	8586	Sikkim
Nanda Devi	7817	Uttarakhand
Saltoro Kangri	7742	Jammu and Kashmir
Kangto	7090	Arunachal Pradesh
Reo Purgyil	6816	Himachal Pradesh
Saramati	3841	Nagaland
Sandakphu	3636	West Bengal
Khayang	3114	Manipur
Anaimudi	2695	Kerala
Dodda Betta	2636	Tamil Nadu

Important Passes

Pass	Location	Connectivity
Karakoram Pass	Jammu and Kashmir	India to China
Zojila Pass	Jammu and Kashmir	Srinagar to Leh
Banihal Pass	Jammu and Kashmir	Jammu to Srinagar
Pirpanjal Pass	Jammu and Kashmir	Jammu to Srinagar
Shipki la Pass	Himachal Pradesh	Shimla to Gartok (Tibet)
Rohtang Pass	Himachal Pradesh	Kullu to Lahaul -Spiti
Nathu la Pass	Sikkim	India to China

Rivers

In India, the rivers are divided into two main groups

(i) Himalayan rivers (Northern India)
(ii) Peninsular rivers (Southern India)

Himalayan Rivers

River	Length (km)	Origin	Falls into
Indus	2880	Near Mansarovar Lake	Arabian Sea
Ganga	2525	Gangotri Glacier	Bay of Bengal
Brahmaputra	2900	Kailash Range	Bay of Bengal

Peninsular Rivers

River	Length (km)	Origin	Falls into
Mahi	583	Vindhyan Range	Arabian Sea
Narmada	1312	Amarkantak	Arabian Sea
Tapi	724	Betul District (MP)	Arabian Sea
Luni	495	Aravalies	Arabian Sea
Mahanadi	857	Foothills of Dandakarnaya (Raipur)	Bay of Bengal
Godavari	1465	Nashik	Bay of Bengal
Krishna	1400	Mahabaleshwar	Bay of Bengal
Cauvery	800	Brahmgiri Range	Bay of Bengal

Important Lakes of India

Name of Lake	State
Chilka Lake	Odisha
Kolleru Lake	Andhra Pradesh
Loktak Lake	Manipur
Lonar Lake	Maharashtra
Pangong Lake	Jammu and Kashmir
Sambhar Lake	Rajasthan
Tso Moriri Lake	Jammu and Kashmir
Vembanad Lake	Kerala
Wular Lake, Dal Lake	Jammu and Kashmir

Water Falls in India

Water Falls	Location
Kunchikal Falls	Karnataka
Berehipani Falls	Odisha
Nohkalikai Falls	Meghalaya
Dudhsagar Falls	Goa
Jog Falls	Karnataka
Hundru Falls	Jharkhand

Important River Projects

Project	River
Bhakra Nangal	Sutlej
Damodar Valley	Damodar

Project	River
Hirakud	Mahanadi
Nagarjunasagar	Krishna
Farakka	Ganga, Bhagirathi
Idukki	Periyar
Indira Gandhi Canal	Sutlej, Beas and Ravi
Kakrapar, Ukai	Tapti
Durgapur Barrage	Damodar
Ramganga Dam	Chisot stream near Kalagarh
Matatila	Betwa
Tehri Dam	Bhagirathi

Soils in India

There are different types of soils found in India. Their distribution and suitability to crops have been mentioned in the given table

Types	States where found
Alluvial	Punjab, Haryana, Uttar Pradesh, Bihar and Jharkhand
Black (Regur soil)	Andhra Pradesh, Madhya Pradesh and Tamil Nadu
Red	Eastern parts of Deccan Plateau, Tamil Nadu, Goa, Odisha and Meghalaya
Laterite	Assam hills, Andhra Pradesh, Karnataka, West Bengal and Odisha
Desert (Aridisol)	West and North-West India, Rajasthan, North Gujarat and Southern Punjab
Saline (Reh,Kallar, Usar, Thur, Rukar) and Alkaline	Bihar, Jharkhand, Uttar Pradesh, Haryana, Punjab, Rajasthan and Maharashtra
Peaty and Marshy	Kerala, Tamil Nadu and Sundarbans of West Bengal

Forests in India

- India has 24.4% of land area under forest and tree cover as per Indian State of Forest Report 2017.
- Madhya Pradesh has the largest forest cover in the country.
- With respect to total Geographical area, Lakshadweep followed by Mizoram has the highest forest cover.

Type of Forest in India

Types	Distribution	Plant Species
Tropical Evergreen Forests	Western Ghats, North-East India, Coastal areas of West Bengal and Odisha, Andaman and Nicobar Islands.	Mahogany, Mahua, Bamboo, Rubber
Tropical Moist Deciduous Forests	Western Ghats, Foothills of Himalayas, Ganga Valley	Sal, Teak, Mulberry, Sandalwood
Tropical Dry Deciduous Forests	Maharashtra, Andhra Pradesh, Punjab, Haryana, Rajasthan, Madhya Pradesh, Tamil Nadu and Uttar Pradesh	Teak, Sal, Bamboo, Shisham
Dry Forests or Arid Forests	Rajasthan, Haryana, Gujarat, Punjab and some parts of South India.	Babool, Date Palm, Cactus
Mangrove Forests	Coastal regions of West Bengal, Odisha, Tamil Nadu, Kerala, Gujarat, Maharashtra, Andhra Pradesh and Andaman and Nicobar Island	Sundari, Palm, Canes, Rhizophora

Important National Parks

National Park	Location	Reserve For
Bandhavgarh National Park	Madhya Pradesh	Cheetal, sambhar, chinkara and wild birds
Bandipur National Park	Karnataka	Elephant, tiger, panther, sambhar, deer and birds
Banerghatta National Park	Karnataka	Elephant, cheetalm, deer
Corbett National Park	Uttarakhand	Tiger, leopard, elephant
Dachigam National Park	Jammu and Kashmir	Kashmiri stag, long tailed marmot, Himalayan serow
Dudhwa National Park	Uttar Pradesh	Tiger, panther, sambar, cheetal, nilgai and barking deer
Gir Forest National Park	Gujarat	India's biggest wildlife sanctuary famous for Gir lions
Jaldapara National Park	West Bengal	Rhinoceros, Elephant
Kaziranga National Park	Asom	One-horned rhinoceros, gaur, elephant
Kanchenjunga National Park	Sikkim	Snow leopard, musk deer and Himalayan boar
Nagarhole National Park	Karnataka	Panther, cheetal, sloth bear and four-horned antelope
Simlipal National Park	Odisha	Tiger, panther, cheetal, nilgai and wild boar

Transportation in India

The most important means of Transport in India are following

Roadways

- It mainly consists of National Highways, State Highways and other district and rural roads.
- The longest National Highway in India is NH-44. It connects Srinagar to Kanyakumari.
- NH-47A is the smallest National Highway in India.
- The Golden Quadrilateral projects connects four major metropolitan cities (Delhi, Mumbai, Chennai and Kolkata).
- Maharashtra has the maximum length of surfaced roads in India.

Railways

- India has the second largest railway network in Asia and fourth largest in the world.
- The first railway line in India was opened in 1853 between Bombay to Thane. It covered a distance of 34 km.
- The first electric train in India was started in 1929 between Bombay to Poona. Its name was 'Deccan Queen'.
- **Vande Bharat Express** is also known as 'Train 18'. It is India's first fully made-in-India train. It is fastest train of India, which runs between Delhi to Varanasi.
- Tejas express in India's first semi-high speed fully air conditioned train introduced by Indian Railways. The inaugural run of Tejas Express was on 24 May, 2017 from Mumbai Chhatrapati Shivaji Maharaj terminus to Karmali, Goa. It covered 552 km in 8 hours and 30 minutes on 2 March, 2019, second Tejas express of the country was flagged off between Chennai Egmore and Madural Junction by Prime Minister Narender Modi. It covered 497 km in 6 hours and 30 minutes.
- The first metro which started in India is Kolkata Metro in 1984. Delhi Metro was started in 2002 between Shahdara to Tees Hazari.

Railway Zones and their Headquarters

Railway Zone	Headquarters
Central	Mumbai (CST)
Eastern	Kolkata
Northern	New Delhi
North-Eastern	Gorakhpur
North-East Frontier	Maligaon-Guwahati
Southern	Chennai
South Central	Secunderabad
South-Eastern	Kolkata
Western	Mumbai (Churchgate)
East Coast	Bhubaneswar
East Central	Hajipur
North Central	Pyayagraj
North-Western	Jaipur
South-Western	Hubli
West Central	Jabalpur
South-East Central	Bilaspur
Kolkata Metro	Kolkata

Note *Southern coastal Railway zone, headquartered at Visakhapatnam (Andhra Pradesh) has been proposed as 18th railway zone of India.*

Air Transport

- JRD Tata was the first person to take a solo flight from Mumbai to Karachi in 1931.
- In 1935, the 'Tata Air Lines' started its operation between Mumbai to Thiruvananthapuram and in 1937 between Mumbai to Delhi.
- In 1953, Indian Airliness and Air India came into existence.
- Vayudoot Limited started in 1981 as a private carries.
- In 2007, both Air India and Indian Airlines have been murged in NACIL.

Major International Airports of India

International Airport	City
Rajiv Gandhi International Airport	Hyderabad
Chhatrapati Shivaji International Airport	Mumbai
Kempegowda International Airport	Bengaluru
Netaji Subhash Chandra Bose International Airport	Kolkata
Lokpriya Gopinath Bordoloi International Airport	Guwahati
Sardar Vallabhbhai Patel International Airport	Ahmedabad
Indira Gandhi International Airport	Delhi
Chennai International Airport	Chennai
Shri Guru Ram Dass Jee International Airport	Amritsar
Cochin International Airport	Kochi

Note *Kerala is the only state in India, which have four international airports.*

Inland Waterways

There are six officially notified Inland National Waterways in India, *which are given below*

	Waterways	Length (km)
NW 1	Prayagaraj to Haldia on Ganges river	1620
NW 2	Sadia to Dhubri on Brahmaputra river	891
NW 3	Kollam to Kottapuram on Champakara Kanal	205
NW 4	Kakinada to Marakkanam along Godavari and Krishna river	1095
NW 5	Mangalgarhi to Paradip and Talcher to Dhamra along Mahanadi and Brahmani river	623
NW 6	Lakhipur to Bhanga along Barak river	121

Ports

- India has about 185 ports including 13 major ports.
- Largest container port of India is Jawaharlal Nehru (Nhava Sheva) port in Mumbai.
- The largest natural port is in Visakhapatnam.
- Kandla port in Gujarat is renamed as Deen Dayal port. It is a tidal port.

Exam Pattern Questions

World Geography

1. Explosion by which universe came into being is called
(a) Universal theory
(b) Solar System theory
(c) Milky Way theory
(d) Big Bang theory

2. In outer space a space man
(a) cannot see star during day time
(b) cannot see stars at all
(c) can see stars during day time opposite Sun
(d) can see stars during day time in all directions

3. The Milky Way Galaxy was first observed by
(a) Galileo (b) Maarten Schmidt
(c) Marconi (d) Newton

4. A group of stars is known as
(a) Galaxy (b) Universe (c) Satellite (d) Planet

5. In which Galaxy our solar system located?
(a) Andromeda (b) Milky Way
(c) Orion (d) Ursa Major

6. What does the study of Universe called?
(a) Cosmology (b) Astrophysics
(c) Cosmography (d) Geophysics

7. Which of the following does not belong to the solar system?
(a) Asteroids (b) Comets
(c) Planets (d) Nebulae

8. Which planet in our solar system is as big as the Earth?
(a) Mercury (b) Max (c) Venus (d) Pluto

9. Nearest planet to Earth is ....
(a) Mars (b) Venus (c) Mercury (d) Jupiter

10. Which planet is known as 'Evening Star'?
(a) Venus (b) Mars (c) Uranus (d) Saturn

11. Farthest planet from Sun is ....
(a) Naptune (b) Uranus (c) Saturn (d) Mars

12. The biggest planet is
(a) Earth (b) Saturn (c) Uranus (d) Jupiter

13. The nearest planet to Sun is
(a) Venus (b) Earth (c) Mars (d) Mercury

14. Which planet is known as the 'Earth's twin'?
(a) Venus (b) Mars (c) Uranus (d) Neptune

15. Which of the following is a cold planet?
(a) Uranus (b) Mars (c) Venus (d) Jupiter

16. Which planet experiences all the seasons as on Earth?
(a) Saturn (b) Uranus (c) Mars (d) Jupiter

17. Which planet does not have satellite?
(a) Jupiter (b) Neptune
(c) Uranus (d) Venus

18. All the planets move around the Sun in a
(a) Circular path (b) Rectangular path
(c) Projectile path (d) Elongated path

19. Which among the following is not a terrestrial planet?
(a) Mercury (b) Jupiter
(c) Venus (d) Earth

20. Among the following which planet takes maximum time for one revolution around the Sun?
(a) Earth (b) Jupiter (c) Mars (d) Venus

21. Which planet looks reddish in the night sky?
(a) Mercury (b) Mars (c) Jupiter (d) Saturn

22. The hottest planet is
(a) Mercury (b) Venus (c) Jupiter (d) Saturn

23. Name of the planet having largest number of natural satellites or Moon?
(a) Jupiter (b) Mars (c) Saturn (d) Venus

24. In how many angle Earth is inclined to its axis?
(a) $66\frac{1}{2}^\circ$ (b) $23\frac{1}{2}^\circ$ (c) 90° (d) 47°

25. What is the reason behind the day and night occur?
(a) Earth rotates to its axis
(b) Earth revolution
(c) Earth rotates with revolution
(d) None of the above

26. International Dateline is situated on
(a) 230° West (b) 180° East and West
(c) 90° East (d) 90° West

27. The time difference between IST and GMT is
(a) 5 hours (b) 5 hours 15 minutes
(c) 5 hours 30 minutes (d) 5 hours 45 minutes

28. Tropic of Cancer is situated in
(a) $23^\circ27'$ North to Equator
(b) $23^\circ27'$ South to Equator
(c) $66^\circ30'$ North to Equator
(d) $66^\circ30'$ South to Equator

29. The latitude which divides the Earth into Northern and Southern hemisphere is
(a) Tropic of Cancer (b) Prime Meridian
(c) Equator (d) Tropic of Capricorn

30. Which among the following eclipse occurs when the Earth comes between Sun and Moon?
(a) Solar eclipse (b) Lunar eclipse
(c) Both (a) and (b) (d) None of these

31. Which divides the world into different time zones?
(a) Latitudes (b) Longitudes
(c) Equinox (d) Solstice

32. On which date Vernal Equinox is observed?
(a) 21st March (b) 21st June
(c) 23rd September (d) 22nd December

33. Longest day on Northern hemisphere is observed on
(a) 22nd June (b) 21st June
(c) 24th June (d) 25th June

34. A knowledge of the Earth interior is obtained from
(a) volcanic eruption
(b) study of the seismic waves
(c) study of deep bores
(d) All of the above

35. Lithosphere is the
(a) upper most part of the Earth
(b) middle part of the Earth
(c) top most layer of the Earth
(d) inner part of the Earth

36. The highly heated fluid rock beneath the crust is termed as
(a) lava (b) magma (c) gabbro (d) rhyolite

37. Weathering is a process by which
(a) river causes erosion
(b) land gets heated
(c) exposed rocks get disintegrated
(d) weather changes take place

38. Marble is the metamorphosed form of
(a) Shale (b) Basalt
(c) Sandstone (d) Lime stone

39. Fossils are commonly found in
(a) Igneous rocks (b) Metamorphic rocks
(c) Sedimentary rocks (d) Volcanic rocks

40. Sedimentary rocks are known to have
(a) stratification (b) fossils
(c) without fossils (d) None of these

41. Which one of the following is igneous rock?
(a) Lime stone (b) Granite (c) Marble (d) Slate

42. Lime stone is a
(a) Intrusive igneous rock
(b) Metamorphic rock
(c) Extrusive Igneous rock
(d) Sedimentary rock

43. Quartzite is a
(a) Metamorphic rock (b) Igneous rock
(c) Sedimentary rock (d) None of these

44. Height of troposphere is ....
(a) 0 to 5 km (b) 0-18 km
(c) 0-25 km (d) 0-30 km

45. Troposphere contains .... % of the gases in the atmosphere
(a) 60 (b) 65 (c) 70 (d) 75

46. Which layer of atmosphere contains the ozone layer?
(a) Troposphere (b) Stratosphere
(c) Mesosphere (d) Exosphere

47. Which is the coldest region of the atmosphere?
(a) Troposphere (b) Mesosphere
(c) Thermosphere (d) Exosphere

48. Due to the presence of ions in this layer, radio waves are reflected back to the Earth.
(a) Troposphere (b) Stratosphere
(c) Mesosphere (d) None of these

49. Maximum height of Mesosphere is
(a) 18 km (b) 50 km
(c) 80 km (d) 200 km

50. Upper part of exosphere is called ......
(a) Magnetosphere (b) Stratosphere
(c) Mesosphere (d) None of these

51. What are cyclones called in 'Northern Australia'?
(a) Hurricanes (b) Typhoon
(c) Cyclones (d) Willy Willies

52. Toranadoes is the name of cyclone of ....
(a) USA (b) Australia
(c) Philippines (d) Indian

53. Willy willies is the name of ....
(a) Cyclones (b) Canals (c) River (d) Deserts

54. Egypt is also called 'Gift of .... river'.
(a) Amazon (b) Kiel (c) Nile (d) Fujiyama

55. Largest river of the world is
(a) Nile (b) Amazon (c) Niger (d) Kiel

56. Hunag Ho is also known as
(a) Green river (b) Blue river
(c) Yellow river (d) Red river

57. Deepest river in the world is ......
(a) Nile (b) Amazon
(c) Yangtze (d) Huang Ho

58. Which of the following deserts found in Iran ....
(a) Barren Desert (b) Sahara
(c) Thar (d) Kalahari

59. Alaska Mountain ranges found in ....
(a) USA (b) Europe
(c) Australia (d) Asia

60. Which mountain range found in Europe?
(a) Andes (b) Alps
(c) Atlal (d) Western Ghat

61. Pustaz grasslands found in ....
(a) Eurasia (b) USA (c) Australia (d) Hungary

62. Name of grasslands found in Brazil ......
(a) Campos (b) Veld (c) Steppe (d) Downs

63. One of the largest Island of the world 'New Guinea' is located in
(a) Denmark (b) Indonesia
(c) Canada (d) Madagascar

64. The longest mountain range of the world 'Andes' is located in which continent?
(a) South America (b) North America
(c) Europe (d) Africa

65. Which lake does not belong to Asia?
(a) Caspian sea (b) Baikal
(c) Aral sea (d) Malawi

66. Which is the second largest continent in the world?
(a) Antarctica (b) Africa
(c) Europe (d) South America

67. Which continent has largest amount of countries?
(a) Asia (b) Africa
(c) South America (d) Europe

68. Which is the highest mountain in Africa?
(a) Atlas mountain (b) Mount Elgon
(c) Mount Kenya (d) Mount Kilimanjaro

69. Mt Kilimanjaro lies in which continent?
(a) North America (b) Europe
(c) Antarctica (d) Africa

70. Europe shares its South boundary with
(a) Arctic ocean (b) Atlantic ocean
(c) Mediterranean sea (d) Ural mountain

71. India accounts for how many percentage of the total geographical land of the world?
(a) 16% (b) 2.4% (c) 4.2% (d) 24%

72. The total geographical area of India is
(a) 15.9 million sq km (b) 3.28 million sq km
(c) 4.67 million sq km (d) None of the above

73. The Southern most latitude of India is
(a) 5°4′ N (b) 6°4′ N
(c) 8°4′ N (d) 10°5′ N

74. What is the share of population of India in the world?
(a) 18% (b) 19% (c) 17.05% (d) 18.55%

75. What is the rank of India in terms of geographical area in the world?
(a) 2nd (b) 5th (c) 3rd (d) 7th

76. The Southern most point of Indian main land is
(a) Kavarati (b) Lakshadweep
(c) Kanyakumari (d) Indira Point

77. Where is the only active volcano of India located?
(a) Lakshadweep
(b) Puducherry
(c) Andaman and Nicobar
(d) Odisha

78. With which among the following countries India shares its longest international border?
(a) Pakistan (b) Nepal (c) Bangladesh (d) China

79. The latitude which divides the country into almost two equal halves is
(a) Tropic of Cancer (b) Tropic of Capricorn
(c) Equator (d) Arctic Circle

80. From how many states of India 'Tropic of Cancer' passes?
(a) Seven (b) Six (c) Four (d) Eight

81. The Southernmost point of India is
(a) Indira Point (b) Indira Col
(c) Kanyakumari (d) Leh

82. Which longitude is taken as the Standard Time Meridian of India?
(a) 82°30' East (b) 82° East
(c) 82°30' West (d) 81°30' East

83. Which of the following Indian state is situated on the border of Nepal?
(a) Himachal Pradesh (b) Arunachal Pradesh
(c) Sikkim (d) Assam

84. Which of the following Indian state is not situated on the border of Pakistan?
(a) Gujarat (b) Rajasthan
(c) Punjab (d) Himachal Pradesh

85. Which of the following Indian state is not situated on the border of Bhutan?
(a) Sikkim (b) Assam
(c) West Bengal (d) Tripura

86. Which of the following Indian state is not situated on the border of Bangladesh?
(a) Assam (b) Meghalaya (c) Tripura (d) Sikkim

87. Which state shares common boundaries with maximum number of other states?
(a) Madhya Pradesh (b) West Bengal
(c) Uttar Pradesh (d) Andhra Pradesh

88. Which country shares its border with maximum number of states in India?
(a) Nepal (b) Pakistan (c) Afghanistan (d) Bhutan

89. India is politically divided into
(a) 29 States 7 Union Territories
(b) 28 States 7 Union Territories
(c) 27 States 7 Union Territories
(d) 29 States 6 Union Territories

90. Which among the following is the highest peak of India?
(a) Mount K-2 (b) Kanchenjunga
(c) Nanda Devi (d) Anaimudi

91. Which among the following is the highest peak of Uttarkhand?
(a) Kanchenjunga (b) Kangro
(c) Saramati (d) Nanda Devi

92. Which among the following is the highest peak of Nagaland?
(a) Sandakphu (b) Saramati
(c) Kangto (d) Nanda Devi

93. Sandakphu is the highest peak of
(a) Sikkim (b) Arunachal Pradesh
(c) Nagaland (d) West Bengal

94. Reo Purgyil is the highest peak of
(a) Himachal Pradesh (b) Arunachal Pradesh
(c) Uttarakhand (d) Manipur

95. Which among the following is not a Himalayan river?
(a) Indus (b) Ganga
(c) Brahmaputra (d) Mahanadi

96. The river Brahmaputra originates from
(a) Mansarovar lake (b) Kailash range
(c) Nashik (d) Gangotri glacier

97. Which among the following is West flowing river in Peninsular India?
(a) Mahanadi (b) Krishna
(c) Godavari (d) Narmada

98. The longest river of Peninsular India is
(a) Tapi (b) Mahanadi
(c) Godavari (d) Mahi

99. From which place Narmada river originates?
(a) Amarkantak (b) Aravalies
(c) Betul (d) Nashik

100. Tapi river falls into
(a) Arabian sea (b) Bay of Bengal
(c) Hemavati (d) Mand

101. Amarkantak is the source of
(a) Cauvery (b) Mahi
(c) Narmada (d) Yamuna

102. Amaravati is the tributaries of
(a) Mahi river (b) Narmada river
(c) Tapi river (d) Cauvery river

103. Which of the following is not a river?
(a) Luni (b) Mahi (c) Indus (d) Aravalies

104. Which among the following dam is located on Periyar river?
(a) Farakka (b) Hirakud (c) Ukai (d) Idukki

105. Which major dam is located on Betwa river?
(a) Tehri dam (b) Matatila
(c) Ukai (d) Indukki

106. Tehri Dam is located on
(a) Betwa (b) Krishna
(c) Bhagirathi (d) Tapi

107. India Gandhi Canal is located on
(a) Sutlej (b) Tapi (c) Damodar (d) Betwa

108. Kakrapar is located on .... river.
(a) Tapti (b) Betwa (c) Sutlej (d) Ravi

109. Bhakra Nangal Dam is located on river.........
(a) Sutlej (b) Damodar
(c) Krishna (d) Ganga

110. Which major dam is located on Krishna river?
(a) Hirakud (b) Nagarjunasagar
(c) Idukki (d) Tehri

111. What per cent of land area of India is under forest and tree cover as per Indian State Forest Report 2017?
(a) 21.7% (b) 21.4% (c) 23.6% (d) 24.4%

112. Which state of India has the largest forest cover?
(a) Uttar Pradesh (b) Uttarakhand
(c) Madhya Pradesh (d) Chhattisgarh

113. Which type of forest in India occupies the largest area?
(a) Montane Wet Temperate forest
(b) Sub - tropical Dry Evergreen forest
(c) Tropical Moist Deciduous forest
(d) Tropical Wet Evergreen forest

114. Most widespread vegetation in India is
(a) Coniferous forest
(b) Tropical Rain forest
(c) Tropical Deciduous forest
(d) Mangrove forest

115. With respect to total Geographical area, which state has the highest forest cover?
(a) Sikkim (b) Mizoram
(c) Uttar Pradesh (d) Nagaland

116. The largest producer of natural rubber is
(a) Tamil Nadu (b) Kerala
(c) Assam (d) Andhra Pradesh

117. In which state largest coal reserves of India are found?
(a) Chhattisgarh (b) Jharkhand
(c) Madhya Pradesh (d) Odisha

118. Which is the largest producer of coal in India?
(a) Bihar (b) Chhattisgarh
(c) Odisha (d) Jharkhand

119. The largest producer of petroleum in India is
(a) Mumbai High (b) Gujarat
(c) Assam (d) Andhra Pradesh

120. The soil formed by the deposition of silt brought by river
(a) Alluvial soil (b) Red soil
(c) Black soil (d) Pod soil

121. Which is the most fertile soil of India?
(a) Black soil (b) Red soil
(c) Alluvial soil (d) Laterite soil

122. The most abundance soil of India is
(a) Black soil (b) Laterite soil
(c) Red soil (d) Alluvial soil

123. Which National Park is famous for Asiatic lions?
(a) Gir (b) Bandhavgarh
(c) Jim Corbett (d) Kaziranga

124. First National Park of India is
(a) Kaziranga (b) Jim Corbett
(c) Simplipal (d) Satpura

125. The only ape of India found in Assam and Nagaland is
(a) Orangutan (b) Gibbon
(c) Chimpanzee (d) Gorilla

126. The longest National Highway of India is
(a) NH 7 (b) NH 44 (c) NH 74 (d) NH 47

127. Which two places are connected by NH 44?
(a) Varanasi to Kanyakumari
(b) Leh to Srinagar
(c) Srinagar to Kanyakumari
(d) Allahabad to Varanasi

128. The transport which provides door to door connectivity is
(a) road transport (b) railways
(c) metro (d) water transport

129. Which project connects four major metropolitan cities (Delhi, Mumbai, Chennai and Kolkata)?
(a) NS-EW Corridor
(b) Golden Quadrilateral
(c) Pradhan Mantri Bharat Jodo Yojana
(d) East-West Corridor

130. What is the position of Indian Railway in Asia?
(a) Second (b) Third
(c) Fouth (d) First

131. When was first railway line opened in India?
(a) 1851 (b) 1852 (c) 1853 (d) 1854

132. The first railway line was opened between
(a) Bombay and Thane
(b) Pune and Bombay
(c) Goa and Pune
(d) Delhi and Agra

133. The first electric train in India started was known by the name
(a) Deccan Queen (b) Deccan Odissi
(c) Shatabdi (d) Maharaja Express

134. Which among the following is the longest railway platform in India?
(a) Gorakhpur (b) Kolkata
(c) Khadakpur (d) New Delhi

135. What is the mascot of Indian Railway?
(a) Misha
(b) Bholu-The guard elephant
(c) Dragon
(d) Waldi

136. Where is the headquarter of Central Railway zone?
(a) Mumbai (b) Jaipur
(c) Kolkata (d) Lucknow

137. The longest train route in India connects
(a) Dibrugarh and Kanyakumari
(b) Srinagar and Chennai
(c) Gujarat and Silchar
(d) Kanyakumari and Bhopal

138. The first metro which started in India in 1984 is
(a) Delhi Metro (b) Mumbai Metro
(c) Kolkata Metro (d) Jaipur Metro

139. In which among the following year Delhi Metro started operating?
(a) 2001 (b) 1998
(c) 2005 (d) 2002

140. In 1937, the 'Tata Air Lines' started its operation between
(a) Mumbai and Delhi
(b) Mumbai and Goa
(c) Goa and Kanyakumari
(d) Mumbai and Thiruvananthapuram

141. Where is Chhatrapati Shivaji International Airport located?
(a) Mumbai (b) Kolkata
(c) Goa (d) Delhi

142. Sardar Vallabhbhai Patel International Airport is in
(a) Guwahati (b) Chennai
(c) Ahmedabad (d) Amritsar

143. National Waterway 1 runs between
(a) Prayagraj to Haldia
(b) Kollam to Kottapuram
(c) Lakhipur to Bhanga
(d) Sadia to Dhubri

144. Which among the following is the longest container port of India?
(a) Vishakhapatnam Port
(b) Mumbai Port
(c) Jawaharlal Nehru Port
(d) Kandla Port

145. Name the port which has been renamed as Deen Dayal Port?
(a) Kandla Port
(b) Mumbai Port
(c) Chennai Port
(d) Vishakhapatnam Port

146. Which is the largest natural port of India?
(a) Paradip (b) Tuticorin
(c) Port Blair (d) Vishakhapatnam

147. Which is the busiest port of India?
(a) Mumbai (b) Kandla
(c) Mangalore (d) Cochin

Answers

1 (d)	2 (c)	3 (a)	4 (a)	5 (b)	6 (a)	7 (d)	8 (c)	9 (b)	10 (a)
11 (a)	12 (d)	13 (b)	14 (a)	15 (a)	16 (c)	17 (d)	18 (d)	19 (b)	20 (b)
21 (b)	22 (b)	23 (a)	24 (b)	25 (a)	26 (b)	27 (c)	28 (a)	29 (c)	30 (b)
31 (b)	32 (a)	33 (b)	34 (d)	35 (a)	36 (b)	37 (c)	38 (d)	39 (c)	40 (a)
41 (b)	42 (d)	43 (a)	44 (b)	45 (d)	46 (b)	47 (b)	48 (d)	49 (c)	50 (a)
51 (d)	52 (a)	53 (a)	54 (c)	55 (b)	56 (c)	57 (c)	58 (a)	59 (a)	60 (b)
61 (d)	62 (a)	63 (b)	64 (a)	65 (d)	66 (b)	67 (b)	68 (d)	69 (d)	70 (c)
71 (b)	72 (b)	73 (c)	74 (c)	75 (d)	76 (c)	77 (c)	78 (c)	79 (a)	80 (d)
81 (a)	82 (a)	83 (c)	84 (d)	85 (d)	86 (c)	87 (c)	88 (a)	89 (a)	90 (a)
91 (d)	92 (b)	93 (d)	94 (a)	95 (d)	96 (b)	97 (d)	98 (c)	99 (a)	100 (a)
101 (c)	102 (d)	103 (d)	104 (d)	105 (b)	106 (c)	107 (a)	108 (a)	109 (a)	110 (b)
111 (d)	112 (c)	113 (c)	114 (c)	115 (b)	116 (b)	117 (b)	118 (d)	119 (a)	120 (a)
121 (c)	122 (d)	123 (a)	124 (b)	125 (d)	126 (b)	127 (c)	128 (a)	129 (b)	130 (a)
131 (c)	132 (a)	133 (a)	134 (a)	135 (b)	136 (a)	137 (a)	138 (c)	139 (d)	140 (b)
141 (a)	142 (a)	143 (a)	144 (c)	145 (a)	146 (d)	147 (a)			

Chapter 04

The Constitution of India

Making of the Constitution

- Firstly, the idea to have a Constitution was given by **MN Roy** (a pioneer of Communist Movement in India) in 1934.
- The Constitution was framed by the **Constituent Assembly** of India, set-up on 16th May, 1946 in accordance with the Cabinet Mission Plan.
- The first meeting of Constituent Assembly was held on 9th September, 1946 under the Chairmanship of Sachchidananda Sinha.
- **Dr Rajendra Prasad** and **HC Mukherjee** were elected as the President and Vice-President respectively on 11th December, 1946.
- BN Rau was appointed as the Constitutional Advisor.
- The Chairman of the Drafting Committee was **Dr BR Ambedkar**, also known as 'the Father of the Indian Constitution'.
- The Constituent Assembly took **2 years, 11 months** and **18 days** to complete the Constitution.
- The Constitution, is adopted on 26th November, 1949, contained a Preamble, 395 Articles divided into 22 Parts and 8 Schedules (presently 12 Schedules).
- The Constitution came into force on 26th January, 1950, known as 'Republic Day of India'.

Sources of the Indian Constitution

UK	Rule of Law, Cabinet System, Prerogative Writs, Parliamentary Government, Bicameral Parliament, CAG Office, Single Citizenship, Law making Procedures
USA	Written Constitution, Fundamental Rights, Supreme Court, Provision of States, Independence of Judiciary and Judicial Review, Idea of Preamble
Erstwhile USSR	Fundamental Duties
Australia	Concurrent List, Joint sitting in the Parliament, language of Preamble
Japan	Procedure established by law
Germany	Suspension of Fundamental Rights during the Emergency
Canada	Scheme of federation with a strong Centre, Distribution of powers between the Centre and the States and placing Residuary Powers with the Centre
Ireland	Concept of Directive Principles of State Policy, Method of election of the President
South Africa	Procedure for amendment of the Constitution and election of member of Rajya Sabha
France	The ideals of liberty, equality and fraternity in the preamble

List of Schedules

First Schedule	Name of States and UTs and their Territorial Extent
Second Schedule	Salaries and emoluments of President, Governor, Chief Judges and Auditor General
Third Schedule	Forms of oath and affirmation of Members of Legislatures, Ministers, Judges and Auditor General
Fourth Schedule	Allocation of seats in the Rajya Sabha
Fifth Schedule	Administration and control of Scheduled Areas and Scheduled Tribes
Sixth Schedule	Administration of Tribal Areas in the States of Assam, Meghalaya, Tripura and Mizoram

Seventh Schedule	Union List, State List and Concurrent List
Eighth Schedule	Languages recognised by Constitution
Ninth Schedule	Validation of certain Acts and Regulations
Tenth Schedule	Anti-Defection Law
Eleventh Schedule	Panchayats (Rural Local Government)
Twelfth Schedule	Municipalities (Urban Local Government)

Fundamental Rights

- The Fundamental Rights are provided in Part-III (Articles 12-35) of the Indian Constitution.
- Originally, there were seven, Fundamental rights but after depletion of right to property, their number reduced to six.

The six Fundamental Rights are given as follows

1. Right to equality (Articles 14-18)
2. Right to liberty (Articles 19-22)
3. Right against exploitation (Articles 23-24)
4. Right to freedom of religion (Articles 25-28)
5. Cultural and educational rights (Articles 29-30)
6. Right to constitutional remedies (Article 32)

Fundamental Duties

- There are 11 Fundamental duties (Earlier was 10) in our Indian Constitution, which are incorporated in Article 51A in Part-IVA of Indian Constitution.
- These were included on the recommendations of Swarna Singh Committee by 42nd Amendment Act in 1976.

Union Legislatures and Executives

Parliament

The Indian Parliament consist of Lok Sabha, Rajya Sabha and President (Article 79).

The Constitution of India has provided for the Parliamentary form of Government.

Rajya Sabha (Article 80)

- It is the Upper House of the Parliament.
- Its maximum strength is 250, out of which 12 members are nominated by President from the fields of science, art, literature and social service.
- Its members are indirectly elected by state legislatures.
- It is a permanent body and is not subject to dissolution.
- 1/3rd of its members retire every second year (their tenure is of 6 years).

Lok Sabha (Article 81)

- It is the Lower House of the Parliament.
- Its maximum strength is 552, of which 530 represents States, 20 represents Union Territories and 2 are nominated by President from Anglo-Indian community.
- Members hold the office for the period of 5 years.
- It is not a permanent body and is subject to dissolution.

Qualifications

For Members of the Parliament Article 84 provides for the eligibility for membership of the Parliament.

The conditions are

(a) citizen of India;

(b) atleast 25 years of age for the Lok Sabha and 30 years of age for the Rajya Sabha; and

(c) possess such other qualifications as may be prescribed by the Parliament.

President

- He is the head of the Union Executive and the first citizen of India.
- President of India is the executive head of Union Government and Supreme Commander of the Armed forces.
- The President is elected indirectly through electoral college consisting of the elected members of both Houses of Parliament and that of state legislative assemblies.
- The oath to the office of President is administered by Chief Justice of India.

Qualifications

- Must be a citizen of India and have completed the age of 35 years. Be qualified for election as a member of Lok Sabha and must not hold any office of profit.

- President can resign from his office by addressing his resignation letter to the Vice-President.
- He can be removed through the process of impeachment on the ground of violation of the Constitution.
- Vice-President acts as a President in case of latter's absence.

Presidents of India

Name	Years
Dr Rajendra Prasad	1950-62
Dr S Radhakrishnan	1962-67
Dr Zakir Hussain	967-69
VV Giri	969
Justice M Hidayat-ul-lah	1969
VV Giri	1969-74
F Ali Ahmed	1974-77
BD Jatti	1977
N Sanjeeva Reddy	1977-82
Giani Zail Singh	1982-87
R Venkataraman	1982-92
Dr SD Sharma	1992-97
KR Narayanan	1997-02
Dr APJ Abdul Kalam	2002-07
Mrs Pratibha Patil	2007-12
Pranab Mukherjee	2012-17
Ramnath Kovind	2017 – till now

Prime Minister

- The Prime Minister elected by Lok Sabha. He is the leader of Lok Sabha.
- As per Article 75 of the Indian Constitution, the Prime Minister shall be appointed by President.
- The term of the Prime Minister's office is not fixed. He remain in office during the pleasure of the President.
- He is administered Oath of the office by President of India.

Prime Ministers of India

Name	Years
Pandit Jawaharlal Nehru	1947-1964
Gulzarilal Nanda	1964
Lal Bahadur Shastri	1964-66
Gulzarilal Nanda	1966
Indira Gandhi	1966-77
Morarji Desai	1977-79
Charan Singh	1979-80
Indira Gandhi	1980-84
Rajiv Gandhi	1984-89
VP Singh	1989-90
Chandra Shekhar	1990-91
PV Narsimha Rao	1991-96
Atal Bihari Vajpayee	1996
HD Deve Gowda	1996-97
IK Gujral	1997-98
Atal Bihari Vajpayee	1998-99
Atal Bihari Vajpayee	1999-04
Dr Manmohan Singh	2004-14
Narendra Modi	2014- till now

Judicial System

Supreme Court of India

- The Supreme Court (SC) stands at the apex of 'The Judicial System of India'.
- Article 124 of the Constitution, deals with the establishment of Supreme Court.
- Under Article 130, the Constitution declares Delhi as the seat of the Supreme Court.
- At present, the Supreme Court consists of 31 judges (including Chief Justice of India).
- Chief Justice of India (CJI) is appointed by the President and other judges of SC are appointed by President after consultation with CJI. Judges holds the office until he attains the age of 6 years.

Qualifications of the Judges

- He should be a citizen of India.
- Must have been a judge of HC for 5 years; or
- Must have been an advocate of a HC for 10 years; or should be distinguished jurist.

High Court

- The Constitution of India provides a High Court for each state, but Parliament can establish a common High Court for two or more or a state and a Union Territory. Presently there are 25 High Courts in India.

- The judges of the High Court are appointed by the President (Article 217).

Qualification of Judges

- He should be a citizen of India. He should have held judicial office in the Territory of India for 10 years; or
- He should have been an advocate of a High Court (or High Courts in succession) for 10 years.
- Governor of a state administers the oath of the office to the judges of High Court.
- A judge of HC holds the office until he attains the age of 62 years.

Local Self Government

Panchayats

(73rd Amendment Act, 1992)

- Panchayats are local self government at rural level.
- Part-IX of the Indian Constitution provides for three tier system of Panchayats, namely :
  - (i) Gram Panchayat (village level)
  - (ii) Panchayat Samiti (intermediate level)
  - (iii) Zila Parishad (district level)
- All the seats in Panchayats are filled by direct elections and the electorate is called 'Gram Sabha'.
- State Election Commission looks after the elections to the Panchayats.
- Rajasthan (Nagaur) is the first state in India to implement Panchayati Raj on 2nd October, 1959 and followed by Andhra Pradesh.

Municipalities (74th Amendment Act)

- Part-IXA provides for local self government in urban areas.
- It deals with the following levels of local self governments.
- **Nagar Panchayat** (for transformed area from rural to urban).
- **Municipal Council** (for smaller urban area).
- **Municipal Corporation** (for larger urban area).

National Symbols of India

National Flag

- Also called 'Tiranga',. It was designed by Pingli Venkayya and adopted on 22nd July, 1947.

National Emblem

- Lion capital of Ashoka at Sarnath was adopted as the National Emblem of India on 24th January, 1950.
- 'Satyameva Jayate', a quote taken from Mundaka Upanishad inscribed below the abacus of Lion capital.

National Anthem

'Jana Gana Mana' was written by Rabindranath Tagore and officially adopted by Constituent Assembly as the Indian National Anthem on 24th January, 1950.

Other Symbols

National Flower	Lotus
National Tree	Banyan
National Animal	Royal Bengal Tiger
National Bird	Indian Peacock
National Calendar	Saka Calendar

Exam Pattern Questions

1. Which country has the largest Constitution?
(a) India (b) America (c) Nepal (d) Japan

2. Who presided over the first meeting of the Indian Constituent Assembly?
(a) Dr Rajendra Prasad (b) Sachidananda Sinha
(c) BR Ambedkar (d) HV Kamath

3. The Constituent Assembly took how many years to complete the Constitution?
(a) 2 years, 11 months, 18 days
(b) 2 years, 11 months, 22 days
(c) 2 years, 11 months, 10 days
(d) 2 years, 11 months, 12 days

4. Who was appointed as the Constitutional advisor of the Assembly?
(a) BN Rau (b) BR Ambedkar
(c) HC Mukherjee (d) MN Roy

5. The Constitution of India was framed by
(a) Working Committee (b) President
(c) Planning Commission
(d) Constituent Assembly

6. Who among the following was the Chairman of the Union Constitution Committee of the Constituent Assembly?
(a) BR Ambedkar
(b) JB Kriplani
(c) Jawaharlal Nehru
(d) Alladi Krishnaswami Ayyar

7. On which day the Constitution of India came into force?
(a) 15th Aug, 1950 (b) 13th Jan, 1952
(c) 26th Jan, 1950 (d) 26th Aug, 1956

8. The Indian Constitution was adopted on
(a) 26th January, 1950 (b) 26th January, 1946
(c) 26th November, 1949(d) 31st December, 1949

9. The first country which adopted Preamble for its written Constitution?
(a) USA (b) India (c) Britain (d) Canada

10. Which of the following term is not used in the Preamble of the Constitution?
(a) Sovereign Democratic (b) Socialist
(c) Secular (d) Federal

11. Fundamental Rights have been adopted from which Constitution?
(a) UK (b) USA (c) Canada (d) Ireland

12. From where have we borrowed the parliamentary form of government?
(a) Russia (b) Ireland
(c) Britain (d) America

13. The directive principle of State policy has been adopted from which Constitution?
(a) US Constitution (b) British Constitution
(c) Irish Constitution (d) French Constitution

14. The National Anthem was adopted by the Constituent Assembly on
(a) 24th May,1949 (b) 24th November,1949
(c) 24th January,1950 (d) 24th June,1950

15. Which Amendment of the Indian Constitution inserted the two words - 'Socialist' and 'Secular' in the preamble?
(a) 28th (b) 40th (c) 42nd (d) 52nd

16. How many schedules (Presently) are there in the Constitution of India?
(a) 9 (b) 10 (c) 11 (d) 12

17. The total number of languages in 8th Schedule of Indian Constitution are
(a) 15 (b) 18 (c) 22 (d) 14

18. How many parts are in Indian Constitution?
(a) 22 (b) 32 (c) 42 (d) 52

19. Which part of the Indian Constitution deals with Fundamental Rights?
(a) Part-I (b) Part-II (c) Part-III (d) Part-IV

20. In how many ways Indian citizenship can be acquired?
(a) Three (b) Four (c) Five (d) Six

21. In which part of the Constitution, details of citizenship are mentioned?
(a) I (b) II (c) III (d) IV

22. Which of these is not included as a Fundamental Right in the Indian Constitution?
(a) Right to Freedom of Speech
(b) Right to Equality before Law
(c) Right to Constitutional remedies
(d) Right to equal wages for equal work

23. In which of the following articles,there is provision of 'Right to Equality'?
(a) Article 14 (b) Article 19
(c) Article 20 (d) Article 21

24. At present in the Constitution of India Right to Property is
(a) Fundamental Right (b) Legal Right
(c) Moral Right (d) Human Right

25. Who is the guardian of Fundamental Rights enumerated in Indian Constitution?
(a) Supreme Court (b) Parliament
(c) Constitution (d) President

26. Which Article of the Indian Constitution did Dr BR Ambedkar term as the 'Heart and Soul of the Indian Constitution'?
(a) Article 14 (b) Article 19
(c) Article 356 (d) Article 32

27. Which of the following has been described as the soul of the Indian Constitution?
(a) Fundamental Rights
(b) Directive Principles of State Policy
(c) Right to Constitutional Remedies
(d) The Preamble

28. In which of the following articles, the interests of minorities are covered?
(a) 14 (b) 19 (c) 29 (d) 32

29. Which of the following writs meaning is - 'to have the body of'?
(a) Habeas Corpus (b) Mandamus
(c) Quo Warranto (d) Certiorari

30. Which writ is issued by a High Court or the Supreme Court to compel an authority to perform a function that it was not performing?
(a) Certiorari (b) Habeas Corpus
(c) Mandamus (d) Quo Warranto

31. How many Fundamental Duties are in the Indian Constitution?
(a) Nine (b) Eleven (c) Twelve (d) Twenty

32. Under which article of the Constitution is the President's rule promulgated in any state in India?
(a) 356 (b) 352 (c) 360 (d) 370

33. Which of the following is not appointed by the President?
(a) Finance Commission
(b) Planning Commission
(c) Commission on Official Languages
(d) UPSC

34. The President of India is elected by the
(a) members of the Lok Sabha
(b) members of both Houses of the Parliament
(c) members of the State Legislature
(d) by an electoral college consisting of elected members of both Houses of Parliament and State assemblies

35. President can forward his resignation to whom?
(a) Speaker of Lok Sabha
(b) Prime Minister
(c) Vice-President
(d) Chief Justice of Supreme Court

36. What is the maximum age limit for the President post of India?
(a) 58 years (b) 60 years (c) 62 years (d) No age limit

37. How many members can be nominated for both Houses of Parliament by the President?
(a) 16 (b) 10 (c) 12 (d) 14

38. Which of the following appointments are not made by President of India?
(a) Speaker of Lok Sabha (b) Chief Justice of India
(c) Chief of Airforce (d) Chief of Army

39. Vice-President is
(a) Member of Lok Sabha
(b) Member of Rajya Sabha
(c) Member of any house
(d) Not a member of any house

40. Which of the following can bring the impeachment motion of Vice-President?
(a) Legislative Council (b) Legislative Assembly
(c) Rajya Sabha (d) Lok Sabha

41. The President can dismiss a member of the Council of Ministers
(a) with the consent of the speaker
(b) only under emergency condition
(c) on the recommendation of the Prime Minister
(d) on his own

42. Who is competent to dissolve the Rajya Sabha?
(a) Chairman of Rajya Sabha
(b) The President
(c) Joint Session of Parliament
(d) None of the above

43. How many members of the Rajya Sabha are elected every two years?
(a) All (b) One fourth
(c) Half (d) One third

44. What is the maximum permissible limit of members in Lok Sabha?
(a) 512 (b) 542
(c) 552 (d) 532

45. What is the minimum age to qualify for the Lok Sabha Elections?
(a) 25 years (b) 30 years
(c) 21 years (d) 18 years

46. Who was the first Speaker of Lok Sabha?
(a) GV Mavalankar
(b) Sarvapalli Radhakrishnan
(c) M Ananthasayanam Ayyangar
(d) Dr. PV Cherian

47. If the Speaker of Lok Sabha wants to resign. To whom does he resign?
(a) President of India
(b) Deputy speaker
(c) Prime Minister
(d) Council of Ministers

48. Who approves a bill as money bill in Lok Sabha?
(a) President (b) Finance Minister
(c) Prime Minister (d) Speaker

49. What is the retirement age of the Judge of Supreme Court?
(a) 60 years (b) 62 years
(c) 64 years (d) 65 years

50. Who holds the power to increase the number of judges in the Supreme Court?
(a) Prime Minister (b) President
(c) Parliament (d) Ministry of Law

51. The Governor does not appoint
(a) Judges of the High Court
(b) Chief Minister
(c) Chairman of the State Public Service Commission
(d) Advocate General of the State

52. Which of the following is related with the Panchayati Raj?
(a) Shah Commission
(b) Nanavati Commission
(c) Balwant Rai Mehta Committee
(d) Librahan Commission

53. 74th Amendment Act is related to
(a) Judicial review (b) Panchayats
(c) Muncipalities (d) State commission

54. Which year is related to 73rd Amendment Act of Indian Constitution?
(a) 1962 (b) 1972 (c) 1982 (d) 1992

55. What is the minimum age required to contest in elections to the panchayats?
(a) 16 (b) 17
(c) 20 (d) 21

56. When was the National Flag adopted?
(a) 22nd July, 1947 (b) 24th January, 1950
(c) 26th January, 1950 (d) 22nd March, 1957

57. When was National Calendar adopted?
(a) 22nd July, 1947 (b) 26th January, 1950
(c) 26th April, 1957 (d) 22nd March, 1957

58. Who composed the song Vande Mataram?
(a) Aurobindo Ghosh
(b) Bankim Chandra Chatterji
(c) Rabindranath Tagore
(d) Satyajit Ray

59. Which is the National Aquatic Animal of India?
(a) Gangetic Dolphine (b) Turtle
(c) Black Cobra (d) None of these

60. What is the name of National Calendar of India?
(a) Vikrama Calendar (b) Hizri Calendar
(c) Saka Calendar (d) None of these

Answers

1 (a)	2 (b)	3 (a)	4 (a)	5 (d)	6 (c)	7 (c)	8 (c)	9 (a)	10 (d)
11 (b)	12 (c)	13 (c)	14 (c)	15 (c)	16 (d)	17 (c)	18 (a)	19 (c)	20 (c)
21 (b)	22 (d)	23 (a)	24 (b)	25 (a)	26 (d)	27 (c)	28 (c)	29 (a)	30 (c)
31 (b)	32 (a)	33 (b)	34 (d)	35 (c)	36 (d)	37 (d)	38 (a)	39 (d)	40 (c)
41 (c)	42 (d)	43 (d)	44 (c)	45 (a)	46 (a)	47 (b)	48 (d)	49 (d)	50 (c)
51 (a)	52 (c)	53 (c)	54 (d)	55 (d)	56 (a)	57 (d)	58 (b)	59 (a)	60 (c)

Chapter 05 Sports

Olympics

- Olympic games were started in 776 BC on Mount Olympus in the honour of Greek God, 'Zeus'.
- The modern Olympic games were started in Athens, the capital of Greece on 6th April, 1896 with great efforts made by French nobleman, Baron Pierre de Coubertin.
- The Olympic Games are organised after every 4 years with the summer and winter games alternative of 2 years.
- The Olympic Flag is made up of white silk and contains five interwined rings as the Olympic Emblem. These five rings coloured blue, yellow, black, green and red represents five continents.
- The official Olympic Motto is Citius, Altius, Fortius, a Latin phrase meaning Swifter, Higher, Stronger.
- The 2016 Olympic games were held in Rio-de-Janerio (Brazil).
- 2020 Summer Olympic will be held in Tokyo, Japan.

India in Olympics

- India first sent a team to the summer Olympic Games in 1920.
- Indian Hockey team won eleven medals in twelve olympics between 1928 to 1980.
- First Individual medal in olympics for India was won by KD Jadhav as a bronze in 1952 Helsinki olympics in wrestling.
- In 2004, Athens olympics Rajyavardhan Singh Rathore won silver medal in shooting.
- In 2008, Beijing Olympics India won first individual gold in shooting by Abhinav Bindra.
- In 2016, Reo Olympics, PV Sindhu won silver medal in Badminton and Sakshi Malik became first Indian woman wrestler to win an Olympic medal (Bronze).

Commonwealth Games

- The first Commonwealth Games were held in 1930 in Hamilton, Canada.
- Since 1930, the games have been conducted every 4 years except for 1942 and 1946 due to World War II.
- 21st Commonwealth Games 2018 was held in Cold Coast City, Queensland, Australia. India finished third in the medals tally at the Commonwealth Games 2018, behind Australia (1st) and England (2nd).
- The 2022 Commonwealth Games will be held at Birmingham (United Kingdom).

Asian Games

- The Asian Games, also called 'Asiad', are a multi-sport event held every 4 years among athletes from all over Asia.
- The games are regulated by the olympic Council of Asia.
- The first Asian Games were held in 1951 in New Delhi (India).
- The 18th Asian Games, 2018 were held in Jakarta and Palembang (Indonesia), India secured 8th position with total 69 medals.
- 19th Asian Games of 2022 will be held at Hangzhou (China).

List of Cups and Trophies

Sport	Trophy
Cricket	Deodhar Trophy, Duleep Trophy, ICC World Cup, Irani Trophy, Ranji Trophy, Vijay Hazare Trophy
Hockey	Sultan Azlan Shah Cup, Agha Khan Cup, Dhyanchand Trophy, Nehru Trophy, Wellington Cup
Football	Durand Cup, Rovers Cup, FIFA World Cup, Kalinga Cup, Santosh Trophy, Subroto Cup
Badminton	European Cup, Malaysian Open, Thomas Cup (Men), Uber Cup (Women)
Table Tennis	Travancore Cup (Women), Swathling Cup (Men), Bama Belleck Cup, Jaylaxmi Cup
Lawn Tennis	Davis Cup, Australian Open, French Open, Wimbledon, US Open
Golf	Augusta Masters, British Open, US Maters, Ryder Cup, Walker Cup
Basketball	Federation Cup, Nehru Cup, FIFA Basketball World Cup

Important Sport Terms

Sport	Term
Cricket	Bye, Draw, Over throw, Duck
Football	Free Kick, Header, Red Card
Hockey	Bully, Striking
Chess	Castle, Promote, Bishop
Boxing	Laying on knock, Upper cut
Badminton	Drop, Love
Polo	Chuker, Bunker
Golf	T, Put, Hole
Billiards	Jigger, Pot, Bolting
Swimming	Breast stroke, Butterfly

Players and their Associated Games

Players	Game	Country
Jaspal Rana	Shooting	India
Geet Sethi	Billiards	India
Pankaj Arjan Advani	Snooker	India
Saina Nehwal, PV Sindhu	Badminton	India
Shikha Tandon	Swimming	India
Ignace Tirkey	Hockey	India
Soma Biswas, Hima Das	Athletics	India
Arjun Singh Atwal	Golf	India
Narayan Karthikeyan	Formula One	India
Sania Mirza	Tennis	India
Ian James Thorpe	Swimming	Australia
Michael J Jordan	Basket Ball	USA
Tiger Woods	Golf	USA
Andi Murray	Tennis	Scotland
Caroline Wozniaciki	Tennis	Den Mark
Victoria Anzarenka	Tennis	Belarus
Serena Williams	Tennis	USA

Famous Stadiums and Related Sports

Stadium	Place	Sport
Netaji Stadium	Kolkata	Football
Wembley Stadium	England	Football
Shivaji Stadium	Delhi	Hockey
Jawaharlal Nehru Stadium	Delhi	Athletics
Bang Bandhu Stadium	Dhaka	Cricket
Wankhede Stadium	Mumbai	Cricket
Green Park Stadium	Kanpur	Cricket
Keenan Stadium	Jamshedpur	Cricket
Nehru Stadium (Chepak)	Chennai	Cricket
Chinnaswamy Stadium	Bengaluru	Cricket
Feroz Shah Kotla Ground	Delhi	Cricket
Eden Garden	Kolkata	Cricket
Oval, Leeds, Lords	England	Cricket
Indraprastha Stadium	Delhi	Indoor Game
Maddison Square Garden	America	Boxing
Forest Hills Flashing Meadows	America	Lawn Tennis

Exam Pattern Questions

1. First Olympic Games held Greek at Mount Olympus in the year
(a) 1896 AD (b) 776 BC (c) 398 AD (d) 400 BC

2. When was the first modern Olympic Games held?
(a) 1888 (b) 1896 (c) 1996 (d) 1998

3. Who among the following is an Olympic medal winner ?
(a) PT Usha (b) Sania Mirza
(c) Mahesh Bhupati (d) Saina Nehwal

4. India won the first olympic Hockey gold at
(a) Amsterdam (b) London
(c) Berlin (d) Los Angeles

5. First Commonwealth Games were played in
(a) 1920 (b) 1930 (c) 1948 (d) 1958

6. 21st Commonwealth Games were held in
(a) 2016 (b) 2017
(c) 2018 (d) 2020

7. The first Asian Games were held in
(a) Tokyo (b) Shanghai
(c) New Delhi (d) Mumbai

8. FIFA Cup 2018 was held in
(a) India (b) Russia
(c) England (d) South America

9. In which year the first ICC World Cup held
(a) 1972 (b) 1974
(c) 1975 (d) 1980

10. Which of the following pairs about the trophies and games is wrong?
(a) Durand Cup : Football
(b) Santosh Trophy : Football
(c) Aga Khan Cup : Hockey
(d) DCM Cup : Hockey

11. Kalinga Cup is related to which sports?
(a) Football (b) Golf
(c) Hockey (d) Badminton

12. Irani Trophy is related with
(a) Cricket (b) Football (c) Golf (d) Hockey

13. Which of the following trophy is related to Badminton?
(a) Davis Cup (b) Ryder Cup
(c) Uber Cup (d) Durand Cup

14. Nehru trophy is associated with
(a) Cricket (b) Football (c) Hockey (d) Baseball

15. 'Bishop' a sport term is used in
(a) Basketball (b) Chess (c) Bridge (d) Golf

16. 'Libero' term is used in
(a) Basket ball (b) Rifle Shooting
(c) Baseball (d) Volleyball

17. The term 'Smash' is related to
(a) Table Tennis (b) Lawn Tennis
(c) Volley Ball (d) Billiards

18. The term 'Butterfly Stroke' is related with which sport?
(a) Swimming (b) Boxing
(c) Wrestling (d) Kabaddi

19. The term 'Grand Slam' is associated with which one of the following game?
(a) Cricket (b) Swimming
(c) Lawn Tennis (d) Badminton

20. 'Cue ball, break shot, pool table' are terms associated with which of the following games ?
(a) Billiards (b) Squash (c) Golf (d) Cricket

21. P Kashyap is related to which sport?
(a) Boxing (b) Athletes
(c) Badminton (d) Cricket

22. Where is Feroz Shah Kotla Stadium located?
(a) Mumbai (b) Kolkata
(c) Delhi (d) Ahmedabad

23. 'Wimbledon' is located in which country?
(a) USA (b) France
(c) Spain (d) UK

Answers

1 (b)	2 (b)	3 (d)	4 (a)	5 (b)	6 (c)	7 (c)	8 (b)	9 (c)	10 (d)
11 (a)	12 (a)	13 (c)	14 (c)	15 (b)	16 (d)	17 (b)	18 (a)	19 (c)	20 (d)
21 (c)	22 (c)	23 (d)							

Chapter 06

Awards and Prizes

INTERNATIONAL AWARDS

Nobel Prize

- Nobel Prize was set-up in 1900 under the will of **Alfred Bernhard Nobel.**
- It is given in the fields of Peace, Literature, Physics, Chemistry, Physiology or Medicine (from 1901) and Economics (from 1969).
- The Swedish Academy of Literature awards the prize in **Literature.**
- The Royal Swedish Academy of Sciences awards the pirze in **Physics** and **Chemitry.**
- The Nobel Assembly of Larolinska Chirugical (Swedan) awards the prize in **Medicine (Physiology).**

Winners of Nobel Prize from India

Winner	Field	Year
Kailash Satyarthi	Peace	2014
Venkatraman Ramakrishnan	Chemistry	2009
VS Naipaul	Literature	2001
Amartya Sen	Economics	1998
Subrahmanyan Chandrasekhar	Physics	1983
Mother Teresa	Peace	1979
Hargobind Khurana	Medicine	1968
CV Raman	Physics	1930
Rabindranath Tagore	Literature	1913

Ramon Magsaysay Awards

- This award was instituted in 1957 named after Ramon Magsaysay, the former President of Philippines.
- The award is given annually on 31st August, the birth anniversary of Magsaysay, for outstanding contributions in public service, community leadership, journalism, literature and creative arts and international understanding.

Grammy Awards

- It is awarded for the outstanding achievements in the music industry by National Academy for Recording Arts and Sciences, America.
- It was started in 1959 and Pt. Ravi Shankar got this award five times.

Oscar Awards

- It was instituted in 1929, these awards are conferred annually by the Academy of Motion Pictures, Arts and Sciences (USA) in recognition of outstanding contribution in the various fields of film making.
- The Indian films nominated for Oscars are Mother India (1957), Salaam Bombay (1988) and Lagaan (2001).
- Bhanu Athaiya was the first Indian to win Oscar Award in 1982 for costume design in 'Gandhi' movie.

Pulitzer Prize

- It was instituted in 1917 and named after US publisher Joseph Pulitzer.
- It is conferred annually in the United States for the accomplishments in journalism and literature

Man Booker Prize

- It is the highest literary award of the world.
- It was instituted in 1968 set-up by the Booker Company and the British Publishers Association along the lines of the Pulitzer Prize of USA.

Gandhi Peace Prize

- It was established in 2nd October, 1994, on the occasion of the 125th birthday anniversary of Mahatma Gandhi, carries a cash prize of ₹ 1 crore.
- Indian Government instituted this annual prize to encourage and promote the significance of Gandhian values over the world.

NATIONAL AWARDS

Bharat Ratna

- Bharat Ratna is India's highest Civilian Award. It was first awarded in 1954. The first recipients of Bharat Ratna were C Rajgopalachari, S Radhakrishnan and CV Raman.
- Bharat Ratna recipients rank seventh in the Indian order of precedence.
- On 25th January, 2019 Nanaji Deshmukh, Bhupen Hazarika and Pranab Mukherjee honoured with Bharat Ratna.

Padma Awards

Padma Awards were instituted in 1954, and announced every year on the occasion of Republic Day. The awards fall in line after the Bharat Ratna.

There are three Padma Awards

- **Padma Vibhushan** is the second highest National Award given for exceptional and distinguished service in any field including service rendered by government employees.
- **Padma Bhushan** is the third highest National Award given for distinguished service in any field.
- **Padma Shri** is the fourth highest award given for distinguished service in any field.

Gallantry Awards

- **Param Vir Chakra** established in 1950. It is the most conspicuous act of bravery or some act of valour or self-sacrifice ill the presence of the enemy, whether on land, at sea or in the air. The medal is made of bronze.
- **Mahavir Chakra** is the second highest gallantry award for acts of conspicuous gallantry in the presence of the enemy whether on land, at sea or in the air. The medal is made of standard silver.
- **Vir Chakra** is awarded for acts of gallantry in the presence of enemy, whether on land, at sea or in the air. The medal is made of standard silver.
- **Ashok Chakra** This is awarded for valour, courageous action or sacrifice, away from the battlefield. It is highest military award during peace time.
- **Kirti Chakra** The decoration is awarded for conspicuous gallantry. It is made of standard silver and is circular in shape.
- **Shaurya Chakra** The decoration is awarded for an act of gallantry during peace time.

Bharatiya Jnanpith Award

- It is instituted in 22nd May, 1961, carries a cash prize of ₹ 11 lakh, a citation and a bronze replica of Vagdevi (Saraswati).
- This award is given for the best literary writing by an Indian citizen in a language listed in 8th Schedule of the Indian Constitution and English.

Sahitya Akademi Award

- This award is a literary honour in India, given by Sahitya Akademi from 1954.
- Annually, confers to the writers of the most outstanding books published in 24 languages, including the 22 listed in 8th Schedule of the Constitution of India along with English and Rajasthani.

Dadasaheb Phalke Award

- It is India's highest award in cinema and instituted in 1969.
- **Devika Rani** was the first recipient of Dadasaheb Phalke Award. This award is given by the Ministry of Information and Broadcasting.

Sports Awards

Rajiv Gandhi Khel Ratna

- It is instituted in 1991-92 with the objective of honouring most outstanding sportsperson to enhance their general status.
- It is the highest award bestowed to a sports person in India. The amount of prize money is ₹ 750000.

Arjuna Award

- It was instituted in 1961 by the Government of India to recognise outstanding achievement in National Sports.
- The award carries a cash prize of ₹ 5 lakh, a bronze statue of Arjuna and a scroll of honour.

Dronacharya Award

- It was instituted in 1985 by the Government of India to recognise excellence in sports coaching.
- The award carries a cash prize of ₹ 5 lakh, a bronze statue of Dronacharya and a scroll of honour.

Dhyanchand Award

- It was instituted in 2002, carries a cash prize of ₹ 5 lakh, a plaque and a scroll of honour.
- This honour is given to those sportspersons who have contributed to sportspersons, and sports by their performance and continue to contribute their promotion for sports even after their retirement from active sporting career.

Exam Pattern Questions

1. Nobel Prize which were started in 1901 by a scientist Alferd Nobel belonged to the country
(a) Sweden (b) Germany (c) Norway (d) England

2. The Nobel Prize is not given in the field of
(a) Literature (b) Economics
(c) Chemistry (d) Mathematics

3. Who was the first recipient of Nobel Prize from India?
(a) CV Raman (b) Rabindranath Tagore
(c) Hargobind Khurana (d) Mother Teresa

4. Who is the first Asian winner of Nobel Prize?
(a) CV Raman (b) Rajiv Gandhi
(c) Rabindranath Tagore (d) Mother Teresa

5. Nobel Prize winner Amartya Sen is known for his work in
(a) Physics (b) Chemistry
(c) Medicine (d) Economics

6. Magsaysay Award for International peace and understanding is given by the country.
(a) India (b) Russia
(c) Philippines (d) Japan

7. Roman Magsaysay Award is constituted in which year
(a) 1957 (b) 1959
(c) 1961 (d) 1963

8. Oscar Award is given in the field of
(a) Cinema (b) Science
(c) Literature (d) Music

9. Which is the highest literary award of the world?
(a) Nobel Prize (b) Man Booker Prize
(c) Pulitzer Prize (d) Magsaysay Award

10. Man Booker Prize is given by institution of which country?
(a) UK (b) USA
(c) India (d) France

11. Bharat Ratna Award was first awarded in
(a) 1920 (b) 1940 (c) 1950 (d) 1954

12. The first recipient of Bharat Ratna was
(a) CV Raman (b) Rajgopalachari
(c) S Radhakrishnan (d) All of these

13. Who is not a recipient of Bharat Ratna 2019?
(a) Nanaji Deshmukh (b) Bhupen Hazarika
(c) Pranab Mukherjee (d) APJ Abdul Kalam

14. Padma Vibhushan is the............ highest National Award.
(a) first (b) second (c) third (d) fourth

15. Who was not the first awardee of Padma Vibhushan in 1954?
(a) Nandlal Bose (b) Zakir Hussain
(c) VK Krishna Menon (d) Abul Kalam Azad

16. Which among the following is India's Highest civilian awards?
(a) Param Vir Chakra (b) Bharat Ratna
(c) Padma Vibhushan (d) Padma Shri

17. Which is the highest gallantry award in India?
(a) Param Vishisht Seva Medal
(b) Param Vir Chakra
(c) Kirti Chakra
(d) Vir Chakra

18. Param Vir Chakra medal is made of
(a) Silver (b) Gold (c) Bronze (d) Steel

19. When was the Param Vir Chakra established?
(a) 1949 (b) 1950 (c) 1952 (d) 1954

20. Who was the first recipient of Param Vir Chakra?
(a) Somnath Sharma (b) Prashan Goyal
(c) MN Singh (d) Ramsunder Das

21. Which is the highest Military Award during peace time?
(a) Ashok Chakra (b) Kirti Chakra
(c) Shaurya Chakra (d) None of these

22. Bharatiya Jnanpith Award was instituted in
(a) 1945 (b) 1951 (c) 1961 (d) 1970

23. What is the cash prize for Jnanpith Award?
(a) ₹ 13 lakh (b) ₹ 11 Lakh
(c) ₹ 10 Lakh (d) ₹ 8 Lakh

24. Maximum Number of Jnanpith Awards are given to which language?
(a) Hindi (b) English
(c) Bengali (d) Malyalam

25. First Sahitya Akademi Award for Hindi language was given to
(a) Makhanlal Chaturvedi
(b) Rahul Sankrityayan
(c) Narendra Dev
(d) Shiv Pujan Sahai

26. The first recipient of Dadasaheb Phalke Award was
(a) Ashok Kumar (b) Devika Rani
(c) Nirupama Rai (d) Guru Dutta

27. The first recipient of Rajiv Gandhi Khel Ratna Award was
(a) K Malleshwari
(b) Viswanathan Anand
(c) Aparna Ghosh
(d) Salim Durrani

28. Rajiv Gandhi Khel Ratna Award was instituted in
(a) 1960-61 (b) 1970-71
(c) 1980-81 (d) 1991-92

29. Arjuna Award is given to
(a) Sportspersons (b) Poets
(c) Scientists (d) Actors

30. The first recipient of Dhyan Chand Lifetime Achievement Award was
(a) Aparna Ghosh (b) Mahavir Singh
(c) A Srinivas Rao (d) Clarence Lobo

Answers

1 (a)	2 (d)	3 (b)	4 (c)	5 (d)	6 (c)	7 (a)	8 (a)	9 (b)	10 (a)
11 (d)	12 (d)	13 (d)	14 (b)	15 (d)	16 (b)	17 (b)	18 (c)	19 (b)	20 (a)
21 (a)	22 (c)	23 (b)	24 (a)	25 (a)	26 (b)	27 (b)	28 (d)	29 (a)	30 (a)

Chapter 07 Indian Armed Forces

Indian Armed forces are divided into three sub categories Indian Army, Indian Airforce and Indian Navy. The President of India is the Supreme Commander of Indian Defence Forces.

Indian Army

Indian Army is the land based and the largest component of the Indian Armed Forces. It is commanded by the Chief of Army Staff. Its headquarter is in New Delhi.

Indian Army Commands

Command	HQ Location
Central Command	Lucknow
Eastern Command	Kolkata
Northern Command	Udhampur
Southern Command	Pune
South-Western Command	Jaipur
Western Command	Chandigarh
Training Command	Shimla

Indian Air Force

The Indian air force is the Air Arm of the Indian Armed Forces. The Chief of Air Staff, an Air Chief Marshal is responsible for operational command of the Air Force.

Indian Air Force Commands

Command	HQ Location
Central Air Command	Prayagraj
Eastern Air Command	Shillong
Southern Air Command	Thiruvananthapuram
South-Western Air Command	Gandhinagar
Western Air Command	New Delhi
Training Command	Bengaluru

Indian Navy

The Indian Navy is the naval branch of the Indian Armed Forces. The chief of Naval staff, a senior flag officer commands the Navy.

Indian Navy Commands

Command	HQ Location
Western Naval Command	Mumbai
Eastern Naval Command	Visakhapatnam
Southern Naval Command	Kochi
Andaman and Nicobar Command	Port Blair

Ranks of Commissioned Officer in Armed Forces

Rank in Army	Rank in Navy	Rank in Air Force
Field Marshal	Admiral of the Fleet	Marshal of the IAF
General	Admiral	Air Chief Marshal
Lt General	Vice Admiral	Air Marshal
Major General	Rear Admiral	Air Vice-Marshal
Brigadier	Commodore	Air Commodore
Colonel	Captain	Group Captain
Lt Colonel	Commander	Wing Commander
Major	Lt Commander	Squadron Leader
Captain	Lieutenant	Flight Lieutenant
Lieutenant	Sub-Lieutenant	Flying Officer

Indian Defence Training Institutions

Training Institution	Place	Estd in
Rashtriya Indian Military College (RIMC)	Dehradun	1922
Army Cadet College (ACC)	Dehradun	1929
Indian Military Academy (IMA)	Dehradun	1932
National Defence Academy (NDA)	Khadakwasla, Pune	1941
College of Defence Management	Secunderabad	1970
Army School of Physical Training (ASPT)	Pune	1978

Training Institution	Place	Estd in
Army Air Defence College (AADC)	Gopalpur (Odisha)	1989
Officers Training Academy	Gaya	2011
Indian National Defence University (INDU)	Gurugram (Haryana)	2013

Paramilitary and Reserve Forces

Assam Rifles	It was established in 1835
Intelligence Bureau (IB)	It was set-up in 1920.
Central Reserve Police Force (CRPF)	It was set-up in 1939.
Territorial Army (TA)	It was established in 1948.
Home Guard	It was established in 1962.
Indo-Tibetan Border Police (ITBP)	It was established in 1962, after the Chinese attack.
Central Bureau of Investigation (CBI)	It was established in 1963.
Border Security Force (BSF)	It was established in 1965.
Central Industrial Security Force (CISF)	It was set-up in 1969 after the recommendations of Justice B Mukherji.

Important Indian Missiles

Name	Class	Range
Agni I	SRBM	750 km
Agni II	MRBM	2500 km
Agni III	IRBM	3500 km-5500 km
Agni IV	IRBM	4000 km
Agni V	ICBM	5000 km-6000 km
Agni VI	ICBM	8000-10000 km
Dhanush	SRBM	350 km
Nirbhay	Subsonic Cruise Missile	1000 km
Brahmos	Supersonic Cruise Missile	290 km
Brahmos 2	Hypersonic Cruise Missile	290 km
Prithvi I	SRBM	150 km
Prithvi II	SRBM	150-350 km
Prithvi III	SRBM	350-600 km
Sagarika	SLBM	700 km
Shaurya	TBM	700 km
Astra	Air to Air Missile	80 km-100 km
Nag	Anti-Tank	7 km
Barak	Long range missile	0.5-12 km

Submarines of the Indian Navy

Submarines	Description
INS Vibhuti	It was India's first indigenously built missile boat launched at Mazgaon Docks in Mumbai.
INS Shakti	It was India's first indigenously built submarine.
INS Kalvari	It is the first of the Indian Navy's Six Kalvari-class submarine being built in India.
INS Arihant	It is a class of nuclear-powered balistic missile submarines built for the Indian Navy.
INS Karanj	It is the third of the six Kalvari-class submarine launched in January, 2018.
INS Arighat	It is second Arihant class submarine to be commissioned in 2019.
INS Vela	It is siath kalvari class submarines to be commissioned in 6 May, 2019.

Warships of the Indian Navy

Warship	Description
INS Vikrant	The first Aircraft carrier of Indian Navy was INS Vikrant.
INS Viraat	It is a centaur class aircraft carrier.
INS Prahar	It is world's fastest missile ship commissioned in 1997.
INS Vikramaditya	It is a kiev class aircraft carrier. On 14th June, 2014 it inducted into Indian Navy.
INS Kavaratti	It is an anti-submarine warfare corvette of the Indian Navy.
INS Kochi	It is the second ship of the Kolkata-class destroyers built of the Indian Navy.
INS Astradharani	It is first totally indigenously-designed and built torpedo, commissioned on 6th October, 2015.
INS Imphal	It is third guided missile destroyer and designed by the Indian Navy. It is launched in April 2019.

Exam Pattern Questions

1. The Supreme Commander of Armed Forces is
(a) Prime Minister (b) President
(c) Field Marshal (d) General

2. Which of the following pairs of forces and their command is wrong?
(a) Army : 7 Command
(b) Airforce : 7 Command
(c) Navy : 3 Command
(d) Army : 4 Command

3. Training command to Indian Army is located at
(a) Pune (b) Jaipur (c) Shimla (d) Lucknow

4. When was the Indian Air Force created ?
(a) 26th Jan, 1950 (b) 8th Oct, 1932
(c) 8th Oct, 1935 (d) 15th Aug, 1947

5. Central command of Indian Air Force is located at
(a) Prayagaraj (b) Shillong
(c) New Delhi (d) Patna

6. Tri Service Theatre command of Indian Armed Forces is located at
(a) Goa
(b) Andaman and Nicobar
(c) Lakshadweep
(d) Mumbai

7. At which of the following places is the headquarters of South-Western Air Command located?
(a) Vadodara (b) Jodhpur
(c) Pune (d) Gandhinagar

8. How many commands are made in Indian Navy?
(a) Two (b) Three
(c) Four (d) Five

9. Where is the Eastern Naval Command's headquarters located?
(a) Mumbai (b) Visakhapatnam
(c) Kochi (d) Port Blair

10. What is the equivalent rank of Lt. Colonel (Army) in Indian Air Force?
(a) Group Captain (b) Wing Commander
(c) Air Commodore (d) Squadron Leader

11. National Defence College was established in
(a) 1970 (b) 1948 (c) 1960 (d) 1961

12. Which one of the following is Nuclear-capable submarine that can launch ballistic missile?
(a) Arihant (b) Shourya
(c) Prithvi (d) Nag

13. 'Arihant' is the name of
(a) an infantry combat vehicle
(b) a ballistic missile
(c) an attack helicopter
(d) a nuclear-powered submarine

14. Which was the first indigenously built missile boat of India?
(a) INS Vinash (b) INS Vibhuti
(c) INS Shakti (d) INS Ajay

15. Who is the first woman Air Marshal of Indian Air Force (IAF)?
(a) Punita Arora
(b) Harita Kaur Deol
(c) Kanchan Chaudhary
(d) Padmavathy Bandopadhyay

16. The Unmanned Aerial Vehicle (UAV) developed by India is called
(a) Udaan (b) Nishant
(c) Maitri (d) Gauri

Answers

1 *(b)*	2 *(d)*	3 *(c)*	4 *(b)*	5 *(a)*	6 *(a)*	7 *(d)*	8 *(b)*	9 *(b)*	10 *(b)*
11 *(c)*	12 *(c)*	13 *(d)*	14 *(b)*	15 *(d)*	16 *(b)*				

Chapter 08

General Knowledge

(Books and Authors, Invention and Discoveries, International Organisation Abbreviations & Terminology etc)

First in the World

First Space Shuttle Launched	Columbia (April 1981)
First Country to make Constitution	America
First Country to start Underground Metro Rail	Britain
First Unmanned Mission on the Moon	LUNA-9
First Spacecraft to carry man on the Moon	Apollo-11
First Country to do Artificial Satellite Experiment	Russia
First Man to climb Mount Everest	Sherpa Tenzing Norgay and Sir Edmund Hillary
First Man to go into Space	Major Yuri Gagarin
First Woman Prime Minister	Sirimavo Bandaranaike (Sri Lanka)
First Woman to cross the Seven Seas	Bula Choudhary

Superlatives in the World

Superlative	Name and Other Information
Largest island	Greenland
Largest fresh water lake (by surface area)	Lake Superior (USA)
Largest country (by area)	Russia
Largest airport (by area)	King Fahd International Airport, Riyadh (Saudi Arabia)
Largest temple	Angkor Wat, Cambodia
Largest inland salt water body	Caspian Sea
Largest delta	Sundarbans
Largest mosque (by area)	Masjid Al-Haram
Highest extinct volcano	Chimborazo
Lake at highest location	Lake Titicaca (Bolivia and Peru)
Longest bridge	Jiaozhou Bay Bridge (China)
Longest railway platform	Gorakhpur, (India)
Tallest office building	Burj Khalifa (UAE)

First in India

Achievement	Name
First church in India	St. Thomas Church, (Kerala)
First person to receive the Param Vir Chakra	Major Somnath Sharma
First person to receive Dadasaheb Phalke Award	Devika Rani
First Indian to receive Magsaysay Award	Vinoba Bhave
First Indian to win the Nobel Prize	Rabindranath Tagore (for Literature)
First Indian to win an Oscar Award	Bhanu Athaiya
First Woman IPS Officer	Kiran Bedi
First Deputy Prime Minister	Sardar Vallabhbhai Patel
First Woman Minister in the Indian Government	Rajkumari Amrit Kaur
First Indian to go into space	Squadron Leader Rakesh Sharma
First Indian satellite	Aryabhatta
First Indian lunar probe	Chandrayaan-I
First state to achieve 100% primary literacy	Kerala
First National Park established	Corbett National Park
First Women Chief Justice of High Court	Leila Seth

Superlatives in India

Superlative	Name and other Information
Largest fresh water lake	Wular lake (J & K)
Largest man-made lake	Govind Vallabh Pant Sagar (Rihand Dam, Uttar Pradesh
Largest dome	Gol Gumbaz, Bijapur (Karnataka)
Largest district	Kutch (Gujarat)
Largest saline water lake	Lake Chilika (Odisha)
Largest animal fair	Sonepur (Bihar)
Largest river island	Majuli (Assam)
Longest river bridge	Bhupen Hazarika Setu (Assam)
Longest national highway	NH 44 (Srinagar to Kanyakumari)
Longest river	Ganga
Longest road tunnel	Chenani-Nashri Tunnel (Jammu and Kashmir)
Longest dam	Hirakud (Odisha)
State with longest coastline	Gujarat
Highest mountain peak	Kanchenjunga
Tallest statue	Statue of Unity, Gujarat
Smallest state in area	Goa
Least populated state	Sikkim
Most populated city	Mumbai (Maharashtra)
Highest dam	Tehri Dam (Uttarakhand)

Major Countries, their Capitals and Currencies

Name of Country	Capital	Currency
Afghanistan	Kabul	Afghani
Argentina	Buenos Aires	Argentine Peso
Australia	Canberra	Australian Dollar
Bangladesh	Dhaka	Taka
Bhutan	Thimphu	Ngultrum
Brazil	Brasilia	Brazilian Real
Canada	Ottawa	Canadian Dollar
China	Beijing	Yuan, Renminbi
Egypt	Cairo	Egyptian Pound
France	Paris	Euro
Germany	Berlin	Euro
India	New Delhi	Indian Rupee (₹)
Italy	Rome	Euro
Japan	Tokyo	Yen (¥)
Malaysia	Kuala Lumpur	Ringgit
Myanmar	Nypyidaw	Kyat
Pakistan	Islamabad	Pakistani Rupee
Russia	Moscow	Ruble
Saudi Arabia	Riyadh	Saudi Riyal
South Korea	Seoul	Won
South Sudan	Juba	Sudanese Pound
Sri Lanka	Colombo/Sri Jayawardenepure Kotte	Sri Lankan Rupee
Switzerland	Bern	Swiss Franc
United Kingdom	London	Pound Sterling (£)
USA	Washington DC	US Dollar ($)
Zimbabwe	Harare	US Dollar

Seven Wonders of the World

Wonders	Location
Pyramid	Chichen Itza, Mexico
Christ Redeemer	Brazil
The Great Wall	China
Machu Picchu	Peru
Petra	Jordan
Roman Colosseum	Italy
The Taj Mahal	India

International Border Lines

Name	In between
Radcliffe Line (1947)	India and Pakistan (Indo-Pak)
McMahon Line (1914)	India and China (Indo-China)
Durand Line (1893)	Pakistan and Afghanistan
Hindenburg Line	Germany and Poland
Maginot Line	France and Germany
Order Neisse Line	Germany and Poland
Siegfride Line	Germany and France
38th Parallel Line	North and South Korea
49th Parallel Line	USA and Canada
17th Parallel Line	North Vietnam and South Vietnam

Nicknames or Pen Names of Famous Personalities

Nickname or Pen Name	Actual Name
Bird Man of India	Salim Ali
Panditji	Jawaharlal Nehru
Deshbandhu	Chittaranjan Das
Flying Sikh	Milkha Singh
Frontier Gandhi and Badshah Khan	Khan Abdul Ghaffar Khan
Gurudev	Rabindranath Tagore
Haryana Hurricane	Kapil Dev
Iron Man of India	Vallabhbhai Patel
Little Master	Sunil Gavaskar
Lokmanya	Bal Gangadhar Tilak
Loknayak	Jayaprakash Narayan
Magician of Hockey and Hockey Wizard	Dhyanchand
Master Blaster	Sachin Tendulkar
Mother Teresa	Agnes Gonxha Bojaxhiu
Netaji	Subhash Chandra Bose
Punjab Kesari	Lala Lajpat Rai
Father of the Nation, Bapu and Mahatma	M.K Gandhi
Swar Kokila	Lata Mangeshkar
Udanpari and Payyoli Express	PT Usha

Crematorium of Famous Persons (India)

Crematorium	Person
Samata Sthal	Jagjivan Ram
Karma Bhumi	Dr Shankar Dayal Sharma
Mahaprayan Ghat	Dr Rajendra Prasad
Raj Ghat	Mahatma Gandhi
Vijay Ghat	Lal Bahadur Shastri
Kisan Ghat	Chaudhary Charan Singh
Smriti Sthal	IK Gujral
Veer Bhumi	Rajiv Gandhi
Ekta Sthal	Giani Zail Singh, Chandra Shekhar, PV Narasimha
Uday Bhumi	KR Narayanan
Shanti Van	Jawaharlal Nehru
Shakti Sthal	Indira Gandhi
Sadaiv Atal	Atal Bihari Vajpayee

Nicknames of Important Indian Places

Nickname	Place
Golden City	Amritsar
Space City/Garden City/ Electronic City	Bengaluru
Pink City	Jaipur
Twin City	Hyderabad-Secunderabad
Steel City	Jamshedpur (Tata Nagar)
City of Joy/Palaces	Kolkata
Manchester of India	Ahmedabad
Venice of the East	Alappuzha
Hollywood of India/ Gateway of India	Mumbai
Heaven of India	Jammu and Kashmir
Pittsburg of India	Jamshedpur
Little Lhasa	Dharamshala
Deccan Queen	Pune

Books and their Authors (International)

Name of Book	Name of Author
A Tale of Two Cities	Charles Dickens
Macbeth, Hamlet, Julius Caesar	William Shakespeare
The Time Machine, The Invisible Man	HG Wells
Adventures of Sherlock Holmes	Arthur Conan Doyle
Das Kapital	Karl Marx
War and Peace, Anna Karenina	Leo Tolstoy
On the Origin of Species	Charles Darwin
The Diary of a Young Girl	Anne Frank
Long Walk to Freedom	Nelson Mandela
Mein Kampf (My Struggle)	Adolf Hitler
Up From Slavery	Booker T Washington
The Adventures of Huckleberry Finn	Mark Twain

Books and their Authors (Indian)

Name of Book	Name of Author
Ram Charit Manas	Tulsidas
Bhagwad Gita, The Mahabharata	Maharshi Ved Vyas
Meghdoot, Kumarasambhava	Kalidas

Name of Book	Name of Author
Arthashastra	Kautilya
Gitanjali	Rabindranath Tagore
Godan	Munshi Premchand
The Discovery of India	Jawaharlal Nehru
My Experiments with Truth	MK Gandhi
The Guide	RK Narayan
Wings of Fire	Dr APJ Abdul Kalam
Kalpana Chawla – A Life	Anil Padmanabhan
The God of Small Things	Arundhati Roy
What Young India Wants, Two States	Chetan Bhagat
Train to Pakistan	Khuswant Singh
The Broken Wing: Songs of Love, Death and Destiny	Sarojini Naidu
Devdas, Parineeta	Saratchandra Chattopadhyay
You Can Win	Shiv Khera
The Sleeping Giant	Swami Vivekananda
A House for Mr. Half-A Life, A Bend in the River	VS Naipaul
The Golden Gate, A Suitable Boy	Vikram Seth
Pinjar, The Other Dimension	Amrita Pritam
A Tunnel of Time : An Autobiography	RK Laxman
A Voice of Freedom	Nayantara Sehgal
Between the Lines	Kuldip Nayar
Exam Warriors	Narendra Modi
The Coalition Years	Pranab Mukherjee
Why I am a Hindu	Shashi Tharoor
The Accidental Prime Minister	Sanjaya Baru
India after Gandhi	Ramachandra Guha

Invention and Discoveries

Invention	Inventory
Telescope	Galileo
Steam Engine	James Watt
Elevator	Elisha Otis
Light Bulb	Thomas Edison
Radio	Guglielmo Marconi
Car	Henry Ford
Aeroplane	Wright Brothers
Barometer	Evanglista Torrecelli
Electronic Computer	Dr. Alam M Turing
Gramophone	Thomas Alva Edison
Machine Gun	James Puckle
Printing Press	Johan Gutenberg
Steam Engines	James Watt
Telegraph	M Lammond

Important-International organisation

United Nations (UN)

- The United Nations (UN) is a world level organisation formed in 1945.
- It came into existence after World War II to create a world level organisation that would help to ensure peace.
- UN comprised of 193 member countries. The 193rd member being the newly created South Sudan.

There are six principle organs of the United Nations, they are

1. General Assembly (HQ-New York, USA)
2. The Security Council (HQ-New York, USA)
3. The Economic and Social Council (HQ-New York, USA)
4. The Trusteeship Council (HQ-New York, USA)
5. The International Court of Justice (HQ- Hague, Netherland)
6. The Secretariat (HQ-New York, USA)

Important United Nation Agencies

Name of Agency	Headquarter	Objective
International Labour Organisation (ILO) (1919)	Geneva	To improve conditions and living standards of workers.
International Monetary Fund (IMF) (1945)	Washington DC	To promotes international monetary cooperation.
Food and Agricultural Organisation (FAO) (1945)	Rome	To improve living conditions of rural population.

Name of Agency	Headquarter	Objective
International Bank for Reconstruction and Development (IBRD) (1944)	Washington DC	To provide funds from different sources.
United Nations International Children's Emergency Fund (UNICEF) (1946)	New York	To promote children's welfare all over the world.

Important International Organisation

Name of Agency	Headquarters
World Trade Organisation (WTO)	Geneva (Switzerland)
World Health Organisation (WHO)	Geneva
South Asian Association for Regional Cooperation (SAARC)	Kathmandu (Nepal)
Asia Pacific Economic Cooperation (APEC)	Singapore
Organisation of the Petroleum Exporting Countries (OPEC)	Vienna (Austria)
United Nations Development Programme (UNDP)	New York
United Nations Educational, Scientific and Cultural Organisation (UNESCO)	Paris

Important Date/Days

9th January	Pravasi Bhartiya Diwas
12th January	National Youth Day (Birthday of Swami Vivekanand)
15th January	Army Day
24th January	Rashtriya Balika (Girl Child) Day
30th January	Martyr's Day (Mahatma Gandhi's Martyrdom Day)
28th February	National Science Day
3rd March	National Defence Day, World Wildlife Day
8th March	International Women's Day
22nd March	World Water Day
7th April	World Health Day
22nd April	World Earth Day
1st May	International Labour Day
31st May	World Anti-Tobacco Day
21st June	World Yoga Day
29th July	International Tiger Day
26th July	Kargil Victory Day
15th August	Independence Day
20th August	Sadbhavana Diwas
29th August	National Sports Day
5th September	Teacher's Day
14th September	Hindi Divas
27th September	World Tourism Day
2nd October	Gandhi Jayanti
8th October	Indian Air Force Day
14th November	Children Day
1st December	World AIDS Day
7th December	Armed Forces Flag Day
10th December	Human Right Day
16th December	Vijay Diwas
23rd December	Kisan Diwas
25th December	Good Governance Day

ABBREVIATIONS

A

ABM	Anti-Ballistic Missiles
ADB	Asian Development Bank
AIDS	Acquired Immuno Deficiency Syndrome
AIIMS	All India Institute of Medical Sciences
ALH	Advanced Light Helicopter
APEC	Asia-Pacific Economic Cooperation
ASAT	Anti-Satellite Weapon
ASIAN	Association of South-East Asian Nations
ASLV	Augmented Satellite Launch Vehicle
ATM	Automated Teller Machine

B

BARC	Bhabha Atomic Research Centre
BBC	British Broadcasting Corporation
BMD	Ballistic Missile Defence System
BHIM	Bharat Interface for Monday
BSF	Border Security Force

C

CBI	Central Bureau of Investigation
CID	Criminal Investigation Department
CISF	Central Industrial Security Force
CNG	Compressed Natural Gas
CRR	Cash Reserve Ratio
CSIR	Council of Scientific and Industrial Research

D

DNA	De-oxyribonucleic Acid
DRDO	Defence Research and Development Organisation

E

ECG	Electrocardiogram
EVM	Electronic Voting Machine

F

FAO	Food and Agriculture Organisation
FDI	Foreign Direct Investment
FBI	Federal Bureau of Investigation
FIR	First Information Report

G

GDP	Gross Domestic Product
GNP	Gross National Product
GPO	General Post Office
GPS	Global Positioning System
GSLV	Global Positioning Satellite Launch Vehicle
GST	Goods and Services Tax

H

HAL	Hindustan Aeronautics Limited
HIV	Human Immunodeficiency Virus
HYV	High Yielding Variety

I

IAS	Indian Administrative Service
IAEA	International Atomic Energy Agency
INS	Indian Naval Ship
ILO	International Labour Organisation
IPC	Indian Penal Code
IRBM	Intermediate Range Ballistic Missile
IRSS	Indian Remote Sensing Satellite
ISRO	Indian Space Research Organisation

J,K,L

JAM	Jandhan Aadhar Mobile
KCC	Kisan Credit Card/Kisan Call Centre
KYC	Know Your Customer
LCA	Light Combat Aircraft
LOC	Line of Control
LPG	Liquified Petroleum Gas

M, N

MSS	Multimedia Message Service
MTCR	Missile Technology Control Regime
NAA	National Airport Authority
NABARD	National Bank for Agriculture and Rural Development
NASA	National Aeronautics and Space Administration
NITI Aayog	National Institution for Transformation India Aayog

O

OCI	Overseas Citizenship of India
OPEC	Organisation of the Petroleum Exporting Countries
ONGC	Oil and Natural Gas Corporation

P

PAN	Permanent Account Number
PIN	Postal Index Number
POTA	Prevention of Terrorism Act
PSLV	Polar Satellite Launch Vehicle
PTI	Press Trust of India

R, S

RBI	Reserve Bank of India
RTI	Right to Information
SAARC	South Asian Association for Regional Cooperation
SBI	State Bank of India
SAIL	Steel Authority of India Limited
SCO	Shanghai Cooperation Organisation
SEBI	Securities and Exchange Board of India
STARS	SatelliteTracking and Ranging Station

T, U

TIN	Tax Identification Number
TRAI	Telecom Regulatory Authority of India
UAV	Unmanned Aerial Vehicle
UNDP	United Nations Development Programme
UPS	Uninterruptible Power Supply

W	
WADA	World Anti-Doping Agency
WFP	World Food Programme
WHO	World Health Organisation
WWW	World Wide Web

Terminologies

Geographical Terms

- **Cartography** The art and science of making maps.
- **Census** An investigation or count of a population.
- **Climate** The long-term trends in weather conditions for an area.
- **Demography** The study of population statistics and trends, such as births, deaths and disease.
- **Floodplain** A flat, low-lying area near a river or stream which is subject to flooding.
- **Epicenter** The point on the Earth's surface directly above the hypocenter, where the energy of an earthquake is first released.
- **Erosion** Forces that shape the Earth's surface. Includes water, wind and ice.
- **Estuary** The wide end of a river when it meets the sea; salty tidal water mixes with the fresh water of the river here.
- **Hemisphere** Half of the Earth's surface.
- **Humidity** The amount of water vapour in the air.
- **Magma** Molten rock that lies beneath the surface of the Earth; once exposed, magma becomes lava.
- **Lithosphere** The soil and rock layer of the Earth.
- **Map** A graphic representation of the Earth's surface.
- **Meteorology** The scientific study of the atmosphere.
- **Monsoon** A wind system in South-East Asia which changes direction seasonally, creating wet and dry seasons.
- **Precipitation** Any form of water that falls from the atmosphere to the surface of the Earth (e.g. rain, snow, sleet and hail).

Economic Terms

- **Bank** A bank is a financial institution that accept deposits from the public and creates credit.
- **Gross Domestic Product** (GDP) is a monetary measure of the market value of all final goods and services produced in a period of time, often annually.
- **Production** It is the creation of goods or services that has value to another individual.
- **Distribution** It is the method of getting the goods to the individuals who will use them.
- **GST** An indirect tax which is a comprehensive multi-stage, destination based tax is levied on every value addition.
- **Consumption** The actual use of the goods that are produced is what is known as 'consumption'. Often times, consumption produces some form of waste.
- **Services** These are the processes that are desired by individuals.
- **Consumer** is the individual who will use the goods or services.
- **Producer** is the individual who will create the goods or services.
- **A government** is a formal body which is in charge of creating and enforcing laws within a state.
- **Money** Anything customarily used as a medium of exchange, a unit of accounting and a store of value.

Legal Terms

- **Counsel** A lawyer or attorney.
- **Defendant** A person, company, etc. who is accused of something and taken to court.
- **Prosecution** The legal team who presents the case in a criminal trial against an individual suspected of breaking the law (the defendant).
- **Testimony** The statement or declaration of a witness under oath.
- **Circumstantial Evidence** Evidence that is implied it.
- **Premeditated Homicide/Murder** A murder that was done on purpose (not accidental) or one that was planned in advance is considered 'premeditated.'
- **Deliberate** To consider carefully.
- **Verdict** The Jury's final decision; the verdict is either 'not guilty' or 'guilty'.
- **Acquitted** Declared 'not guilty' (found innocent).
- **Hung Jury** A jury that cannot agree on a verdict.

Exam Pattern Questions

1. Who among the following was the first lady Prime Minister in the world?
(a) Golda Meir (b) Indira Gandhi
(c) Mary Engenia Charles
(d) Shrimavo Bhandaranaika

2. Who was the first woman President of the Central Assembly of UNO?
(a) Vijay Laxmi Pandit (b) Rajkumari Amrit Kaur
(c) S Bandarnaika (d) Sarojini Naidu

3. Who was the first man to land on Moon?
(a) Neil-Armstrong (b) Edwin
(c) Gagarin (d) John Collins

4. Who was the first US President to be assassinated?
(a) Abraham Lincoln (b) Richard Nixon
(c) John Adams (d) None of these

5. Which among the following is the first country to impose Carbon Tax?
(a) New Zealand (b) Sweden
(c) America (d) Russia

6. The first person to reach South pole
(a) Robert Peary (b) Amundsen
(c) Sherpa Tenzing (d) Helmer Hanssen

7. First country to appoint Lokpal was
(a) Germany (b) Britain
(c) Sweden (d) India

8. First country to launch artificial satellite in the space
(a) USA (b) UK (c) Germany (d) Russia

9. The first spacecraft to reach on Mars is
(a) Columbia (b) Voyager
(c) New Horizons (d) Viking-I

10. The first person to travel twice to space is
(a) Robert Blacksmith (b) Charles Simonyi
(c) David Kellermann (d) None of these

11. Which among the following is the longest railway platform?
(a) Prayagaraj (b) New Delhi
(c) Gorakhpur (d) Mumbai

12. Sri Ranganathaswamy Temple, the largest temple in India is located in
(a) Tamil Nadu (b) Maharashtra
(c) Gujarat (d) Mumbai

13. Largest fresh water lake in the world is
(a) Baikal lake (b) Superior lake
(c) Wular lake (d) Vembanad lake

14. The largest man-made canal in the world is
(a) Rhine canal (b) Panama canal
(c) Suez canal (d) Baltic White sea canal

15. Which is the highest located airport in the world?
(a) Bangda Airport, Tibet
(b) Daocheng Yading, Tibet
(c) EL Alto, Bolivia
(d) Shigatse Peace Airport, China

16. The name of world's tallest statue is
(a) Spring Temple Buddha (b) Laykyun Sekkya
(c) Sendai Daikannon (d) Statue of Unity

17. Which is the deepest ocean in the world?
(a) Indian ocean (b) Atlantic ocean
(c) Pacific ocean (d) Arabian sea

18. Which of the following is the largest country by area?
(a) Russia (b) China
(c) USA (d) Brazil

19. Largest country of Asia
(a) Mangoli (b) Myanmar (c) China(d) India

20. The first Indian to join the ICS was
(a) Romesh Dutt (b) Surendranath Banerjee
(c) Behari Lal Gupta (d) Satyendranath Tagore

21. The first Indian to get Nobel Prize
(a) Dr CV Raman (b) Rabindranath Tagore
(c) Amartya Sen (d) Mahatma Gandhi

22. Who was the first speaker of the Lok Sabha?
(a) Dr S Radhakrishnan (b) G V Mavalankar
(c) Sukumar Sen (d) Abul Kalam Azad

23. The first fully Indian Bank is
(a) Canara Bank (b) Punjab National Bank
(c) State Bank of India (d) Central Bank of India

24. First Atomic Reactor of India was named as
(a) Aryabhatta (b) Tara
(c) Apsara (d) Dhruva

25. The first foreigner to receive Bharat Ratna Award?
(a) Nelson Mandela
(b) Khan Abdul Ghaffar Khan
(c) Mother Teresa (d) Martin Luther King

26. First woman judge of Supreme Court of India was
(a) R Bhanumati (b) MS Fatima Bibi
(c) Sujata Manohar (d) Gyan Sudha Misra

27. Who was the first woman Chairperson of Union Public Service Commission?
(a) Roze Millian Bethew (b) Sushma Chawla
(c) Leela Seth (d) CB Muthamma

28. The first Lady Governor of Independent India was
(a) Vijayalaxmi Pandit (b) Shanti Devi
(c) Sarojini Naidu (d) None of these

29. Who was the first Indian to be appointed President of the International Court of Justice?
(a) Nagendra Singh (b) Bhagat Singh
(c) Dr Hardayal (d) None of these

30. Yen is the currency of
(a) Germany (b) France
(c) Japan (d) South Korea

31. Berlin is the capital of
(a) Germany (b) France
(c) Switzerland (d) Italy

32. 'Amman' is the capital city of
(a) Lebanon (b) Jordan
(c) Yemen (d) Bahrain

33. The currency of Myanmar is known as
(a) Rufiyaa (b) Kyat (c) Peso (d) Rupiah

34. Lira is the currency of which European country?
(a) Italy (b) Greece (c) Finland (d) Austria

35. Lima is the capital of
(a) Peru (b) Sudan (c) Libya (d) Italy

36. Currency of Saudi Arabia is
(a) Dinar (b) Lira (c) Riyal (d) None of these

37. Euro is not the currency of
(a) Italy (b) France
(c) Germany (d) Switzerland

38. Which of the following is not among the Seven Wonders of the World?
(a) The Great Wall of China
(b) Petra
(c) The Taj Mahal
(d) Pyramid of Egypt

39. One of the Seven wonders of the world 'Machu Picchu' is located in
(a) Peru (b) Brazil (c) India (d) Mexico

40. Which of the following is called 'Blue Mountains'?
(a) Himalayas (b) Shivaliks
(c) Nilgiri hills (d) Western Ghats

41. Land of Rising Sun is
(a) Japan (b) China (c) India (d) Sri Lanka

42. The International Border between India and China is known by the name
(a) Radcliffe line (b) Durand line
(c) McMahon line (d) Siegfried line

43. 'Hindenburg Line' is the international border between which among the following countries?
(a) Germany and Poland
(b) France and Germany
(c) USA and Canada
(d) North and South Korea

44. Name the parallel which divides USA and Canada.
(a) 38th parallel line (b) 17th parallel line
(c) 24th parallel line (d) 49th parallel line

45. Who is the author of book 'The Time Machine'?
(a) Leo Tolstoy (b) HG Wells
(c) Karl Marx (d) Homer

46. Who is known as 'Iron Man of India'?
(a) Vardhaman (b) Vallabhbhai Patel
(c) Narendranath Dutta (d) Rabindranath Tagore

47. Mother Teresa's area of work was
(a) Charity (b) Religion
(c) Author (d) Philosopher

48. 'Samta Sthal' is the crematorium of which famous personality?
(a) I K Gujral (b) Jagjivan Ram
(c) Rajiv Gandhi (d) Indira Gandhi

49. 'Sadaiv Atal' is the crematorium of which famous personality?
(a) Jagjivan Ram (b) Lal Bahadur Shastri
(c) K R Narayanan (d) Atal Bihari Vajpayee

50. What is the name of crematorium of Mahatma Gandhi?
(a) Veer Bhumi (b) Ekta Sthal
(c) Shanti Van (d) Raj Ghat

51. 'Faizabad' is the old name of which of the following cities?
(a) Prayagaraj (b) Ayodhya
(c) Gurgaon (d) Mysore

52. Changed name of 'Allahabad' is
(a) Prayagraj (b) Atal Nagar
(c) Palghat (d) Vidisha

53. Which city is known as 'Pink City'?
(a) Amritsar (b) Kolkata
(c) Jaipur (d) Mumbai

54. Which place is called 'Manchester of India'?
(a) Coimbatore (b) Ahmedabad
(c) Mumbai (d) Khajjiar

55. Jamshedpur is also known as
(a) Steel City (b) City of Joy
(c) City of Temples (d) Golden City

56. Who wrote the book 'Anand Math?
(a) Bankim Chandra Chatterjee
(b) Abul Fazal
(c) Kalidas
(d) Sarat Chand Chattopadhyay

57. 'The Accidental Prime Minister', a book written by
(a) Martin Luther King (b) Sanjaya Baru
(c) Mahatma Gandhi (d) Kuldip Nayyar

58. Which of the following book was written by Dr. Rajendra Prasad?
(a) India Wins Freedom
(b) India Divided
(c) India of Our Dreams (d) Discovery of India

59. 'A Bend in the River' is the renowned book written by
(a) Charles Dickens (b) RK Narayan
(c) VS Naipaul (d) Khuswant Singh

60. The famous book 'Meghdoot' is written by
(a) Kalidas (b) Maharishi Ved Vyas
(c) Tulsidas (d) Kautilya

61. 'A Voice for Freedom' is a book written by
(a) Corazon Aquino (b) Nayantara Sahgal
(c) Aung San Suu Kyi (d) Benazir Bhutto

62. Which of the following book has been written by Vikram Seth?
(a) My God Died Young (b) Look Back in Anger
(c) A Suitable Boy (d) Islamic Bomb

63. Which of the following is not written by Munshi Premchand?
(a) Gaban (b) Godan (c) Guide (d) Manasarovar

64. Who is the author of the book 'Guide'?
(a) VS Naipaul (b) RK Narayan
(c) Rabindranath Tagore (d) Chales Dickens

65. 'Apsara' is the name of India's first?
(a) Railway Locomotive (b) Helicopter
(c) Nuclear Reactor (d) Unmanned Aircraft

66. Where is Vikram Sarabhai Space Centre located?
(a) Thiruvananthapuram (b) Ahmedabad
(c) Thumba (d) Mumbai

67. What is the name of first Indian Research Station in the Arctic?
(a) Himadri (b) Maitri
(c) Bharati (d) Dakshin Gangotri

68. Where is Satish Dhawan Space Centre located?
(a) Sriharikota (b) Chandipur
(c) Thumba (d) Bengaluru

69. What was the name of the first satellite launched into space?
(a) Sputnik 1 (b) Explorer 1
(c) A4 Rocket (d) Jupiter 1

70. What was the first spacecraft to reach the Moon's surface?
(a) Apollo 11 (b) Luna 9
(c) Surveyor 1 (d) Luna 2

71. Which was the first successful mission to land on the surface of Mars?
(a) Viking 1 (b) Mars 3
(c) Curiosity rover (d) Pathfinder

72. India's first Defence Industrial Park was set up in
(a) Dehradun (Uttarakhand)
(b) Ottapalam (Kerala)
(c) Visakhapatnam (Andhra Pradesh)
(d) Pune (Maharashtra)

73. When was United Nations (UN) formed?
(a) 1945 (b) 1946
(c) 1947 (d) 1944

74. UNICEF was established in which year?
(a) 1946 (b) 1948
(c) 1950 (d) 1958

75. Headquarter of World Health Organisation is located in
(a) London (b) Kathmandu
(c) New York (d) Geneva

76. National Voter's Day is observed on which date?
(a) 25th January (b) 26th January
(c) 15th August (d) 26th November

77. Which one of the following days is observed as the World Environment Day?
(a) 28th February (b) 4th March
(c) 5th June (d) 16th September

78. National Sports Day' celebrated on
(a) 9th February (b) 14th April
(c) 29th August (d) 27th September

79. On which date, National Science Day is celebrated?
(a) 30th January (b) 28th February
(c) 31st May (d) 5th June

80. Which day is observed as Human Right Day?
(a) 24th October (b) 4th July
(c) 10th December (d) None of these

81. World Health Day is celebrated
(a) 7th April (b) 7th May
(c) 1st April (d) 1st May

82. APEC stands for
(a) Atlantic and Pacific Economic Community
(b) Asia-Pacific Economic Cooperation
(c) Australia-Panama Economic Cooperation
(d) Pan African Economic Community

83. FAO is the abbreviation of
(a) Fibre and Agricultural Organisation
(b) Food and Agricultural Organisation
(c) Free Arbitration Organisation
(d) Free and Allowed Open Software

84. VAT stands for
(a) Value Added Tax (b) Very Added Tax
(c) Very Average Tax (d) Very AverageTerm

85. An investigation of count of a population is known as
(a) Climate (b) Equator (c) Census (d) Desert

86. Animal life present in particular region is known as
(a) Flora (b) Fauna (c) Fault (d) Globe

87. The Scientific study of the atmosphere is
(a) Magma (b) Lava
(c) Pangea (d) Meteorology

Answers

1 (d)	2 (a)	3. (a)	4 (a)	5 (b)	6 (b)	7 (c)	8 (d)	9 (d)	10 (b)
11 (c)	12 (a)	13 (b)	14 (c)	15 (b)	16 (d)	17 (c)	18 (a)	19 (c)	20 (d)
21 (b)	22 (b)	23 (b)	24 (c)	25 (b)	26 (b)	27 (a)	28 (c)	29 (a)	30 (c)
31 (c)	32 (b)	33 (b)	34 (b)	35 (a)	36 (c)	37 (d)	38 (d)	39 (a)	40 (c)
41 (a)	42 (c)	43 (a)	44 (d)	45 (b)	46 (b)	47 (a)	48 (b)	49 (d)	50 (d)
51 (b)	52 (a)	53 (c)	54 (b)	55 (a)	56 (a)	57 (b)	58 (b)	59 (c)	60 (a)
61 (b)	62 (c)	63 (c)	64 (b)	65 (c)	66 (a)	67 (a)	68 (a)	69 (a)	70 (d)
71 (a)	72 (b)	73 (a)	74 (a)	75 (d)	76 (a)	77 (c)	78 (c)	79 (b)	80 (c)
81 (a)	82 (b)	83 (b)	84 (a)	85 (c)	86 (b)	87 (d)			

LOGICAL REASONING

Logical Reasoning

Series

Series is a sequential order of letters, numbers or both arranged such a way that each term in the series is obtained according to some specific rules. These rules can be based on mathematical operations, place of letters in alphabetical order etc.

In this type of questions, a series consisting of numbers/alphabets or letters is given. One or two elements of the series are kept hidden and it is denoted by '?'. Candidates have to fill up the appropriate number/alphabets or letters from the options by observing the series carefully.

Example 1 Find the next number in the series.

2, 15, 41, 80, ?

(a) 111 (b) 120 (c) 121 (d) 132

Sol. (*d*) Here, there is an increment of consecutive multiples of 13 in consecutive terms.

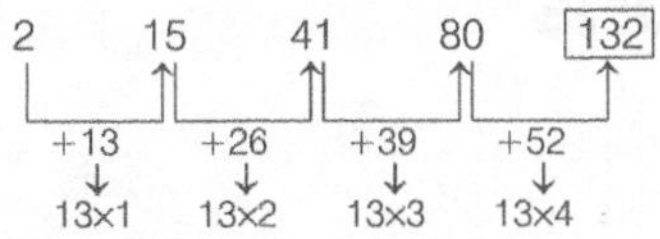

Example 2 Find the next term of the given series.

S, O, K, G, ?

(a) C (b) N
(c) O (d) D

Sol. (a) Here, every next term is obtained by subtracting 4 from the corresponding position of its previous term (letter).

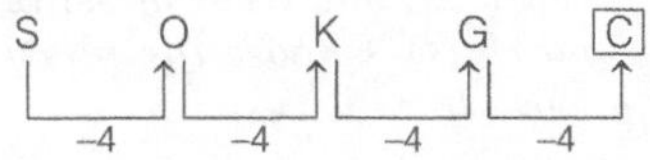

Example 3 Which of the alternatives, complete the series _cb_ca_bacb_ca_bac_d.

(a) addddb
(b) addbbb
(c) bddddb
(d) bbbddd

Sol. (a) The pattern of the series is acbd/cadb/acbd/cadb/acbd ⇒ addddb

The sequence is made of repetition of two blocks 'acbd' and 'cadb', alternatively.

Objective Questions

Directions (Q. Nos. 1-6) *In each of the following questions, a number series is given with one term missing. Choose the correct alternative that will continue the same pattern in place of question mark(?).*

1. 10, 100, 200, 310, ?
(a) 400 (b) 410
(c) 420 (d) 430

2. 0, 2, 6, 12, ?, 30
(a) 20 (b) 23
(c) 24 (d) 25

3. 28, 33, 31, 36, ?, 39
(a) 32 (b) 34
(c) 38 (d) 40

4. 125, 80, 45, 20, ?
(a) 5 (b) 8
(c) 10 (d) 12

5. 1, 5, 13, 25, 41, ?
(a) 51 (b) 57 (c) 61 (d) 63

6. 1, 4, 9, 16, 25, ?
(a) 35 (b) 36 (c) 48 (d) 49

Directions (Q. Nos. 7-11) *In each of the following questions, one term in the number series is wrong. Find out the wrong term.*

7. 1, 5, 9, 16, 25, 37, 49
(a) 16 (b) 9
(c) 25 (d) 37

8. 3, 10, 27, 4, 16, 64, 5, 25, 125
(a) 3 (b) 4 (c) 10 (d) 27

9. 1, 3, 7, 15, 27, 63, 127
(a) 7 (b) 15 (c) 27 (d) 63

10. 3, 2, 8, 9, 13, 22, 18, 32, 23, 42
(a) 8 (b) 9 (c) 13 (d) 22

11. 89, 78, 86, 80, 85, 82, 83
(a) 83 (b) 82 (c) 86 (d) 78

Directions (Q.Nos. 12-16) *In each of the following questions, various terms of a letter series are given with one term missing as shown by question mark (?). Choose the missing term out of the given alternatives.*

12. U, O, I, ?, W
(a) E (b) C (c) S (d) G

13. A, B, D, G, ?
(a) M (b) L (c) K (d) H

14. Z, U, Q, ?, L
(a) I (b) K (c) M (d) N

15. B, D, F, I, L, P, ?
(a) R (b) S (c) T (d) U

16. U, B, I, P, W, ?
(a) D (b) F (c) Q (d) Z

Directions (Q.Nos. 17 and 18) *In the following questions, which of the alternatives will complete the series?*

17. _ _ dan_ _ nda_dand_
(a) dnadna (b) ndanda
(c) andana (d) danndn

18. b_y_ _ by_b_yt
(a) bgtbt (b) btbtb (c) atbbt (d) cbbtc

Answers

1 *(d)*	2 *(a)*	3 *(b)*	4 *(a)*	5 *(c)*	6 *(b)*	7 *(a)*	8 *(c)*	9 *(c)*	10 *(b)*
11 *(c)*	12 *(b)*	13 *(c)*	14 *(d)*	15 *(c)*	16 *(a)*	17 *(c)*	18 *(b)*		

Hints & Solutions

1. (d) 10, 100, 200, 310, [430]
+90, +100, +110, +120

2. (a) 0, 2, 6, 12, [20], 30
+2, +4, +6, +8, +10

3. (b) 28, 33, 31, 36, [34], 39
+3, +3 (28 → 31 → 34)
+3, +3 (33 → 36 → 39)

4. (a) 125, 80, 45, 20, [5]
−45, −35, −25, −15

5. (c) 1, 5, 13, 25, 41, [61]
+4, +8, +12, +16, +20

6. (b) 1, 4, 9, 16, 25, [36]
$1^2 \rightarrow 2^2 \rightarrow 3^2 \rightarrow 4^2 \rightarrow 5^2 \rightarrow 6^2$

7. (a) 1, 5, 9, [17], 25, 37, 49
$(1)^2$, (2^2+1), $(3)^2$, (4^2+1), $(5)^2$, (6^2+1), $(7)^2$

Hence, 16 is the wrong term, it should be $4^2 + 1 = 17$

8. (c) 3 [9] 27 | 4 16 64 | 5 25 125
3^1 3^2 3^3 | 4^1 4^2 4^3 | 5^1 5^2 5^3

Hence, 10 is the wrong term and it should have been 9.

9. (c) 1, 3, 7, 15, [31], 63, 127
×2+1, ×2+1, ×2+1, ×2+1, ×2+1, ×2+1

Hence, 27 is the wrong term and it should be 31.

10. (b)

+5 +5 +5 +5

3 2 8 [12] 13 22 18 32 23 42

+10 +10 +10 +10

Hence, 9 is the wrong term, it should be 2 + 10 = 12.

11. (c)

−2 −2 −2

89 78 [87] 80 85 82 83

+2 +2

Hence, 86 is the wrong term, it should be89 − 2 = 87.

12. (b) U O I [C] W

↓ ↓ ↓ ↓ ↓

21 15 9 3 23

−6 −6 −6 −6

13. (c) A B D G [K]

+1 +2 +3 +4

14. (d) Z U Q [N] L

−5 −4 −3 −2

15. (c) B D F I L P [T]

+2 +2 +3 +3 +4 +4

16. (a) U B I P W [D]

+7 +7 +7 +7 +7

17. (c) a nd/an d/a nd/a n d/and/a ⇒ andana

18. (b) bbyt | bbyt | bbyt ⇒ btbtb

Analogy

Analogy means similarity or correspondence, i.e. having similar features.

In questions based on Analogy, a particular relationship between words/letters/numbers is given and another similar relationship has to be identified from the alternatives provided.

Example 1. Pitch is related to Cricket, in the same way as Arena is related to …… .

(a) Tennis (b) Gymnastic

(c) Badminton (d) Wrestling

Sol. (d) As, Cricket is played on Pitch, similarly, Wrestling is played in Arena.

Example 2. In this question, find out the relationship between the first two words and choose the word from the given alternatives which have the same relationship with the third word, as between the first two.

Reading : Knowledge : : Work : ?

(a) Experience (b) Engagement

(c) Employment (d) Experiment

Sol. (a) By Reading we get the Knowledge, similarly by Work we get Experience.

Example 3. Complete the second pair in the same way as first pair.

14 : 9 : : 26 : ?

(a) 12 (b) 13 (c) 15 (d) 31

Sol. (c) As, in first pair,

$$(14 \div 2) + 2 = 7 + 2 = 9$$

Similarly, in second pair,

$$(26 \div 2) + 2 = 13 + 2 = 15$$

Example 4. Complete the second pair in the same way as first pair.

EGIK : LJHF : : SUWY : ?

(a) ZXVT (b) TVXZ (b) LNPR (d) MOQS

Sol. (a) Here, in first pair the letters are written in reverse order after moving one step forward according to English alphabetical order.

As,

5 7 9 11 → 12 10 8 6

E G I K → L J H F

(+1, +1, +1, +1)

Similarly,

19 21 23 25 → 26 24 22 20

S U W Y → [Z X V T]

(+1, +1, +1, +1)

Objective Questions

1. Hare is related to Burrow, in the same way Owl is related to ....
(a) Hole (b) Hive (c) Nest (d) Barn

2. College is related to Student, in the same way as Hospital is related to ....
(a) Doctor (b) Nurse
(b) Medicine (d) Patient

3. Smell is to Flower, in the same way as Taste is to ....
(a) Tongue (b) Water (c) Sweet (d) Food

Directions (Q. Nos. 4-12) *In each of the following questions, select the related word/words pair/number/letters group from the given alternatives.*

4. Son : Nephew : : Daughter : ?
(a) Niece (b) Sister-in-law
(c) Sister (d) Mother

5. Ring : Ear : : ? : Wrist
(a) Pendant (b) Chain
(c) Bangle (d) Ribbon

6. Fragile : Crack
(a) Cemetery : Death (b) Pliable : Bend
(c) Hydro : Water (d) Irreducible : Reduce

7. Border : Country
(a) Pen : Cap (b) Book : Cover
(c) Handle : Space (d) Frame : Picture

8. 7 : 28 : : 2 : ?
(a) 8 (b) 12
(c) 16 (d) 24

9. 5 : 30 : : 7 : ?
(a) 54 (b) 50 (c) 49 (d) 56

10. EFG : IJK : : MNO : ?
(a) PQR (b) OPQ
(c) QRS (d) NOP

11. RAT : TAR : : PIT : ?
(a) BIT (b) CAT
(c) TIP (d) TOP

12. GREAT : 25 : : NUMBER : ?
(a) 36 (b) 38 (c) 27 (d) 24

Answers

1 (d)	2 (d)	3 (d)	4 (a)	5 (c)	6 (b)	7 (d)	8 (a)	9 (d)	10 (c)
11 (c)	12 (a)								

Hints & Solutions

1. (d) Burrow is the dwelling place of Hare. Similarly, Barn is the dwelling place of Owl.

2. (d) In the College, education is given to Students, in the same way, treatment is given to Patient in Hospital.

3. (d) Smell comes from Flower, in the same way, Taste comes from Food.

4. (a) As, Son is related to Nephew. Similarly, Daughter is related to Niece.

5. (c) As, Ring or Earring is worn in the Ear. Similarly, Bangle is put on Wrist.

6. (b) A Fragile things crack easily, in the same way, Pliable articles bend easily.

7. (d) Border makes the boundary of the Country, in the same way, Frame makes the boundary of the Picture.

8. (a) As, 7 and $7 \times 4 = 28$

Similarly, 2 and $2 \times 4 = 8$

$\therefore ? = \boxed{8}$

9. (d) As, $5 \times 5 + 5 = 25 + 5 = 30$

Similarly, $7 \times 7 + 7 = 49 + 7 = \boxed{56}$

10. (c)

As,
E $\xrightarrow{+4}$ I
F $\xrightarrow{+4}$ J
G $\xrightarrow{+4}$ K

Similarly,
M $\xrightarrow{+4}$ Q
N $\xrightarrow{+4}$ R
O $\xrightarrow{+4}$ S

11. (c) As,

R A T —Reverse Sequence→ T A R

Similarly,

P I T —Reverse Sequence→ T I P

∴ ? = TIP

Coding-Decoding

Coding means to hide the meaning of any message and decoding means to understand the actual meaning of that message.

In questions based on coding-decoding, a word or sentence is coded in a particular way and the candidates are asked to code other word or sentence in the same way or to decode the word or sentence.

Example 1. If EARN is written as GCTP, how NEAR can be written in that code?

(a) CTGP (b) GPTC
(c) PGCT (d) PCGT

Sol. (c) Here, each letter of the word is moved two steps forward to obtain the code

As, E —+2→ G Similarly, N —+2→ P
A —+2→ C E —+2→ G
R —+2→ T A —+2→ C
N —+2→ P R —+2→ T

Example 2. If CUP = 40, then KITE = ?

(a) 10 (b) 20
(c) 30 (d) 45

Sol. (d) Using forward letter positions

As, C (3) U (21) P (16) = 3 + 21 + 16 = 40

Similarly, K (11) I (9) T (20) E (5) = 11 + 9 + 20 + 5 = 45

Example 3. In a certain coded language, STRING is written as '% = * – $ ÷' and PRAISE as '? * @ – % ×'. How will the word SPRING is coded?

(a) % ? – * $÷ (b) ? % – * ÷ $
(c) % ? * – $ ÷ (d) % % * – ÷ $

Sol. (c) Given codes,

S	T	R	I	N	G
%	=	*	–	$	÷

and

P	R	A	I	S	E
?	*	@	–	%	×

Therefore,

S	P	R	I	N	G
%	?	*	–	$	÷

Example 4. If 'water' is 'called' 'food', 'food' is called 'tree', 'tree' is called 'sky', 'sky' is called 'well' and 'well' is called 'pond', then which of the following would yield (produce) fruits?

(a) Sky (b) Food (c) Well (d) Tree

Sol. (a) As, we all know that, tree yields fruits and according to the code tree is called sky. So, sky yield fruits.

Example 5. In a certain coded language, 'food is good' is written as 'ho na ta', 'eat food regularly' is written as 'sa ta la', 'keep good health' is written as 'da na ja'. How is 'eat' written in that code?

(a) sa or la
(b) sa
(c) la
(d) ja

Sol. (a) According to the question,

food is good ⟶ ho na ta ...(i)

eat food regularly ⟶ sa ta la ...(ii)

keep good health ⟶ da na ja ...(iii)

From Eqs. (i) and (iii), good → na
From Eqs. (i) and (ii), food → ta
From Eq. (i) is → ho
So, the code for 'eat' must be either 'sa' or 'la'.

Objective Questions

1. If DELHI can be coded as CCIDD, how would you code BOMBAY?
(a) AJMTVT (b) AMJXVS
(c) MJXVSU (d) WXYZAX

2. If TRUTH is coded as SUQSTVSUGI, then the code of FALSE will be
(a) EGZBKMRDE (b) EGZKMRTDF
(c) EGZBKMRTDF (d) FGZBKNRTDF

3. If BOMBAY is written as MYMYMY, how will TAMILNADU be written in that code?
(a) TIATIATIA (b) MNUMNUMNU
(c) IATIATIAT (d) ALDALDALA

4. If MADRAS can be written as ARSMDA, how can ARKONAM be written in the code?
(a) ROAAKNM (b) ROAKANM
(c) ROAKNNM (d) ROAKNAM

5. If HEALTH is written as GSKZDG, then how will NORTH be written in that code?
(a) OPSUI (b) GSQNM
(c) FRPML (d) IUSPO

6. In a certain code BEAN in written as ABNE and SALE is written as LSEA. How in NEWS written in that code?
(a) SNEW (b) SNWE (c) WNES (d) WNSE

7. If the word EARTH be written as QPMZS in coded form, how can HEART be written following the same coding?
(a) SQPZM (b) SQMPZ
(c) SPQZM (d) SQPMZ

8. In a certain code, FIRE is written as QHOE and MOVE as ZMWE. Following same rule of coding, what should be the code for the word OVER?
(a) MWED (b) MWEO (c) MWOE (d) MWZO

9. If BASKET is written as TEKSAB, how can PILLOW be written in that code?
(a) LOWPIL (b) WOLLIP
(c) LOWLIP (d) WOLPIL

10. In a certain code, TOPPER is written as POTREP. In that code, which word will be written as RUBREG?
(a) BURGER (b) BLURBE
(c) BURGET (d) BEURGR

11. If LAME is written as ODPH, how can MALE be written in that code?
(a) PDOH (b) HOPD (c) DOPH (d) OPDH

12. If TALENT is written as LATENT, how EXOTIC can be written in the codes?
(a) OXOTIC (b) TEXTIC
(c) OXETIC (d) EXOTIC

13. In a certain code, the word DEAL is coded as 4 – 5 – 1 – 12. Following the same rule of coding, what should be the code for the word LADY?
(a) 12 – 4 – 1 – 25 (b) 12 – 1 – 4 – 25
(c) 10 – 1 – 4 – 23 (d) 12 – 1 – 4 – 22

14. If A = 2, M = 26 , Z = 52, then BET is equal to
(a) 44 (b) 54
(c) 64 (d) 72

15. If A = 26, SUN = 27, then CAT is equal to
(a) 24 (b) 27
(c) 57 (d) 58

16. In a certain code, 'BASKET' is written as '5$3%#1' and 'TRIED' is written as '14★#2'. How is 'SKIRT' written in that code?
(a) 3%★41 (b) 3★%41
(c) 3%#41 (d) 3#4%1

17. If 'oranges' are 'apples', 'bananas' are 'apricots', 'apples' are 'chillies', 'apricots' are 'oranges' and 'chillies' are 'bananas', then which of the following are green in colour?

(a) Apricots (b) Apples (c) Chillies (d) Bananas

18. If 'blue' is called 'black', 'black' is called 'green', 'green' is called 'white', 'white' is called 'red', 'red' is called 'yellow' and 'yellow' is called 'gray', then what is the colour of milk?

(a) White (b) Blue
(c) Red (d) Yellow

19. In a certain code language, 'go for morning walk' is written as '$ * ? #', 'good for health' is written as '£ ? @' and 'good to walk fast' is written as '+ @ ↑ #', then what is the code for 'health' in that code language?

(a) + (b) # (c) £ (d) ?

20. In a certain code, '975' means 'throw away garbage', '528' means 'give away smoking' and '213' means 'smoking is harmful'. Which digit in that code means 'smoking'?

(a) 5 (b) 8 (c) 2 (d) 3

Answers

1 *(b)*	2 *(c)*	3 *(b)*	4 *(a)*	5 *(b)*	6 *(d)*	7 *(d)*	8 *(b)*	9 *(b)*	10 *(a)*
11 *(a)*	12 *(c)*	13 *(b)*	14 *(b)*	15 *(c)*	16 *(a)*	17 *(d)*	18 *(c)*	19 *(c)*	20 *(c)*

Hints & Solutions

1. (b) As, D E L H I → (−1, −2, −3, −4, −5) → C C I D D

Similarly, B O M B A Y → (−1, −2, −3, −4, −5, −6) → A M J X V S

2. (c) Each letter in the word is replaced by a set of two letters, one preceding it and the other following it in the code.

Thus, T is replaced by SU, R is replaced by QS and so, on.

∴ FALSE = EGZBKMRTDF

3. (b) The letters at the third and sixth places are repeated thrice to code BOMBAY as MYMYMY. Similarly, the letters at the third, sixth and ninth placed are repeated thrice to code TAMILNADU as MNUMNUMNU.

4. (a) As,

1 2 3 4 5 6
M A D R A S

A R S (even position letters) M D A (odd position letters)

⇒ ARSMDA

Similarly,

1 2 3 4 5 6 7
A R K O N A M

R O A (even position letters) A K N M (odd position letters)

5. (b) H E A L T H → G S K Z D G (each −1)

Similarly, N O R T H → G S Q N M (each −1)

6. (d) That pattern is as follows,

1 2 3 4 → 3 1 4 2
B E A N → A B N E

Similarly,

1 2 3 4 → 3 1 4 2
S A L E → L S E A

Therefore,

1 2 3 4 → 3 1 4 2
N E W S → W N S E

7. (d) According to the question,

Letters	E	A	R	T	H
Code	Q	P	M	Z	S

Therefore, H E A R T → S Q P M Z

8. (b) According to the question,

Letters	F	I	R	E	M	O	V	E
Code	Q	H	O	E	Z	M	W	E

Therefore, O V E R → M W E O

9. (b) Letters are written in reverse order.

∴ B A S K E T → T E K S A B

Similarly,

P I L L O W → W O L L I P

10. (a) First half letters and second half letters are coded in reverse order.

∴ T O P P E R → P O T R E P

Similarly, R U B R E G → B U R G E R

11. (a) As,

L $\xrightarrow{+3}$ O
A $\xrightarrow{+3}$ D
M $\xrightarrow{+3}$ P
E $\xrightarrow{+3}$ H

Similarly,

M $\xrightarrow{+3}$ P
A $\xrightarrow{+3}$ D
L $\xrightarrow{+3}$ O
E $\xrightarrow{+3}$ H

12. (c) As, TAL ENT $\xrightarrow[\text{sequence}]{\text{Reverse}}$ LAT ENT

Similarly, EXO TIC $\xrightarrow[\text{sequence}]{\text{Reverse}}$ OXE TIC

13. (b) Clearly, each letter is coded by the numeral denoting its position in the English alphabet.

Thus, A is coded as 1, B as 2, C as 3, D as 4, ..., L as 12, M as 13, ..., Y as 25, Z as 26. So, the code for LADY is 12 – 1 – 4 – 25

14. (b) Clearly, each letter is assigned a numerical value which is twice the numeral denoting its position in the English alphabet.

B, E and T are 2nd, 5th and 20th letters respectively.

So, BET = B + E + T =

$(2 \times 2) + (5 \times 2) + (20 \times 2) = 54$

15. (c) Clearly, each letter is represented by the numeral denoting its position from the end of the English alphabet i.e. Z = 1, Y = 2, ..., M = 14, ..., B = 25, A = 26

Then, SUN = S + U + N = 8 + 6 + 13 = 27

So, CAT = C + A + T = 24 + 26 + 7 = 57

16. (a) As, B A S K E T → 5 $ 3 % # 1

and T R I E D → 1 4 ⋆ # 2

Similarly, S K I R T → 3 % ⋆ 4 1

17. (d) 'Green' in colour ⇒ 'Chillies'

But, according to the question,

Chillies are bananas

Therefore, 'Green' in colour ⇒ 'Bananas'

18. (c) The colour of Milk ⇒ 'White'.

But, according to the question,

'White' ⇒ 'Red'

Therefore, the colour of Milk ⇒ Red

19. (c) According to the given information,

go for morning walk ⇒ $*?# ...(i)

good for health ⇒ £ ? @ ...(ii)

good to walk fast ⇒ + @↑ # ...(iii)

From Eqs. (i) and (ii), we get

'for' ⇒ '?'

From Eqs. (ii) and (iii), we get

'good' ⇒ '@'

By elimination in Eq. (ii), we get

'health' ⇒ '£'

20. (c) According to the given information,

9 7 5 → throw away garbage ...(i)

5 2 8 → give away smoking ...(ii)

2 1 3 → smoking is harmful ...(iii)

From Eqs. (ii) and (iii),

smoking → 2

Word, Number & Alphabet Test

As the name says, this test is related to the English alphabets and numbers. Questions asked in this test are based on the alphabetical order of letters, formation of words either meaningful or meaningless various arrangements of letters and numbers etc.

Example 1. Find the 11th letter to the left of 20th letter from left in the English alphabet.

(a) D (b) J
(c) K (d) I

Sol. (*d*) Here,

1	2	3	4	5	6	7	8	9	10	11	12	13	14	15	16	17	18	19	20	21	22	23	24	25	26
A	B	C	D	E	F	G	H	(I)	J	K	L	M	N	O	P	Q	R	S	T	U	V	W	X	Y	Z

To the left: 11th ← 20th
From left: → 20th

Hence, 11th letter to the left of 20th letter from left is I.

Alternate Method

In English alphabet, 11th letter to the left of 20th letter from left = (20 − 11)th letter from left = 9th letter from left = I

Example 2. If the letters in the word FATHER are written in alphabetical order, then how many letters will not change their position?

(a) None (b) One
(c) Two (d) Three

Sol. (*b*)

Word	F	A	T	H	E	R
In alphabetical order	A	E	F	H	R	T

There is only one such alphabet.

Example 3. Choose one word out of the given alternatives, which cannot be formed from the letters of the word 'CONSULTATION'.

(a) CONSTANT (b) NATION
(c) SALUTE (d) STATION

Sol. (*c*) Carefully looking at the words, we find that the word 'CONSULTATION' does not contain the letter 'E'.
So, the word 'SALUTE' cannot be formed.

Example 4. How many even numbers are there in the following series of numbers, each of which is preceded by an odd number, but not followed by an even number?

5 3 4 8 9 7 1 6 5 3 2 9 8 7 3 5

(a) 0 (b) 1 (c) 2 (d) 3

Sol. (*d*) 5 3 4 8 9 7 1 [6] 5 3 [2] 9 [8] 7 3 5

There are three such even numbers 6, 2 and 8 each of which is preceded by an odd number and not followed by an even number.

Objective Questions

1. Find the 8th letter to the left of 20th letter from left in the English alphabet.
(a) D (b) J (c) K (d) L

2. If 1st half of the English alphabet is written in backward order, then what will be the 7th letter to the left of the 10th letter from your right?
(a) C (b) E (c) D (d) J

3. How many letters are there between 8th letter from left and 7th letter from right in the English alphabet?
(a) 7 (b) 11 (c) 8 (d) 9

4. How many such pairs of letters are there in the word 'CLEARING' each of which has as many letter between them in the word as also in English alphabet?
(a) One (b) Two (c) Three (d) Four

5. If the letters in the word 'UNDERTAKING' are rearranged in the alphabetical order, which one will be in the middle in order after the rearrangement?
(a) G (b) I
(c) K (d) N

6. If first and second letters in the word 'COMMUNICATIONS' were interchanged, also the third and the fourth letters, the fifth and sixth letters, and so on. Which letter would be the tenth letter counting from your right?
(a) U (b) A
(c) T (d) N

7. If every alternate letter in the word 'SOLITARY' starting from the 1st letter is replaced by the previous letter and each of the remaining letters is replaced by the next letter in the English alphabet, which of the following will be the 3rd letter from the right end after the substitution?

(a) B (b) S (c) Z (d) K

8. Select the word from the given alternatives which cannot be formed using the letters of the given word.

KNOWLEDGE

(a) WEDGE (b) GODOWN
(c) KLEEN (d) GOLDEN

9. Select the word from the given alternatives which cannot be formed using the letters of the given word.

Milestone

(a) Lemon (b) Some (c) Mist (d) Million

10. Select the word which can be formed using the letters of the given word.

PRAGMATIC

(a) Guitar (b) Game
(c) Magic (d) Race

11. Select the word which can be formed using the letters of the given word.

EXAMINATION

(a) National
(b) Animal
(c) Animation
(d) Examiner

12. How many '8' are followed by even number and preceded by an odd number?

18438148328784856878418 6

(a) 3 (b) 4
(c) 9 (d) 5

Answers

1 (d)	2 (c)	3 (b)	4 (b)	5 (c)	6 (d)	7 (a)	8 (b)	9 (d)	10 (c)
11 (c)	12 (b)								

Hints & Solutions

1. (d) Let us see

1 2 3 4 5 6 7 8 9 10 11 12 13 14 15 16 17 18 19 20 21 22 23 24 25 26
A B C D E F G H I J K (L) M N O P Q R S T U V W X Y Z

To the left — 8th; From left — 20th

Hence, 8th letter to the left of 20th letter from left is L.

Alternate Method

In English alphabet 8th letter to the left of 20th letter of your left = (20 – 8) th letter from left = 12 th letter from left = L

2. (c) Let us see

13 12 11 10 9 8 7 6 5 4 3 2 1 14 15 16 17 18 19 20 21 22 23 24 25 26
M L K J I H G F E (D) C B A N O P Q R S T U V W X Y Z

To the left — 7th; From right — 10th

∴ The 7th letter to the left of 10th letter from our right is D.

3. (b) Let us see

1 2 3 4 5 6 7 8 9 10 11 12 13 14 15 16 17 18 19 20 21 22 23 24 25 26
A B C D E F G H I J K L M N O P Q R S T U V W X Y Z

From left — 8th; 11 Letters; From right — 7th

∴ There are 11 letters between 8th letter from left and 7th letter from right.

4. (b) C L E A R I N G

Two such pairs are there.

5. (c) UNDERTAKING

Rearranged A D E G I K N N R T U

Clearly, K lies in the middle.

6. (d) According to the question,

Given word C O M M U N I C A T I O N S

New word O C M M N U C I T A O I S N

10th from right

Hence, required letter is N.

7. (a) After making the change as given in the question, we get the following arrangement

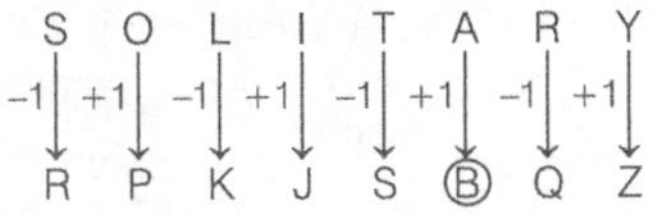

Hence, the 3rd letter from the right end is 'B'.

8. (b) The word 'Godown' cannot be formed from the letters of the given word as there is only one 'o' in the given word.

9. (d) The word 'Million' cannot be formed from the letters of the given word as there is only one 'i' as well as only one 'l' in the given word.

10. (c) From the letters of the given word, the word 'magic' can be formed.

11. (c) The word 'animation' can be formed by using the letters of the given word.

12. (b) 1[8]4381 483287[8]485687[8]41[8]6

There are four such 8's which are followed by even number and preceded by an odd number.

Blood Relations

Blood relation means any relation between two or more persons which is acquired by them by the virtue of their birth. It would be easy to solve these questions through generation flow chart, generation chart between two or more persons clears a picture of the relation that they have.

In order to solve these questions one should have adequate knowledge of 'blood relations'. Different types of relations are given below

1. Relations from Paternal Side

- Father's father → Grandfather
- Father's mother → Grandmother
- Father's brother → Uncle
- Father's sister → Aunt
- Children of uncle or aunt → Cousin
- Wife of uncle → Aunt
- Husband of aunt → Uncle

2. Relations from Maternal Side

- Mother's father → Maternal grandfather
- Mother's mother → Maternal grandmother
- Mother's brother → Maternal uncle
- Mother's sister → Aunt
- Children of maternal uncle or aunt → Cousin
- Wife of maternal uncle → Maternal aunt
- Husband of maternal aunt → Maternal uncle

Example 1. Pointing to a man Deepak said, "His only brother is the father of my daughter's father". How is the man related to Deepak?

(a) Grandfather (b) Father
(c) Uncle (d) Brother-in-law

Sol. (c) According to the question,

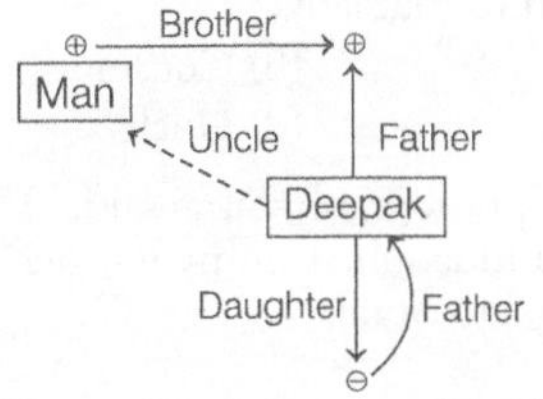

Deepak's daughter's father will be deepak himself. So, the brother of the Man is the father of Deepak. Hence, we can say that the man is the uncle of Deepak.

Example 2. If A × B means A is the brother of B and A + B means that A is the father of B, then which one means that 'M is the nephew of N'?

(a) N + M × K (b) N × K + M
(c) M × K + N (d) None of these

Sol. (d)

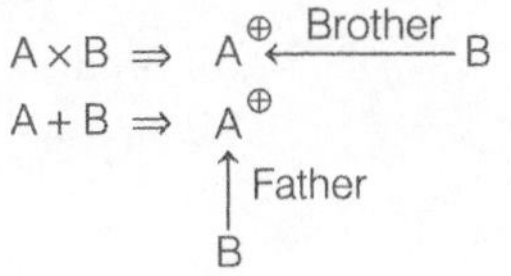

From option (a) N + M × K

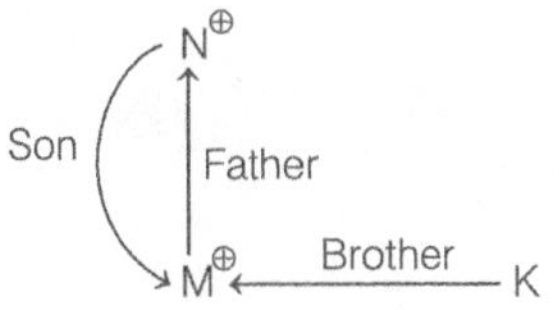

Here, M is the, son of N.

From option (b), N × K + M

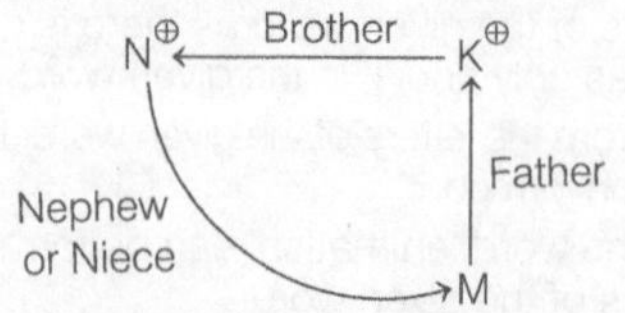

Here, the gender of M is not clear, so N is nephew or niece of M.

From option (c), M × K + N

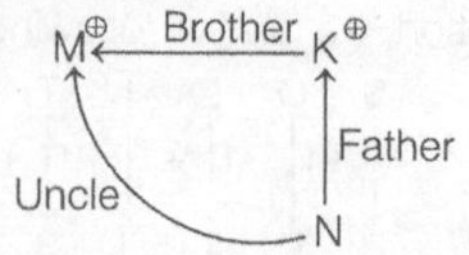

Here, M is the uncle of N.
Thus, none of the above is correct option.

Objective Questions

1. Vijay says "Ananda's mother is the only daughter of my mother." How is Ananda related to Vijay?
(a) Brother (b) Father
(c) Nephew (d) Grandfather

2. Showing the lady in the park, Vineet said, "She is the daughter of my grandfather's only son". How is Vineet related to that lady?
(a) Brother (b) Cousin
(c) Father (d) Uncle

3. Pointing to a photograph, Suraj said, "His daughter Shobha is granddaughter of my mother". How is Shobha related to Suraj?
(a) Aunt
(b) Sister
(c) Daughter
(d) Cannot be determined

4. Pointing to Satish, Ashok said, "He is the son of my sister's only brother". How is Satish related to Ashok?
(a) Son (b) Grandson
(c) Nephew (d) None of these

5. Deepak is brother of Ravi. Rekha is sister of Atul. Ravi is son of Rekha. How is Deepak related to Rekha?
(a) Son (b) Brother
(c) Nephew (d) Father

6. A is B's sister. C is B's mother. D is C's father. E is D's mother. Then, how is A related to D?
(a) Grandmother
(b) Grandfather
(c) Daughter
(d) Granddaughter

Directions (Q. Nos. 7 and 8) *Study the following information carefully to answer these questions.*

(i) 'P ★ Q' means 'P is father of Q'.
(ii) 'P # Q' means 'P is sister of Q'.
(iii) 'P + Q' means 'P is brother of Q'.
(iv) 'P − Q' means 'P is mother of Q'.
(v) 'P/Q' means 'P is son of Q'.
(vi) 'P = Q' means 'P is daughter of Q'.

7. Z ★ X − Y is given, then which of the following is true?
(a) Z is maternal uncle of Y
(b) Z is maternal grandfather of Y
(c) X is nephew of Z
(d) Z is grandmother of Y

8. Which of the following means 'Z has two children'?
(a) Z + Y + X (b) Z ★ Y # X
(c) Z # Y − X (d) Z + X/Y

Answers

1 (c)	2 (a)	3 (d)	4 (a)	5 (a)	6 (d)	7 (b)	8 (b)

Direction Sense Test

Direction is the measurement of position of one object with respect to another object.

In this chapter, we deal with questions in which a successive follow-up of directions is formulated and the candidate is required to ascertain the final direction or the distance between two points.

Main Directions and Cardinal Directions

There are four main directions i.e. North (N), South (S), East (E) and West (W) and four cardinal directions (directions between two adjacent main directions) i.e. North-East (N-E), South-East (S-E), South-West (S-W) and North-West (N-W).

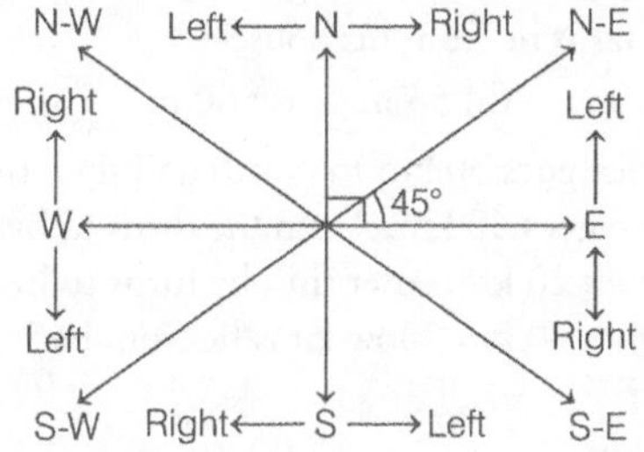

Example 1. Ritu is going Northwards. She turns right, moves some distance and again turns to her right. After moving some distance she turns to her left. In which direction now is she going?

(a) East (b) West (c) South (d) North

Sol. (a) According to the question, the direction diagram can be drawn as,

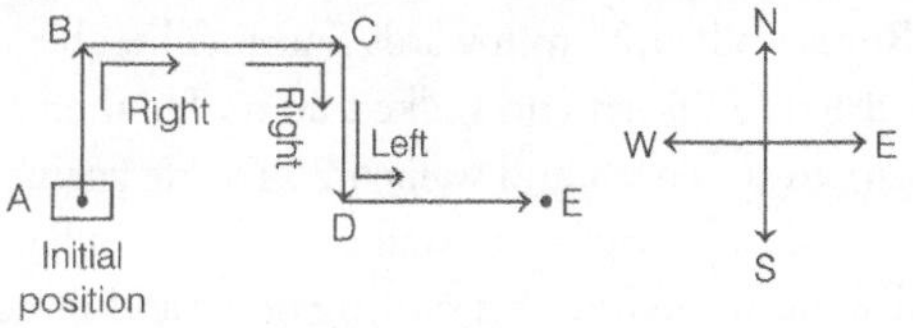

Clearly, Ritu is going towards East.

Example 2. A man walks 30 m in South direction and then turned towards his right and walks 20 m. Again, he turned towards his right and walks 30 m. How far is he from his starting point?

(a) 30 m (b) 20 m (c) 50 m (d) 10 m

Sol. (b) According to the question, the direction diagram can be drawn as

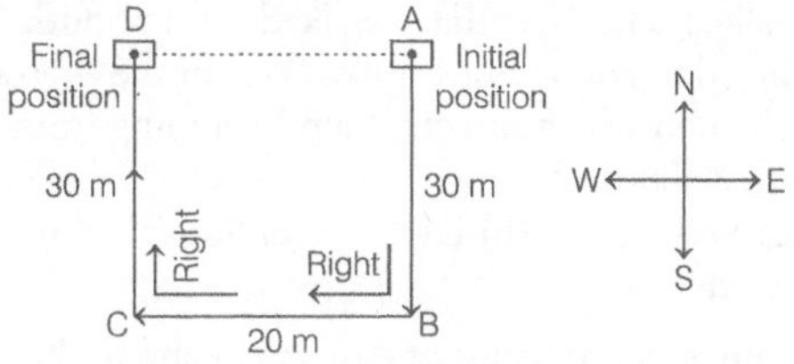

∴ Required distance, AD = BC [as, AB = CD = 30 m]

∴ AD = 20 m

Example 3. Point M is 5 m to the West of point D. Point F is 3 m to the South of point D and point J is 4 m to the East of point F. How far and in which direction is point J with respect to point D?

(a) 5 m, South-East (b) 7 m, North-West

(c) 1 m, East (d) 5 m, South

Sol. (a) The direction diagram can be drawn as,

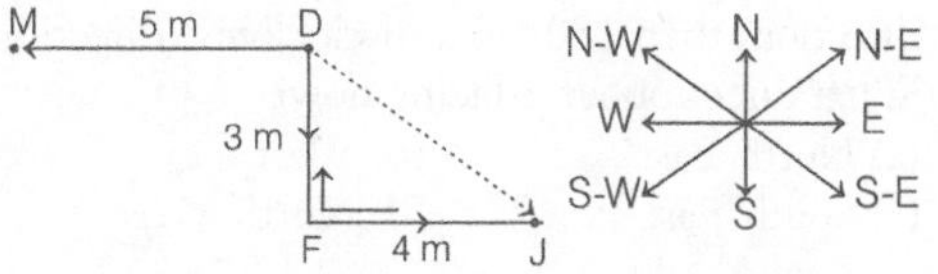

Distance between D and J can be calculated using Pythagoras theorem,

$$DJ = \sqrt{(DF)^2 + (FJ)^2}$$

$$= \sqrt{3^2 + 4^2} = \sqrt{9 + 16} = \sqrt{25} = 5\text{m}$$

Also, J is to the South-East of D.

∴ J is 5m to the South-East of point D.

Objective Questions

1. A boy goes in South direction, then he turns towards left and travels for some distance. After that he turns right and moves certain distance. At last he turns left and travel again for some distance. Now, in which direction is he moving?
   (a) South (b) West
   (c) East (d) North
2. I was facing East from where I turned to my left and walked 12 ft, then I turned towards right and walked 6 ft, After that I walked 6 ft in South direction and at last I walked 6 ft in the West. Then, in which direction am I standing from the original point?
   (a) West (b) East (c) South (d) North
3. Ram is to the South of Aishwarya and to the West of Rani. If Priyanka is to the South of Ram, then in which direction is Priyanka with respect to Rani?
   (a) South (b) North-East
   (c) South-West (d) North
4. There are four roads. I have come from the South and want to go the temple. The road to the right leads me towards the coffee house while straight road leads to the college. In which direction is the temple?
   (a) North (b) East (c) South (d) West
5. I am facing North. I turn 135° in clockwise direction, then 180° in anti-clockwise direction. What direction am I facing now?
   (a) North-East (b) West
   (c) South-East (d) North-West
6. Rama is facing East. He turns 90° in clockwise direction, and then 135° in anti-clockwise direction and then again 90° in clockwise direction. Which direction is she facing now?
   (a) South-East (b) South
   (c) North-East (d) South-West
7. A person walks away from his house at 8:00 am and observes his shadow to his right. Then, he turns towards his left and then again towards his right. Which direction is he facing now?
   (a) West (b) South
   (c) North (d) East
8. One day, during Sunset, two friends Sudhir and Amit were talking, facing each other. If Amit's shadow was on his right, then in which direction is Aman facing, if Aman faces the direction opposite of what Sudhir is facing?
   (a) North (b) West (c) East (d) South
9. The time in a clock is quarter past twelve. If the hour hand points to the East, then towards which direction the minute hand is pointing?
   (a) South-West (b) South
   (c) West (d) North
10. A house faces North. A man coming out of his house walked straight for 10 m, turned left and walked 25 m. He then turned right and walked 5 m and again turned right and walked 25 m. How far is he from his house?
    (a) 15 m (b) 55 m (c) 60 m (d) 65 m
11. A cyclist goes 30 km to North and then turning East he goes 40 km. Again, he turns to his right and goes 20 km. After this, he turns to his right and goes 40 km. How far is he from his starting point?
    (a) 6 km (b) 10 km
    (c) 25 km (d) 40 km
12. A boat moves from port towards East. After sailing for 9 miles, she turns towards right and covers another 12 miles. If she wants to go back to the port, what is the shortest distance now from her position?
    (a) 21 miles (b) 20 miles
    (c) 18 miles (d) 15 miles
13. Rohit walked 25 m towards South. Then he turned to his left and walked 20 m. He then turned to his left and walked 25 m. He again turned to his right and walked 15 m. At what distance is he from his starting point and in which direction?
    (a) 35 m, East
    (b) 35 m, North
    (c) 40 m, East
    (d) 60 m, East

14. Starting from a point P, Rohan walked 20 m towards South. He turned left and walked 30 m. He then turned left and wallked 20 m. He again turned left and walked 40m and reached point Q. How far and in which direction is the point Q from the point P?

(a) 20 m, West (b) 10 m, East
(c) 10 m, West (d) 10 m, North

15. Mohan left for his office in his car. He drove 15 km towards North and then 10 km towards West. He then turned to the South and covered 5 km. Further he turned to the East and moved 8 km. Finally, he turned right and drove 10 km. How far and in which direction is he from his starting point?

(a) 2 km, West (b) 5 km, East
(c) 3 km, North (d) 6 km, South

Answers

1 *(c)*	2 *(d)*	3 *(c)*	4 *(d)*	5 *(d)*	6 *(a)*	7 *(b)*	8 *(a)*	9 *(b)*	10 *(a)*
11 *(b)*	12 *(d)*	13 *(a)*	14 *(c)*	15 *(a)*					

Hints & Solutions

1. (c) The direction diagram is as follows,

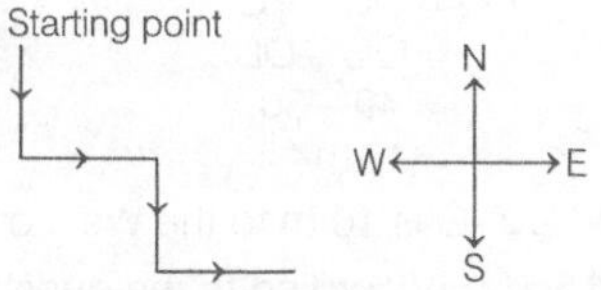

Clearly, he is moving towards East direction.

2. (d) The direction diagram is as follows,

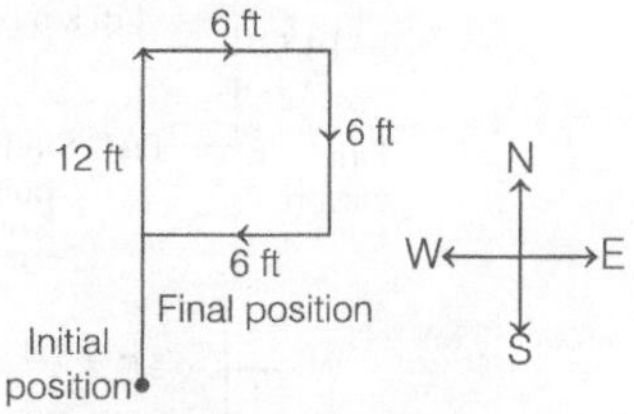

Clearly, the person is towards North from his initial position.

3. (c) According to the question,

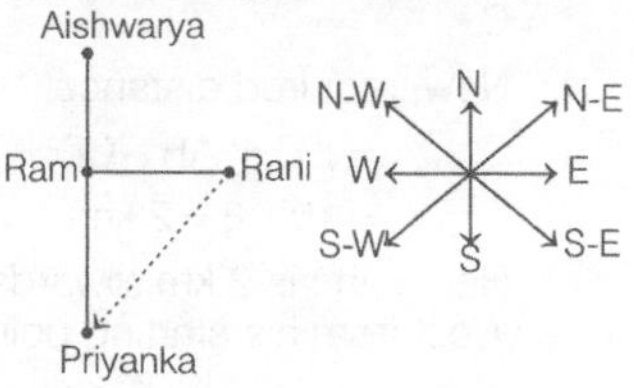

Clearly, Priyanka is towards South-West of Rani.

4. (d) According to the question,

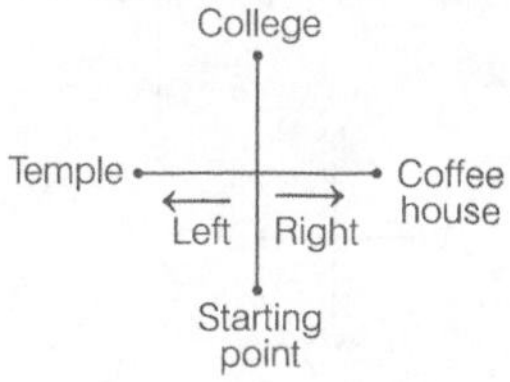

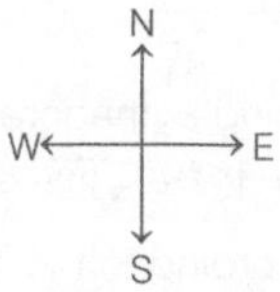

Clearly, temple is towards West.

5. (d) Difference in degrees

$= 180° - 135°$

$= 45°$

anti-clockwise.

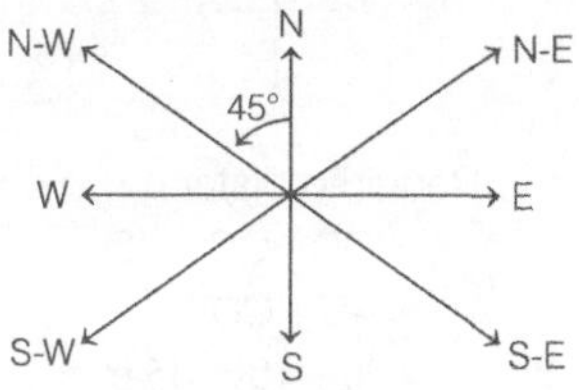

Hence, now I am facing in North-West direction.

6. (a) Clockwise turn $= 90° + 90°$

$= 180°$

Anti-clockwise turn

$= 135°$

Difference $= 180° - 135°$

$= 45°$ clockwise

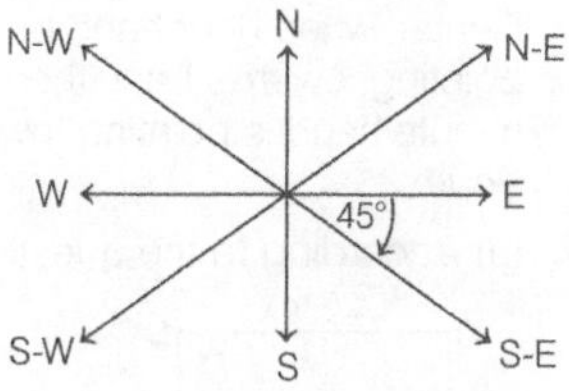

Hence, now Rama is facing in South-East direction.

7. (b) According to the question, the shadow is towards his right at 8:00 am that means the person is walking towards South direction.

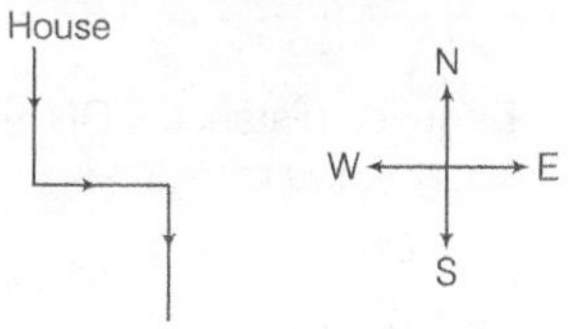

Clearly, he is facing South direction.

8. (a) According to the question, at Sunset Amit's shadow is towards his right that means he is facing North.
Now, Sudhir is standing in front of him that means Sudhir is facing South. Now, Aman faces the direction opposite of Sudhir.
∴ Aman is facing North direction.

9. (b) Time quarter past twelve means that the time is 12 : 15.

Original position

After shifting

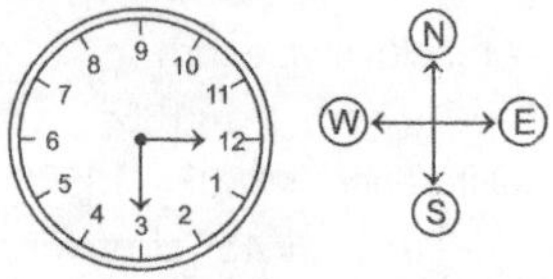

Hence, when hour hand is pointing towards East, then the minute hand is pointing towards South.

10. (a) According to the question,

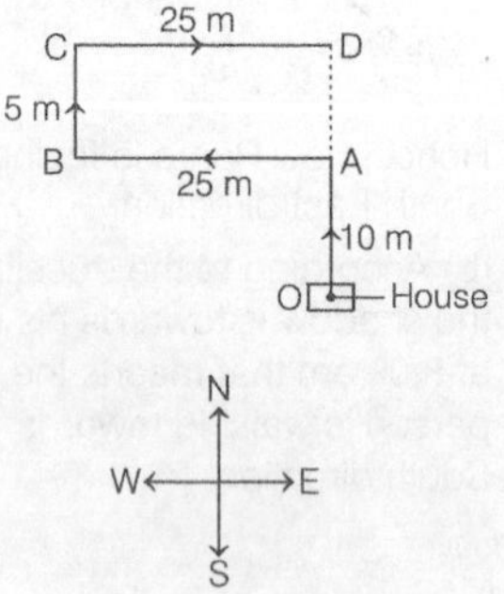

∴ Required distance = OD
= OA + AD
= OA + BC
= 10 + 5
= 15 m

11. (b) According to the question,

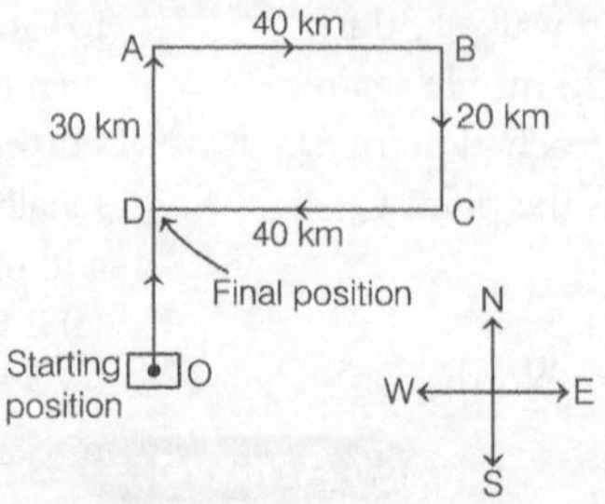

∴ Required distance
= OD = OA − AD = OA − BC
= 30 − 20 = 10 km

12. (d) According to the question,

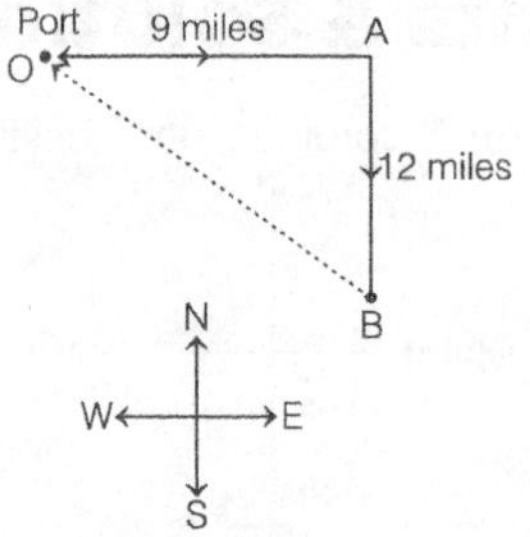

∴ Required distance = OB
$= \sqrt{OA^2 + AB^2}$
[using Pythagoras theorem]
$= \sqrt{9^2 + 12^2} = \sqrt{225} = 15$ miles

13. (a) According to the question,

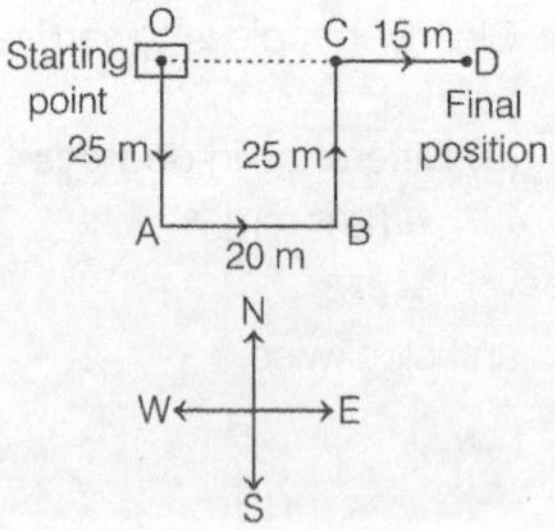

∴ Required distance
= OD = OC + CD
= AB + CD
= 20 + 15 = 35 m

Also, point D is to the East of point O.
∴ He is 35 m towards East from his starting point.

14. (c) According to the question,

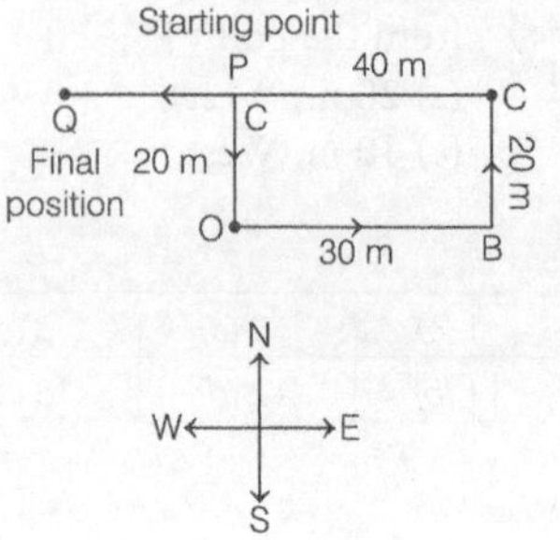

We can see that point 'Q' is to the West of point 'P'.
Now,
Required distance,
PQ = QC − PC
= QC − OB
= 40 − 30
= 10 m
∴ Q is 10 m to the West of P.

15. (a) According to the question,

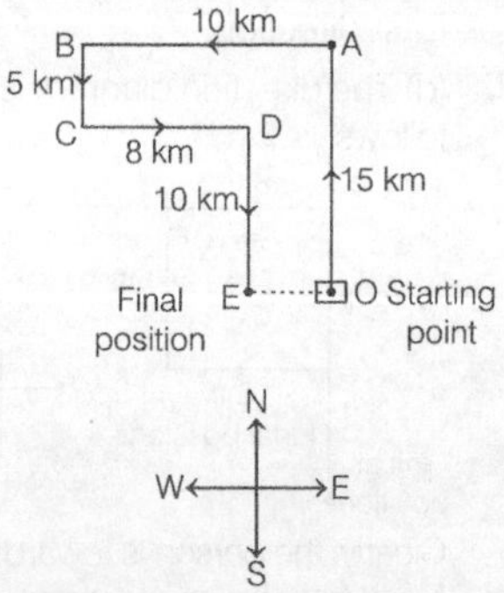

Point E is to the West of point O.
Now, required distance
= EO = AB − CD
= 10 − 8 = 2 km
Hence, he is 2 km towards West from his starting point.

MATHEMATICS

Chapter 01

Number System

The system in which we study to write or represent and their properties of various type of numbers, is called number system.

Types of Numbers

- **Natural Numbers** Natural numbers are counting numbers started from 1.
  e.g. 1, 2, 3, 4, ...
- **Whole Numbers** Whole numbers is a set of all natural numbers and zero.
  e.g. 0, 1, 2, 3, ...
- **Integers** Integers is a set of whole numbers and negative numbers.
  e.g. $\ldots, -4, -3, -2, -1, 0, 1, 2, 3, 4, \ldots$
- **Prime Numbers** Prime numbers are those counting numbers which has exactly two factors, 1 and itself.
  e.g. 2, 3, 5, 7, 11, ...
- **Composite Numbers** Composite numbers are non-prime natural numbers.
  e.g. 4, 6, 8, 9, ...
- **Coprimes** Two natural numbers are coprimes, if their HCF is 1. e.g. (7,9), (8, 11)
- **Rational Numbers** Rational numbers are those numbers which can be expressed as p/q, where p and q are integers and $q \neq 0$.
  e.g. $-2, 4, \frac{8}{3}, \frac{9}{7}$, etc.
- **Irrational Numbers** Irrational numbers are those numbers which cannot be expressed as p/q, where p and q are integers and $q \neq 0$.
  e.g. $\sqrt{41}, \sqrt{31}, \sqrt{7}, \sqrt{3}$
- **Real Numbers** Real numbers include rational and irrational numbers both.
  e.g. $-3, -8, \frac{8}{7}, \sqrt{31}, \sqrt{3}$
- 1 is neither prime nor composite number.
- π is an irrational number.

Divisibility Tests

Number	Condition of Divisibility
2	The last digit of the number must be 0, 2, 4, 6, 8.
3	The sum of digits of number must be divisible by 3.
4	The number formed by last two digits of given number must be divisible by 4 or the last two or three digits of the number must be zero.
5	The last digit of the number must be either 0 or 5.
6	The number must be divisible by 2 and 3.
7	The difference between the number formed by the digits other than the unit's digit and twice the unit digit is either zero or multiple of 7. e.g. 665 is divisible by 7 as $66 - 2 \times 5 = 56$ and 56 is divisible by 7.
8	The number formed by the last three digits of given number must be divisible by 8.
9	The sum of digits of given number must be divisible by 9.
11	The difference between 'sum of digits at even place' and 'sum of digits at odd place' is either zero or divisible by 11. e.g. 2865423 is divisible by 11 as sum of digits at odd place $(O) = 2 + 6 + 4 + 3 = 15$ Sum of digits at even place $(E) = 8 + 5 + 2 = 15$ $\because\ O - E = 0 (15 - 15 = 0)$ $\therefore$ Number is divisible by 11.

Division of Numbers

If we divide a number by another number, then
Dividend = (Divisor × Quotient) + Remainder.

Digit of Unit's Place of an Expression

- If the unit's digit number are 0, 1, 5 and 6, then the resultant unit's digit remains same.
  e.g. $(576)^{43}$, its unit digit is 6.

- If unit's digit is 9 and if the power of 9 is odd, then unit's digit will be 9 and if the power of 9 is even, then unit's digit will be 1.

  e.g. $(19)^{17}$, then unit digit = 9

  $(39)^{12}$, then unit digit = 1

- If unit's digit number are 2, 3, 4, 7, 8, then the power of the number is represented in the form of multiple of 4.

  e.g. Unit digit of $3^{21} = 3^{(4\times5+1)} = (3^4)^5 \times 3^1$

  $= 3^4 \times 3 = 81 \times 3$

  $\Rightarrow$ Unit digit is 3

- To find the unit's digit of product of two or more numbers, we take unit digit of every number and then multiply them.

  e.g. Unit digit of $207 \times 781 \times 39 \times 4$

  $= 7 \times 1 \times 9 \times 4 = 7 \times 36$

  Again take unit digits $= 7 \times 6 = 42$

  Hence, unit digit of the product = 2

Sum of Numbers

1. Sum of first n natural numbers $= \dfrac{n(n+1)}{2}$
2. Sum of first n odd numbers $= n^2$
3. Sum of first n even numbers $= n(n+1)$
4. Sum of squares of first n natural numbers $= \dfrac{n(n+1)(2n+1)}{6}$
5. Sum of cubes of first n natural numbers $= \left[n\left(\dfrac{n+1}{2}\right)\right]^2$

Arithmetic Progression (AP)

The progression of the form $a, (a+d), (a+2d), (a+3d), \ldots$ is known as an arithmetic progression, where $a = 1$ st term, $d =$ common difference

(i) nth term $= a + (n-1)d$

(ii) Sum of n terms $= \dfrac{n}{2}[(2a + (n-1)d)]$

(iii) Sum of n terms $= \dfrac{n}{2}(a + l)$, here l = last term

Geometric Progression (GP)

The progression of the form $a, ar\ ar^2, ar^3, \ldots$ is known as a geometric progression where, $a = 1$ st term, $r =$ common ratio

(i) nth term $= ar^{n-1}$

(ii) Sum of n terms $= \dfrac{a(1-r^n)}{(1-r)}$, here $r < 1$

(iii) Sum of n terms $= \dfrac{a(r^n - 1)}{(r-1)}$, here $r > 1$

Exam Pattern Questions

1. Which of the following numbers is not a rational number?

(a) $\dfrac{8^{\frac{1}{3}} \times 2^{\frac{1}{2}}}{18^{\frac{1}{2}}}$ (b) $2^{\frac{1}{2}} \times 8^{\frac{1}{2}} \times 8^{\frac{1}{3}}$

(c) $\dfrac{125^{\frac{1}{3}} \times 16^{\frac{1}{4}}}{2^{\frac{1}{2}}}$ (d) None of these

2. The difference between the greatest and least prime numbers which are less than 100, is

(a) 95 (b) 97 (c) 96 (d) 94

3. The smallest number of 6 digits which is divisible by 111 is

(a) 111111 (b) 110011 (c) 100011 (d) 10001

4. What least number must be added to 1056 so that the sum is completely divisible by 23?

(a) 2 (b) 3 (c) 18 (d) 21

5. If the number 481 * 673 is completely divisible by 9, then smallest whole number in place of will be

(a) 2 (b) 3
(c) 4 (d) 7

6. Find the unit place digit in the given expression. $(153)^{144} - (115)^{123} - (111)^{510} + (216)^{25}$

(a) 1 (b) 5 (c) 6 (d) 3

Answers

1. (c)	2. (a)	3. (c)	4. (a)	5. (d)	6. (a)

Solutions

1. (c) From option (a),

$$\frac{8^{1/3} \times 2^{1/2}}{(18)^{1/2}} = \frac{2 \times \sqrt{2}}{(\sqrt{2}) \times 3}$$

$= \frac{2}{3}$ is a rational number

From option (b)

$2^{1/2} \times 8^{1/2} \times 8^{1/3}$

$= \sqrt{2} \times 2\sqrt{2} \times 2 = 4 \times 2$

$= 8$ is a rational number

From option (c) $\frac{125^{1/3} \times 16^{1/4}}{2^{1/2}}$

$= \frac{5 \times 2}{\sqrt{2}} = \frac{10}{\sqrt{2}}$

$= 5\sqrt{2}$ is a irrational number

2. (a) Greatest prime number $= 97$

Least prime number $= 2$

$\therefore$ Required difference $= 97 - 2 = 95$

3. (c) The smallest number of 6 digits $= 100000$

$$\begin{array}{r} 111)100000(9 \\ \underline{999} \\ 100 \end{array}$$

$\therefore$ Required number

$= 100000 + (111 - 100)$

$= 100011$

4. (a)

$$\begin{array}{r} 23)1056(46 \\ \underline{92} \\ 136 \\ \underline{138} \end{array}$$

Number, whose divisibile by 23

$= 1056 + (138 - 136)$

$= 1056 + 2 = 1058$

Hence, 2 must be added.

5. (d) Given number $= 481 * 673$

Let x will be come in place of * in the given number. We know that any number is completely divisible by 9, when sum of its digits is divisible by 9.

$\therefore$ Sum of digits of given number

$= 4 + 8 + 1 + x + 6 + 7 + 3 = 29 + x$

Hence, value of x should be 7 to completely divisible by 9.

$\therefore \quad 29 + x = 29 + 7 = 36$

Which is divisible by 9.

$\therefore \quad x = 7$

Hence, number 7 will be come in place of * in the given number.

6. (a) Unit place digit in

$(153)^{144} - (115)^{123} - (111)^{510} + (216)^{25}$

= Unit digit in

$[(3)^{4 \times 36 + 0} - (5)^{4 \times 30 + 3} - (1)^{4 \times 127 + 2} + (6)^{4 \times 6 + 1}]$

= Unit digit in

$[3^4 - 5^3 - 1^2 + 6^1]$

= Unit digit in $[81 - 125 - 1 + 6]$

$= 1 - 5 - 1 + 6 = 1$

Chapter 02 Fraction & Decimal

A fraction is a number which represents a ratio or division of two whole numbers. It is represented by $\frac{a}{b}$, $b \neq 0$. In this, a and b are called numerator and denominator of the fraction, respectively.

Fractions such as $\frac{3}{4}, \frac{2}{3}, \frac{41}{57}$ are called common or vulgar fractions.

Types of Fraction

1. A **proper fraction** is one whose numerator is less than its denominator, such as $\frac{2}{3}$.
2. An **improper fraction** is one whose numerator is greater than its denominator, such as $\frac{3}{2}$.
3. A **mixed fraction** is one which has integral as well as a fractional part, such as $3\frac{1}{3}$.
4. A **compound fraction** is a fraction of a fraction, such as $\frac{3}{5}$ of $\frac{2}{7} = \frac{3}{5} \times \frac{2}{7} = \frac{6}{35}$.
5. A **complex fraction** is one having numerator or denominator or both as fraction.

6. **Equivalent fractions** are those which represent the same ratio or number.
7. The form of following fraction is called **continued or ladder fractions.**

$3+\frac{2}{1+7}; 5+\frac{1}{2}$

Comparison of Fractions

1. Convert the fractions into decimal and compare them. e.g. which fraction is bigger in $\frac{1}{7}$ and $\frac{2}{9}$.

$\frac{1}{7}=0.14$ and $\frac{2}{9}=0.22$

It is clear that $0.22>0.14$ or $\frac{2}{9}>\frac{1}{7}$ i.e. $\frac{2}{9}$ is bigger fractions.

2. Convert the fractions into the fractions of equal denominator by taking LCM of denominators, then compare the numerators of the fractions. e.g. which fraction is smaller in $\frac{4}{3}$ and $\frac{5}{4}$. LCM of denominators (3 and 4)=12

$\therefore \frac{4}{3}=\frac{4}{3}\times\frac{4}{4}=\frac{16}{12}$ and $\frac{5}{4}=\frac{5}{4}\times\frac{3}{3}=\frac{15}{12}$

It is clear that $16>15$. So, $\frac{15}{12}<\frac{16}{12}$ or $\frac{5}{4}<\frac{4}{3}$

i.e. $\frac{5}{4}$ smaller fraction.

Decimal Fraction

A fraction has denominator in the form of powers of 10, is called decimal fraction. e.g. 0.4, 0.31, etc.

Recurring Decimals

A decimal fraction in which a digit or a group of digits is repeated successively is called a recurring or periodic decimal. A decimal fraction in which all the digits after the decimal point are repeated, is called a pure recurring decimal, *i.e.*, 0.3333 and a decimal fraction in which only some of its digits is repeated while remaining digits don't, is called a mixed recurring decimal.

Exam Pattern Questions

1. Find the smallest of the following fractions.
(a) 5/6 (b) 23/37 (c) 51/49 (d) 43/54

2. Find the largest of the following fractions.
(a) 453/584 (b) 231/339 (c) 759/894 (d) 352/478

3. What is the ascending order of the fractions $\frac{-7}{10},\frac{5}{-8},\frac{2}{-3}$?
(a) $\frac{-7}{10},\frac{2}{-3},\frac{5}{-8}$ (b) $\frac{-7}{10},\frac{5}{-8},\frac{2}{-3}$
(c) $\frac{5}{-8},\frac{-7}{10},\frac{2}{-3}$ (d) $\frac{2}{-3},\frac{5}{-8},\frac{-7}{10}$

4. Simplify $\frac{7}{16}\div\frac{28}{32}\div\frac{4}{8}$.
(a) 1 (b) 2 (c) 4 (d) 8

5. If $\frac{1}{x}=4$ and $\frac{1}{y}=7$, find $x+y$.
(a) 11 (b) 28 (c) $\frac{11}{28}$ (d) 3

6. Which of the following equal 1?
(a) $\frac{0.404}{4.04\times0.1}$ (b) $\frac{0.404}{4.04\times0.01}$
(c) $\frac{0.404}{404\times0.1}$ (d) $\frac{0.404}{40.4\times0.1}$

7. What is the value of $9\frac{7}{20}$ in form of decimal fraction ?
(a) 9.05 (b) 9.53 (c) 9.26 (d) 9.35

8. Choose the fraction equation to 0.125.
(a) $\frac{1}{8}$ (b) $\frac{2}{5}$ (c) $\frac{3}{5}$ (d) $\frac{3}{8}$

9. The rational number with recurring decimal expansion $0.\overline{12}$ is
(a) $\frac{3}{22}$ (b) $\frac{4}{33}$ (c) $\frac{6}{43}$ (d) $\frac{7}{53}$

10. The vulgar fraction of $0.\overline{3939}$ is
(a) $\frac{15}{33}$ (b) $\frac{11}{39}$ (c) $\frac{17}{39}$ (d) $\frac{13}{33}$

11. The value of $(0.\overline{63}. + 0.\overline{37})$ is

(a) 1 (b) 100/99
(c) 100/999 (d) 1000/999

12. The difference of $5.\overline{76}$ and $2.\overline{3}$ is

(a) $2.\overline{54}$ (b) $3.\overline{73}$
(c) $3.\overline{46}$ (d) $3.\overline{43}$

Answers

1. (b)	2. (c)	3. (a)	4. (a)	5. (c)
6. (a)	7. (d)	8. (a)	9. (b)	10. (d)
11. (b)	12. (d)			

Solutions

1. (b) $\because \frac{5}{6} = 0.83, \frac{23}{37} = 0.62$

$\frac{51}{49} = 1.04, \frac{43}{54} = 0.79$

$\therefore$ Smallest fraction $= \frac{23}{37}$

2. (c) $\because \frac{453}{584} = 0.77$

$\frac{231}{349} = 0.66$

$\frac{759}{894} = 0.84, \frac{352}{478} = 0.73$

$\therefore$ Largest fraction $= \frac{759}{894}$

3. (a) $-\frac{7}{10} = -0.7, -\frac{5}{8} = -0.62$

$-\frac{2}{3} = -0.66$

$\because -0.7 < -0.66 < -0.62$

$\therefore$ Required ascending order

$= -\frac{7}{10}, -\frac{2}{3}, -\frac{5}{8}$

4. (a) Here, $\frac{7}{16} \div \frac{28}{32} \div \frac{4}{8}$

$= \frac{7}{16} \times \frac{32}{28} \times \frac{8}{4} = 1$

5. (c) Given, $\frac{1}{x} = 4$ and $\frac{1}{y} = 7$

$\therefore \frac{1}{x} \times \frac{1}{y} = 4 \times 7$

$\Rightarrow \frac{1}{xy} = 28$

$\Rightarrow xy = \frac{1}{28}$

$\therefore \frac{(x+y)}{xy} = \frac{1}{x} + \frac{1}{y}$

$\Rightarrow (x+y) = xy\left(\frac{1}{x} + \frac{1}{y}\right)$

$\Rightarrow (x+y) = \frac{1}{28}(4+7)$

$\Rightarrow (x+y) = \frac{11}{28}$

6. (a) From option (a),

$\frac{0.404}{4.04 \times 0.1} = \frac{404 \times 1000}{404 \times 1 \times 1000} = 1$

7. (d) $9 + \frac{7}{20} = \frac{180+7}{20}$

$= \frac{187}{7} = 9.35$

8. (a) $0.125 = \frac{125}{1000} \approx \frac{1}{8}$

9. (b) Let $x = 0.\overline{12}$ ...(i)

$\therefore 100x = 12.\overline{12}$ ...(ii)

In order to rationalise we will subtract Eq. (i) from Eq. (ii),

$100x - x = 12.\overline{12} - 0.\overline{12}$

$\Rightarrow 99x = 12$

$\Rightarrow x = \frac{12}{99} = \frac{4}{33}$

10. (d) $0.39\overline{39} = \frac{3939-39}{9900}$

$= \frac{3900}{9900} = \frac{39}{99} = \frac{13}{33}$

11. (b) $0.\overline{63} + 0.\overline{37}$

$= \frac{63}{99} + \frac{37}{99} = \frac{100}{99}$

12. (d) $5.\overline{76} - 2.\overline{3} = 5 + \frac{76}{99} - \left(2 + \frac{3}{9}\right)$

$= 5 - 2 + \frac{76}{99} - \frac{3}{9}$

$= 3 + \frac{76-33}{99}$

$= 3 + \frac{43}{99} = 3.\overline{43}$

Chapter 03

Square Root and Cube Root

Square Root The square root of a number is that number, the square of which is equal to the given number. It is denotoed by the sign '$\sqrt{\ }$'. e.g. $\sqrt{36} = 6$ and -6 because $(6)^2 = 36$ and $(-6)^2 = 36$.

Methods to Calculate the Square Root

(i) Prime Factorisation Method

- First, express the given number as the product of prime factors.
- Take the product of these prime factors taking one out of every pair of the same primes. This product gives us the square root of the given number.

Sol. e.g. Find the square root of 14400.

2	14400
2	7200
2	3600
2	1800
2	900
2	450
3	225
3	75
5	25
5	5
	1

$\therefore 14400 = 2 \times 2 \times 2 \times 2 \times 2 \times 2 \times 3 \times 3 \times 5 \times 5$

[express as the product prime factor form]

$\Rightarrow \sqrt{14400}$

$= \sqrt{\underline{2 \times 2} \times \underline{2 \times 2} \times \underline{2 \times 2} \times \underline{3 \times 3} \times \underline{5 \times 5}}$

$= 2 \times 2 \times 2 \times 3 \times 5$

[taking one number from each pair]

$= 120$

(ii) Division Method

Sol. e.g. Find the square root of 99856.

	316
3	$\overline{9}\,\overline{98}\,\overline{56}$
	9
61	98
	61
626	3756
	3756
	×

$\therefore \quad \sqrt{99856} = 316$

Square Root of Decimal Numbers

If in a given decimal number, the number of digits after decimal are not even, then we put a 0 (zero) at the extreme right. Now, mark off the periods and try to calculate the square root applying the division method.

e.g. Find the square root of 3.025.

Sol.

	1.739
1	$\overline{3}.\overline{02}\,\overline{50}$
	1
27	202
	189
343	1350
	1029
3469	32100
	31221
	879

$\therefore \quad \sqrt{3.025} = 1.739$

Cube Root The cube root of a given number is the number whose cube is the given number. It is denoted by sign $\sqrt[3]{\ }$. e.g. $\sqrt[3]{27} = 3$ because $(3)^3 = 27$.

Method to Calculate the Cube Root

Prime Factorisation Method

- First, express the given number as the product of prime factors.
- Take the product of these prime factors taking one out of each group of three of the same primes. This product gives us the cube root of the given number.

e.g. Find the cube root of 1728.

Sol.

2	1728
2	864
2	432
2	216
2	108
2	54
3	27
3	9
3	3
	1

$1728 = 2\times2\times2\times2\times2\times2\times3\times3\times3$

[express as the product prime factor form]

$\therefore\ \sqrt[3]{1728} = \sqrt[3]{\overline{2\times2\times2}\times\overline{2\times2\times2}\times\overline{3\times3\times3}}$

$= 2\times2\times3$ [taking one number from each group of three of the same primes]

$= 12$

Exam Pattern Questions

1. Which of the following is not a perfect square?
(a) 9602
(b) 1369
(c) 6241
(d) 3136

2. The smallest whole number that is to be multiplied with 59535 to make a perfect square number is x. The sum of digits of x is
(a) 4
(b) 5
(c) 6
(d) 7

3. What is the least number that should be added to the product $11\times12\times13\times14$ to make it a perfect square?
(a) 1 (b) 311
(c) 5 (d) 0

4. What is the square of 0.5?
(a) 2.5 (b) 0.025 (c) 25 (d) 0.25

5. $\sqrt{248\sqrt{52+\sqrt{144}}} = ?$
(a) 14 (b) 16 (c) 16.6 (d) 18.8

6. The value of $\sqrt[3]{\frac{7}{875}}$ is
(a) $\frac{1}{3}$ (b) $\frac{1}{15}$ (c) $\frac{1}{4}$ (d) $\frac{1}{5}$

7. $\sqrt[3]{512} = ?$
(a) 4 (b) 8 (c) 9 (d) 11

Answers

1. (a)	2. (c)	3. (a)	4. (d)	5. (b)
6. (d)	7. (b)			

Solutions

1. (a) Except 9602 all are the perfect square of any natural number because the unit digit of perfect square of any number is not 2.

2. (c)

3	59535
3	19845
3	6615
3	2205
3	735
5	245
7	49
7	7
	1

$59535 = 3 \times 3 \times 3 \times 3 \times 3 \times 5 \times 7 \times 7$

Here, 5 and 3 are to be multiplied with 59535 to make it a perfect square number.

$\therefore$ Required sum $= (15 = 1 + 5) = 6$

3. (a) $11 \times 12 \times 13 \times 14 = 24024$

Nearest square $= (155)^2 = 24025$

Hence, minimum number $= 24025 - 24024 = 1$

4. (d) $\therefore$ Square of 0.5 $= (0.5)^2 = 0.5 \times 0.5 = 0.25$

5. (b) $\sqrt{248 + \sqrt{52 + \sqrt{144}}}$

$= \sqrt{248 + \sqrt{52 + 12}}$

$= \sqrt{248 + \sqrt{64}}$

$= \sqrt{248 + 8}$

$= \sqrt{256} = 16$

6. (d) $\sqrt[3]{\frac{7}{875}} = \sqrt[3]{\frac{7}{5 \times 5 \times 5 \times 7}}$

$= \sqrt[3]{\frac{1}{5 \times 5 \times 5}} = \frac{1}{5}$

7. (b) $\sqrt[3]{512}$

$= \sqrt[3]{\underline{2 \times 2 \times 2} \times \underline{2 \times 2 \times 2} \times \underline{2 \times 2 \times 2}}$

$= 2 \times 2 \times 2 = 8$

Chapter 04 HCF and LCM

Highest Common Factor (HCF)

The greatest number which divides given two or more numbers, is called HCF of given numbers.

e.g. HCF of 36 and 84

By prime factorisation method,

$\because \quad 36 = 2 \times 2 \times 3 \times 3$ and $84 = 2 \times 2 \times 3 \times 7$

$\therefore$ HCF of 36 and 84 $= 2 \times 2 \times 3 = 12$

Least Common Multiple (LCM)

The least number which is divisible by two or more given numbers is called LCM of given numbers.

e.g. LCM of 24 and 112

By prime factorisation method,

2	24, 112
2	12, 56
2	6, 28
2	3, 14
3	3, 7
7	1, 7
	1, 1

LCM of 24 and 112 $= 2 \times 2 \times 2 \times 2 \times 3 \times 7 = 336$

Product of two numbers = HCF of Numbers × LCM of Numbers

LCM and HCF of Fractions

$$\text{LCM of fractions} = \frac{\text{LCM of Numerators}}{\text{HCF of Denominators}}$$

$$\text{HCF of fractions} = \frac{\text{HCF of Numerators}}{\text{LCM of Denominators}}$$

Exam Pattern Questions

1. Select the most appropriate option. Find the LCM of 15, 30 and 24.
(a) 60 (b) 240
(c) 180 (d) 120

2. If $P = 2^3 \times 3^{10} \times 5$ and $Q = 2^5 \times 3 \times 7$, then HCF of P and Q is
(a) $2 \times 3 \times 5 \times 7$ (b) 3×2^3
(c) $2^2 \times 3^7$ (d) $2^3 \times 3^{10} \times 5 \times 7$

3. The smallest positive number which is exactly divisible by 450, 600 and 900, is
(a) 1800 (b) 3600
(c) 5400 (d) 2100

4. Four bells ring at the intervals of 5, 6, 8 and 9 respectively. All the bells ring simultaneously at same time. They will again ring simultaneously after
(a) 12 min (b) 6 min (c) 24 min (d) 18 min

5. Three bells toll at intervals of 9, 12 and 15 min, respectively. All the three began to toll at 8 am. At what time will they toll together again?
(a) 8:45 am (b) 10:30 am
(c) 11:00 am (d) 1:30 am

Answers

1.	2.	3.	4.	5.
(d)	*(b)*	*(a)*	*(b)*	*(c)*

Solutions

1. (d)

2	15, 30, 24
2	15, 15, 12
2	15, 15, 6
3	15, 15, 3
5	5, 5, 1
	1, 1, 1

So, LCM of 15, 30 and 24
$= 2 \times 2 \times 2 \times 3 \times 5 = 120$

2. (b) $P = 2^3 \times 3^{10} \times 5$
$Q = 2^5 \times 3 \times 7$

HCF of P and $Q = 2^3 \times 3$

3. (a) For smallest such number we need to find LCM of the given numbers.
$450 = 2 \times 3 \times 3 \times 5 \times 5$
$600 = 2 \times 2 \times 2 \times 3 \times 5 \times 5$
$900 = 2 \times 2 \times 3 \times 3 \times 5 \times 5$
So, LCM of 450, 600 and 900
$= 2 \times 2 \times 2 \times 3 \times 3 \times 5 \times 5$
$= 1800$

4. (b) Time of bells ring simultaneously
= LCM of 5, 6, 8 and 9 s = 360 sec
$= \frac{360}{60}$ min
$\left[\because 1 \text{ sec} = \frac{1}{60} \text{min}\right]$
= 6 min

5. (c) First we find LCM of 9, 12 and 15
$9 = 3 \times 3$
$12 = 2 \times 2 \times 3$
$15 = 3 \times 5$
$\therefore$ LCM of 9, 12 and $15 = 2 \times 2 \times 3 \times 3 \times 5$
= 180 min
$= \frac{180}{60}$ hour
= 3 hour
So, the bell ring together again
= 8 am + 3 hour
= 11 am

Chapter 05

Simplification

Simplification is a process of reducing a complex expression into a simpler form.

Approximation is also a process of reducing a complex expression which includes decimal values numbers into simpler form by calculating the nearest (round off) values.

VBODMAS Rule

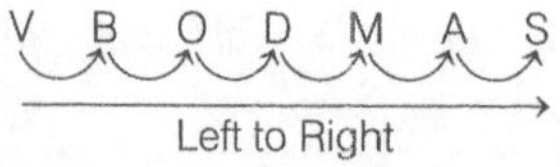

We must follow the below order very strictly.

(i) V - Viniculum or Bar '–'

(ii) B - Brackets '[{( )}]'

(iii) O - of (×)

(iv) D- Division

(v) M - Multiplication

(vi) A - Addition

(vii) S - Subtraction

Order of Removing Brackets

First - Small Brackets '( )'

Second - Curly Brackets '{ }'

Third - Square Brackets '[ ]'

Improtant Formulae

1. $(a+b)^2 = a^2 + 2ab + b^2$
2. $(a-b)^2 = a^2 - 2ab + b^2$
3. $a^2 - b^2 = (a+b)(a-b)$
4. $(a+b)^3 = a^3 + b^3 + 3ab(a+b)$
5. $(a-b)^3 = a^3 - b^3 - 3ab(a-b)$
6. $a^3 + b^3 = (a-b)(a^2 - ab + b^2)$

Exam Pattern Questions

1. The simplified value of $\frac{4}{15}$ of $\frac{5}{8} \times 6 + 15 - 10$ is

(a) 6 (b) 3 (c) 5 (d) 4

2. The value of

$$3 \div \left[(8-5) \div \left\{(4-2) + \left(2 + \frac{8}{13}\right)\right\}\right] \text{ is}$$

(a) $\frac{15}{17}$ (b) $\frac{13}{17}$ (c) $\frac{15}{19}$ (d) $\frac{60}{13}$

3. The value of $5\frac{1}{3} \div 1\frac{2}{9} \times \frac{1}{4}\left(10 + \frac{3}{1 - \frac{1}{5}}\right)$ is

(a) 15 (b) $\frac{67}{25}$ (c) $\frac{128}{11}$ (d) $\frac{128}{99}$

4. The value of

$$3\frac{1}{2} - \left[2\frac{1}{4} \div \left\{1\frac{1}{4} - \frac{1}{2}\left(1\frac{1}{2} - \frac{1}{3} - \frac{1}{6}\right)\right\}\right] \text{ is}$$

(a) $\frac{1}{2}$ (b) $2\frac{1}{2}$

(c) $3\frac{1}{2}$ (d) $9\frac{1}{2}$

5. The value of

$25 - 5\,[2 + 3\,(2 - 2\,(5-3) + 5) - 10] \div 4$ is

(a) 5 (b) 23.25

(c) 23.75 (d) 25

Answers

1. (a)	2. (d)	3. (a)	4. (a)	5. (c)

Solutions

1. (a) $\frac{4}{15}$ of $\frac{5}{8}\times 6+15-10$

$=\frac{4}{15}\times\frac{5}{8}\times 6+15-10=1+5=6$

2. (d) $3\div\left[(8-5)\div\left\{(4-2)+\left(2+\frac{8}{13}\right)\right\}\right]$

$=3\div\left[3\div\left\{2+\frac{34}{13}\right\}\right]=3\div\left[3\div\left\{\frac{60}{13}\right\}\right]$

$=3\div\left[3\times\frac{13}{60}\right]=3\div\frac{13}{20}=3\times\frac{20}{13}=\frac{60}{13}$

3. (a) $5\frac{1}{3}\div 1\frac{2}{9}\times\frac{1}{4}\left(10+\frac{3}{1-\frac{1}{5}}\right)$

$=\frac{16}{3}\div\frac{11}{9}\times\frac{1}{4}\left(10+\frac{3\times 5}{4}\right)$

$=\frac{16}{3}\times\frac{9}{11}\times\frac{1}{4}\left(\frac{40+15}{4}\right)$

$=\frac{12}{11}\times\frac{55}{4}=3\times 5=15$

4. (a) $3\frac{1}{2}-\left[2\frac{1}{4}\div\left\{1\frac{1}{4}-\frac{1}{2}\left(1\frac{1}{2}-\frac{1}{3}-\frac{1}{6}\right)\right\}\right]$

$=\frac{7}{2}-\left[\frac{9}{4}\div\left\{\frac{5}{4}-\frac{1}{2}\left(\frac{3}{2}-\frac{1}{3}-\frac{1}{6}\right)\right\}\right]$

$=\frac{7}{2}-\left[\frac{9}{4}\div\left\{\frac{5}{4}-\frac{1}{2}\left(\frac{9-2-1}{6}\right)\right\}\right]$

$=\frac{7}{2}-\left[\frac{9}{4}\div\left\{\frac{5}{4}-\frac{1}{2}\right\}\right]$

$=\frac{7}{2}-\left[\frac{9}{4}\div\left\{\frac{5-2}{4}\right\}\right]$

$=\frac{7}{2}-\left[\frac{9}{4}\times\frac{4}{3}\right]=\frac{7}{2}-\frac{3}{1}=\frac{7-6}{2}=\frac{1}{2}$

5. (c) $25-5\,[2+3\,(2-2\,(5-3)+5)-10]\div 4$

$=25-5\,[2+3\,(2-2\times 2+5)-10]\div 4$

$=25-5\,[2+3\,(2+1)-10]\div 4$

$=25-5\,[2+9-10]\div 4$

$=25-\frac{5\times 1}{4}=\frac{100-5}{4}=\frac{95}{4}=23.75$

Chapter 06 Average

An average of given quantities is the sum of the given quantities divided by number of quantities.

$$\text{Average}=\frac{\text{Sum of given quantities}}{\text{Number of quantities}}$$

Properties of Average

1. If all the given numbers are added, subtracted, multiplied or divided by a non-zero number *a*, then their average will be also added, subtracted, multiplied or divided respectively by *a*.
2. If '0' is one of the observation of a given data, then that 0 will also be included while calculating average.

Important Formulae

1. Average of n natural numbers from 1 to n is $\left(\frac{n+1}{2}\right)$.
2. Average of even natural numbers from 1 to n is $\left(\frac{n}{2}+1\right)$.
3. Average of odd natural numbers from 1 to n is $\left(\frac{n+1}{2}\right)$.
4. Average of consecutive numbers $=\frac{\text{First number}+\text{Last number}}{2}$.
5. Average of n multiples of any number $=\frac{\text{Number}\times(n+1)}{2}$

Exam Pattern Questions

1. Find the average, 112, 118, 126, 132, 142 and 156
(a) 131 (b) 127
(c) 130 (d) 129

2. The average of squares of first 20 consecutive even number is
(a) 282 (b) 375
(c) 574 (d) 589

3. What will be the average of the first 5 positive even numbers divisible by 9?
(a) 50 (b) 54
(c) 48 (d) 62

4. Of the three numbers, the first is twice the second and is also thrice the third. The average of the numbers is 88. The difference between the first and the third number is
(a) 48 (b) 24 (c) 96 (d) 72

5. 7 kg of tea costing ₹ 280 per kg is mixed with 9 kg of tea costing ₹ 240 per kg. The average price per kg of the mixed tea is
(a) ₹ 257.50
(b) ₹ 255.80
(c) ₹ 267.20
(d) ₹ 267.50

6. If the average weight of 30 men is 65 kg and that of 20 women is 52 kg, then what is the average weight of all 50 persons together ?
(a) 57 kg (b) 60 kg
(c) 67 kg (d) 50 kg

Answers

1. (a)	2. (c)	3. (b)	4. (c)	5. (a)
6. (b)				

Solutions

1. (a) Required average

$$= \frac{\text{Total of Numbers}}{\text{Number of Numbers}} = \frac{112 + 118 + 126 + 132 + 142 + 156}{6}$$

$$= \frac{786}{6} = 131$$

2. (c) Sum of square of first 20 even numbers

$$= \frac{2n(n+1)(2n+1)}{3}$$

$$= \frac{40 \times 21 \times 41}{3} = \frac{34440}{3}$$

$$= 11480$$

∴ Required average

$$= \frac{\text{Sum of Numbers}}{\text{Number of Numbers}} = \frac{11480}{20} = 574$$

3. (b) First 5 even numbers, divisible by 9

= 18, 36, 54, 72, 90

∴ Required average

$$= \frac{\text{Total of Numbers}}{\text{Number of Numbers}}$$

$$= \frac{18 + 36 + 54 + 72 + 90}{5}$$

$$= \frac{270}{5} = 54$$

4. (c) Let three numbers are x, y, z then according to the question.

$x = 2y$ and $x = 3z \Rightarrow y = \frac{x}{2}$

and $z = \frac{x}{3}$ ...(i)

Now average $= \frac{\text{Sum of Numbers}}{\text{Number of Numbers}}$

$$88 = \frac{x + y + z}{3}$$

$$88 = \frac{x + \frac{x}{2} + \frac{x}{3}}{3} \quad [\because \text{from eq (i)}]$$

$$88 \times 3 = \frac{6x + 3x + 2x}{6}$$

$$88 \times 3 \times 6 = 11x$$

$$\Rightarrow \quad 8 \times 3 \times 6 = x$$

then $z = \frac{x}{3} = \frac{8 \times 3 \times 6}{3} = 8 \times 6$

Required

$$x - z = 8 \times 3 \times 6 - 8 \times 6$$

$$= 8 \times 6(3 - 1) = 8 \times 6 \times 2 = 96$$

5. (a) Average price of mixed tea

$$= \frac{\text{Total Price}}{\text{Amount of Tea}}$$

$$= \frac{280 \times 7 + 240 \times 9}{7 + 9}$$

$$= \frac{1960 + 2160}{16} = \frac{4120}{16}$$

= ₹ 257.50 per kg

6. (b) Total weight of 30 men

$= 30 \times 65 = 1950$ kg

and total weight of 20 women

$= 20 \times 52 = 1040$ kg

∴ Average weight of 50 persons

$$= \frac{\text{Total Weight}}{\text{Number of Person}}$$

$$= \frac{1950 + 1040}{30 + 20}$$

$$= \frac{2990}{50} = \frac{299}{5}$$

$$\Rightarrow 59.8 \approx 60 \text{ kg}$$

Chapter 07

Ratio and Proportion

Ratio

It is denoted by (:). Ratio of a and b is denoted by $a : b$. Here, a is known as prior term (antecedent) and b is known as post term (consequent).

Types of Ratio

1. **Compound Ratio** If $\frac{a}{b}$, $\frac{c}{d}$ and $\frac{e}{f}$ are three ratios, then their compound ratio $= \frac{a \times c \times e}{b \times d \times f}$
2. **Duplicate Ratio** If $a : b$ is a ratio, then duplicate ratio $= \frac{a^2}{b^2}$.
3. **Sub-duplicate Ratio** If $a : b$ is a ratio, then sub-duplicate ratio $= \sqrt{a} : \sqrt{b}$.

Proportion

Proportion is the equality of two ratios. As $a : b = c : d$, we write $a : b :: c : d$ and a, b, c and d are in proportion. Here, a and d are extremes and b and c are means.

$\therefore \quad a \times d = b \times c$

Here, d is also known as fourth proportional.

If a, b and c are in proportion, then $\frac{a}{b} = \frac{b}{c}$

$\Rightarrow \quad b^2 = ac$

Here, b is known as mean proportional and c is known as third proportional.

Basic Operations on Proportion

(i) Invertendo $= b : a :: d : c$

(ii) Alternendo $= a : c :: b : d$

(iii) Componendo $= (a + b) : b :: (c + d) : d$

(iv) Dividendo $= (a - b) : b :: (c - d) : d$

(v) Componendo and Dividendo $= (a + b) : (a - b) :: (c + d)\,(c - d)$

Ratio Division

If a quantity P is distributed in the ratio of $a : b : c$, then

First part $= \frac{a}{a + b + c} \times P$

Second part $= \frac{b}{a + b + c} \times P$

Third part $= \frac{c}{a + b + c} \times P$

Exam Pattern Questions

1. If $A : B = 2 : 1$ and $A : C = 1 : 3$, then $A : B : C =$

(a) 1 : 3 : 2 (b) 3 : 2 : 1 (c) 2 : 1 : 6 (d) 1 : 2 : 6

2. If $A = \frac{2}{3}$ of B and $B = \frac{4}{5}$ of C then, $A : B : C$ is

(a) 15 : 10 : 8 (b) 6 : 4 : 5
(c) 10 : 15 : 12 (d) 8 : 12 : 15

3. Two numbers A and B are such that the sum of 5% of A and 4% of B is two-third of the sum of 6% of A and 8% of B. Find the ratio of $A : B$

(a) 1 : 2 (b) 2 : 3 (c) 4 : 3 (d) 3 : 4

4. The sum of three numbers is 392. The ratio of first and second number is 2 : 3 and that of second and third number is 5 : 8. Then, the first number is

(a) 80 (b) 120 (c) 60 (d) 100

5. A bag contains ₹ 55 in the denominations of ₹ 1, 50 paise and 25 paise coins. The coins are in the ratio 1 : 2 : 3 respectively. Find the number of 50 paise coins.

(a) 41 (b) 42 (c) 40 (d) 38

6. If ₹ 672 is divided in the ratio 5 : 3, then the greater part will be.
(a) ₹ 252 (b) ₹ 420
(c) ₹ 572 (d) ₹ 602

7. Divide 94 into two parts in such a way that fifth part of the first and eight part of the second are in the ratio of 3 : 4 is
(a) 20, 44
(b) 30, 64
(c) 35, 69
(d) 34, 60

8. The income of X, Y and Z are in the ratio of 3 : 4 : 2 and their expenses in the ratio 5 : 5 : 2. If X saves ₹ 3000 out of an income of ₹ 18000, then what will be the savings of Y?
(a) 4500 (b) 9000
(c) 6000 (d) 7500

Answers

1. (c)	2. (d)	3. (c)	4. (a)	5. (c)
6. (b)	7. (b)	8. (b)		

Solutions

1. (c) Given,

$$A : B = 2 : 1$$
$$B : A = 1 : 2$$
$$A : C = 1 : 3$$
$$\therefore \quad B : A : C = 1 : 2 : 6$$
$$A : B : C = 2 : 1 : 6$$

2. (d) Given, $A = \frac{2}{3}B$

and $B = \frac{4}{5}C \Rightarrow C = \frac{5B}{4}$

$$A : B : C = \frac{2B}{3} : B : \frac{5B}{4}$$
$$= \frac{2}{3} : 1 : \frac{5}{4}$$
$$= \frac{2}{3} \times 12 : 1 \times 12 : \frac{5}{4} \times 12$$
$$= 8 : 12 : 15$$

3. (c) According to the question,

$$A \times \frac{5}{100} + B \times \frac{4}{100} = \frac{2}{3}\left(A \times \frac{6}{100} + B \times \frac{8}{100}\right)$$
$$\Rightarrow \quad 5A + 4B = \frac{2}{3}(6A + 8B)$$
$$\Rightarrow \quad 15A + 12B = 12A + 16B$$
$$\Rightarrow \quad 15A - 12A = 16B - 12B$$
$$\Rightarrow \quad 3A = 4B \Rightarrow \frac{A}{B} = \frac{4}{3}$$
$$\Rightarrow \quad A : B = 4 : 3$$

4. (a) Let the three numbers are a, b and c

According to the question,

$$a + b + c = 392 \quad \ldots(i)$$
$$a : b = 2 : 3$$
$$b : c = 5 : 8$$

Equating the ratios

$$a : b : c = 10 : 15 : 24$$

Let three numbers are $10x$, $15x$ and $24x$

Then, $a + b + c = 392$

$$10x + 15x + 24x = 392$$
$$49x = 392$$
$$x = 8$$

Now, first number $= 10x$
$$= 10 \times 8 = 80$$

5. (c) From question,

$$\frac{\text{Number of ₹ 1 coins}}{1} = \frac{\text{Number of 50 paise coins}}{2} = \frac{\text{Number of 25 paise coins}}{3} = x \quad \text{(say)}$$

$\therefore$ Number of ₹ 1 coins $= x$
Number of 50 paise coins $= 2x$
Number of 25 paise coins $= 3x$
According to the question,

$$x + \frac{2x}{2} + \frac{3x}{4} = 55$$
$$4x + 4x + 3x = 55 \times 4$$
$$\therefore \quad x = \frac{55 \times 4}{11} = 20$$

$\therefore$ Number of 50 paise coins.
$$= 2x = 2 \times 20 = 40$$

6. (b) Greater part $= 672 \times \frac{5}{5+3}$
$$= 672 \times \frac{5}{8} = 84 \times 5 = ₹\,420$$

7. (b) Let, first part be x, then second part is $(94 - x)$.

$$\therefore \; x \times \frac{1}{5} : (94 - x) \times \frac{1}{8} = 3 : 4$$
$$\Rightarrow \quad \frac{8x}{5(94 - x)} = \frac{3}{4}$$
$$\Rightarrow \quad 32x = 15(94 - x)$$
$$\Rightarrow \quad 32x + 15x = 1410$$
$$x = \frac{1410}{47} = 30$$

$\therefore$ 30 and 64 is the answer.

8. (b) Given ratio of income of X, Y, Z is 3 : 4 : 2.

Let there income is $3x$, $4x$, $2x$ respectively also given that

$$3x = ₹\,18000$$
$$\Rightarrow \quad x = \frac{18000}{3} = ₹\,6000$$

Then income of
$Y = 4 \times 6000 = ₹\,24000$
Income of $Z = 2 \times 6000$
$= ₹\,12000$

Given ratio of expenses
$= 5 : 5 : 2$ of XYZ
Let there expenses are $5a$, $5a$ and $2a$ respectively
Now given expenses of X
$=$ Income $-$ Savings
$= 18000 - 3000 = ₹\,15000$
Then $5a = 15000$

$$a = \frac{15000}{5} = ₹\,3000$$

Then expenses of Y
$= 5 \times a = 5 \times 3000$
$= ₹15000$

Savings of Y = Income $-$ expenses
$= 24000 - 15000$
$= ₹\,9000$

Chapter

08 Percentage

The meaning of term **per cent** is per hundred or hundredth part.

"Per cent is a fraction whose denominator is 100 and numerator of the fraction is called the **rate per cent**". Per cent is denoted by the symbol '%'. e.g.

Meaning of 35% is $\frac{35}{100}$ i.e. 35 parts out of 100 parts.

Percentage

$$= \frac{\text{[The quantity to be expressed in percentage]}}{\text{[2nd quantity (in respect of which the per cent has to be obtained)]}} \times 100\%$$

Important Formulae

1. When a quantity A is increased or decreased by $b\%$, then new quantity will be $= \frac{100 \pm b}{100} \times A$
2. When a is $x\%$ more/less than b, then b is less/more than a by $= \left[\frac{x}{100 \pm x} \times 100\right]\%$
3. If value of an object P is successively changed by $x\%$, $y\%$ and then $z\%$, then final value $= P\left(1 \pm \frac{x}{100}\right)\left(1 \pm \frac{y}{100}\right)\left(1 \pm \frac{z}{100}\right)$

Exam Pattern Questions

1. Select the most appropriate option. What is 12% of 35?

(a) 4.6 (b) 4.4
(c) 4.2 (d) 4.05

2. Find 24% of 75.

(a) 28 (b) 32 (c) 18 (d) 30

3. The length of a rectangle is decreased by 10% but the area remains the same. Then, percentage increase in the breadth of the rectangle is

(a) $11\frac{1}{9}\%$

(b) $12\frac{1}{3}\%$

(c) $13\frac{1}{9}\%$

(d) $14\frac{1}{9}\%$

4. If the price of a television set is increased by 25%, then by what percentage should the new price be reduced to bring the price back to the original level?

(a) 15% (b) 25% (c) 20% (d) 30%

5. The population of a small village increases by 8% annually. If its present population is 23328, then the population 2 yrs ago was

(a) 18900 (b) 19880
(c) 20000 (d) 21268

6. Ratio of boys and girls in a school is 3 : 2. 20% boys and 25% girls have scholarships. What is the total percentage of students. Who have scholarship?

(a) 21% (b) 22% (c) 23% (d) 24%

Answers

1. (c)	2. (c)	3. (a)	4. (c)	5. (c)
6. (b)				

Solutions

1. (c) 12% of 35 = $35 \times \frac{12}{100} = 4.2$

2. (c) 24% of 75 = $75 \times \frac{24}{100} = 18$

3. (a) Let the length and breadth of rectangle be l and b respectively.

Area of rectangle = Length × Breadth = $l \times b$

Again, new length $= l \times \frac{(100-10)}{100} = \frac{9l}{10}$

According to the question,

$l \times b = \frac{9l}{10} \times \frac{b \times (100+x)}{100}$

[∵ x = increased percentage]

$= \frac{9}{10} \times \frac{(100+x)}{100}$

$\Rightarrow \quad x = \frac{1000}{9} - 100$

$= \frac{1000-900}{9}$

$= \frac{100}{9} = 11\frac{1}{9}\%$

4. (c) Let the price of television = ₹ 100

∵ Price of television is increased by 25%

∴ New price of television $= \frac{100 \times 125}{100} = ₹\,125$

∴ We have to reduce ₹ 25 to bring the price back to original level.

Let we have to reduce x%.

∴ $125 \times x\% = 25 \Rightarrow x = 20$

∴ We have to reduce price by 20%.

5. (c) Let the population 2 yr ago be x.

Present population = 23328

Rate of increment = 8%

Population after n year = Present population $\times \left(1 + \frac{\text{Rate}}{100}\right)^{\text{Time}}$

∴ $23328 = x\left(1 + \frac{8}{100}\right)^2$

$23328 = x \times \frac{108}{100} \times \frac{108}{100}$

$\Rightarrow \quad x = \frac{23328 \times 100 \times 100}{108 \times 108}$

$\Rightarrow \quad = 20000$

Chapter 09 Profit, Loss and Discount

Cost price (CP) The price at which an article is purchased is called the cost price.

Selling price (SP) The price at which an article is sold, is called the selling price.

Marked Price (MP) The price on the label of an article is called the marked price or list price.

Profit When an article is sold at a price more than its cost price, then profit or gain is earned.

Loss When an article is sold at a price lower than its cost price, then loss is incurred.

Discount Discount is defined as the amount of discount given on a fixed price.

Important Formulae

Here, CP = Cost Price, MP = Marked Price, SP = Selling Price

1. Profit = SP − CP
2. Loss = CP − SP
3. Profit percentage $= \frac{\text{Profit}}{\text{CP}} \times 100\%$
4. Loss percentage $= \frac{\text{Loss}}{\text{CP}} \times 100\%$
5. $\text{CP} = \frac{\text{SP} \times 100}{(100 + \text{Profit }\%)}$ or $\frac{\text{SP} \times 100}{(100 - \text{Loss }\%)}$
6. $\text{SP} = \frac{\text{CP} \times (100 + \text{Profit }\%)}{100}$ or $= \frac{\text{CP} \times (100 - \text{Loss }\%)}{100}$
7. Discount% $= \frac{\text{MP} - \text{SP}}{\text{MP}} \times 100$
8. $\text{MP} = \frac{\text{SP} \times 100}{(100 - \text{D }\%)}$
9. Single equivalent discount of three discounts, $r_1\%$, $r_2\%$ and $r_3\%$

$$= \left[1 - \left(1 - \frac{r_1}{100}\right)\left(1 - \frac{r_2}{100}\right)\left(1 - \frac{r_3}{100}\right)\right] \times 100\%$$

Exam Pattern Questions

1. If a person incurs a loss of 25% by selling a product at ₹150, the cost price of the product is
(a) ₹125 (b) ₹175
(c) ₹ 200 (d) ₹ 225

2. Rahul purchases a watch for ₹ 250 and sells it for ₹ 500. His profit percentage is
(a) 200% (b) 50%
(c) 300% (d) 100%

3. If the ratio of cost price to selling price is 10 : 11, then profit per cent is
(a) 1.1% (b) 1%
(c) 10% (d) 0.1%

4. Surabhi sold 80 kg of wheat. She sold the first 20 kg at a profit of 20%, but the rest at a loss of 10%. What was her overall profit or loss percentage?
(a) 10% profit (b) 2.5% loss
(c) 5% loss (d) 2.5% profit

5. By selling 12 kg of potatoes for ₹ 63, a shopkeeper gains 5%. What does his gain or loss per cent by selling 50 kg of the same potatoes for ₹ 247.50?
(a) 2.5% loss
(b) 1% loss
(c) 1% profit
(d) No profit no loss

6. A merchant has 1000 kg sugar, part of which he sells at 8% profit and the rest at 18% profit. He gains 14% on the whole. The quantity sold at 8% profit is
(a) 560 kg (b) 600 kg
(c) 640 kg (d) 400 kg

7. A book seller sells a book at a profit of 10%. If he had bought it at 4% less and sold it for ₹ 6 more, he would have gained $18\frac{3}{4}$%. The cost price of the book is
(a) ₹130 (b) ₹140
(c) ₹150 (d) ₹160

8. Dinesh bought two radios for ₹1920. He sold one at profit of 20% and the other at a loss of $6\frac{2}{3}$%. If the selling price of both radios are same, the cost prices of the two radios are
(a) ₹ 800 and ₹1120
(b) ₹ 840 and ₹1080
(c) ₹ 860 and ₹1060
(d) ₹ 900 and ₹1020

9. Kewal sells two tape recorders at the same price. On one, he gains 10% and on the other he loses 10%. The total gain or loss in the transaction is
(a) 1% gain
(b) 1% loss
(c) No loss or gain
(d) 2% loss

10. A dishonest dealer professes to sell his goods at the cost price but uses a false weight of 850 g instead of 1 kg. His gain per cent is
(a) $17\frac{12}{17}$% (b) $17\frac{11}{17}$%
(c) $71\frac{11}{17}$% (d) $11\frac{11}{17}$%

11. After allowing 15% discount, the selling price of radio becomes ₹255. The marked price, is
(a) ₹ 400 (b) ₹ 300
(c) ₹ 600 (d) ₹ 500

12. The list price of an electric fan is ₹300. If two successive discounts of 15% and 10% are allowed its selling price would be
(a) ₹ 227.50 (b) ₹ 229.50
(c) ₹ 225 (d) ₹ 230

Answers

1. (c)	2. (d)	3. (c)	4. (b)	5. (b)
6. (d)	7. (c)	8. (b)	9. (b)	10. (b)
11. (b)	12. (b)			

Solutions

1. (c) Selling price = ₹ 150

Loss = 25%

$\therefore$ Cost price $= \dfrac{\text{SP} \times 100}{100 - \text{Loss\%}}$

$= \dfrac{150}{100-25} \times 100$

$= \dfrac{150}{75} \times 100 = ₹\, 200$

2. (d) $\therefore$ Profit percentage

$= \dfrac{\text{SP} - \text{CP}}{\text{CP}} \times 100$

$= \dfrac{500-250}{250} \times 100 = 100\%$

3. (c) Let CP and SP are respectively ₹ $10x$ and ₹ $11x$.
Then, profit percentage

$= \left(\dfrac{\text{SP} - \text{CP}}{\text{CP}} \times 100\right)$

$= \left(\dfrac{11x - 10x}{10x} \times 100\right)\%$

$= \dfrac{x}{10x} \times 100\% = 10\%$

4. (b) Let CP of 1 kg Wheat = ₹ 1

$\therefore$ CP of 80 kg Wheat = ₹ 80

SP of 20 kg Wheat

$= 20 \times \dfrac{120}{100} = ₹\, 24$

SP of rest 60 kg Wheat

$= 60 \times \dfrac{90}{100} = ₹\, 54$

Total SP = 24 + 54 = ₹ 78

$\therefore$ Loss per cent

$= \dfrac{\text{CP} - \text{SP}}{\text{CP}} \times 100$

$= \dfrac{80-78}{80} \times 100$

$= \dfrac{2}{80} \times 100 = \dfrac{5}{2} = 2.5\%$

5. (b) SP of 1 kg potatoes

$= \dfrac{63}{12} = ₹\, 5.25$

CP of 1 kg potatoes

$= \dfrac{5.25 \times 100}{(100+5)} = \dfrac{525}{105} = ₹\, 5$

New SP of 1 kg potatoes

$= \dfrac{247.50}{50} = ₹\, 4.95$

$\because$ CP > SP

$\therefore$ Loss percentage

$= \dfrac{5 - 4.95}{5} \times 100$

$\left[\because \dfrac{(\text{SP} - \text{CP})}{\text{CP}} \times 100\right]$

$= 0.05 \times 20 = 1\%$

6. (d) Let he sold x kg of sugar at 8% profit

According to the question,

$x \times \dfrac{(100+8)}{100} + \dfrac{(1000-x) \times (100+18)}{100}$

$= \dfrac{1000 \times (100+14)}{100}$

$\Rightarrow 108x + 118000 - 118x = 114000$

$\Rightarrow 4000 = 10x$

$\Rightarrow x = 400$

Hence, the quantity sold at 8% profit = 400 kg

7. (c) Let the CP of book be ₹ x.

According to the question,

$x \times \dfrac{(100+10)}{100} + 6$

$= x \times \dfrac{(100-4)}{100} \times \dfrac{\left(100 + 18\frac{3}{4}\right)}{100}$

$\Rightarrow x \times \dfrac{110}{100} + 6 = x \times \dfrac{96}{100} \times \dfrac{\left(100 + \frac{75}{4}\right)}{100}$

$\Rightarrow \dfrac{110x}{100} + 6 = x \times \dfrac{96}{100} \times \dfrac{475}{400}$

$\Rightarrow 110x + 600 = x \times 114$

$\Rightarrow 4x = 600$

$\therefore x = ₹\, 150$

8. (b) Let the CP of radio sold on gain and loss be ₹ x and ₹ $(1920 - x)$, respectively.

According to the question, SP of both the radios are equal.

$\Rightarrow x \times \dfrac{(100+20)}{100} = 1920 - x \times \dfrac{\left(100 - \frac{20}{3}\right)}{100}$

$\Rightarrow \dfrac{6x}{5} = 1920 - x \times \dfrac{280}{300}$

$\Rightarrow \dfrac{6x}{5} = (1920 - x) \times \dfrac{14}{15}$

$\Rightarrow 18x = 26880 - 14x$

$\Rightarrow 32x = 26880$

$\therefore x = 840$

CP of Ist radio = ₹ 840

IInd radio

= ₹ (1920 − 840) = ₹ 1080

9. (b) Let the SP of both the tape recorders are ₹ x.

CP of Ist tape recorder

$= \dfrac{\text{SP} \times 100}{100 + \text{Profit\%}}$

$= \dfrac{x \times 100}{110} = ₹\, \dfrac{10}{11}x$

CP of IInd tape recorder

$= \dfrac{x \times 100}{90} = ₹\, \dfrac{10x}{9}$

$\therefore$ Total CP $= ₹\left(\dfrac{10x}{11} + \dfrac{10x}{9}\right)$

$= ₹\, \dfrac{200}{99}x$

$\therefore$ Total SP = ₹ $(x + x)$ = ₹ $2x$

$\because$ CP > SP, then loss occurs.

$\therefore$ Loss percentage

$= \dfrac{\text{CP} - \text{SP}}{\text{CP}} \times 100$

$= \dfrac{\frac{200x}{99} - 2x}{\frac{200x}{99}} \times 100$

$= \dfrac{200x - 198x}{200x} \times 100 = 1\%$

10. (b) ∴ Gain percentage

$$= \frac{\text{True weight} - \text{False weight}}{\text{False weight}} \times 100\%$$

$$= \frac{1000 - 850}{850} \times 100$$

$$= \frac{150}{850} \times 100 = 17\frac{11}{17}\%$$

11. (b) Discount given = 15%

∴ Marked price

$$= \frac{SP}{100 - \text{discount}\%} \times 100$$

$$= \frac{255}{(100 - 15)} \times 100$$

$$\Rightarrow \frac{255}{85} \times 100 = ₹\,300$$

12. (b) Total discount

$$= 15 + 10 - \frac{15 \times 10}{100} = 23.5\%$$

∴ Selling price after discount

$$= 300 - 300 \times \frac{23.5}{100}$$

$$= 300 - 70.5 = ₹\,229.50$$

Chapter 10 Simple and Compound Interest

Interest When a person borrows some amount of money from another person, then the person borrwing money pays some extra money during repayment that extra money during repayment is called interest.

Principal (P) Principal is the money borrowed or deposited for a certain time.

Amount (A) The Sum of principal and interest is called amount.

Rate of Interest (R) It is the rate at which the interest is charged on principal.

Simple Interest (SI) If the interest is calculated on the original principal for any length of time, then it is calculated simple interest.

Important Formulae

1. Simple Interest (SI)

$$= \frac{\text{Principal} \times \text{Rate} \times \text{Time}}{100} = \frac{P \times r \times t}{100}$$

2. Amount = Principal + SI $\Rightarrow A = P\left(1 + \frac{rt}{100}\right)$

Compound Interest (CI) If after the completion of a specific period, interest is accrued on the principal as well as the interest due on the principal. This interest is known as compound interest.

1. Compound interest (CI) $= P\left[\left(1 + \frac{r}{100}\right)^n - 1\right]$

2. $A = P\left(1 + \frac{r}{100}\right)^n$, here n = time period

3. If interest is compounded half-yearly,

then Amount $= P\left(1 + \frac{r}{2 \times 100}\right)^{2n}$

4. If interest is compounded quarterly,

then Amount $= P\left(1 + \frac{r}{4 \times 100}\right)^{4n}$

5. When rate of interest for three consecutive years are r_1 %, r_2 % and r_3 % respectively, then

$$A = P\left(1 + \frac{r_1}{100}\right)\left(1 + \frac{r_2}{100}\right)\left(1 + \frac{r_3}{100}\right)$$

6. If interest is compounded annually but time is in fraction

(suppose time $= n\frac{a}{b}$ yr), then

$$A = P\left(1 + \frac{r}{100}\right)^n \left(1 + \frac{\left(\frac{a}{b}\right) \times r}{100}\right)$$

7. Difference between CI and SI.

(i) For 2 yr, CI − SI $= P\left(\frac{r}{100}\right)^2$

(ii) For 3 yr, CI − SI $= \frac{Pr^2(300 + r)}{(100)^3}$

Exam Pattern Questions

1. ₹ 25000 was invested at a particular rate of simple interest for a period of 5 yr. If the interest earned at the end of the term was ₹ 7500, what was the rate of interest per annum?
(a) 7.5% (b) 5% (c) 6% (d) 10%

2. How long will a sum of money invested at 5% per annum SI take to increase its value by 50%?
(a) 10 yr (b) 12 yr (c) 15 yr (d) 7 yr

3. The simple interest on an amount at the rate of 5% per annum for 2 yr and 3 yr are respectively ₹ 100 and ₹ 150 Find principal amount.
(a) ₹ 5000 (b) ₹ 8000
(c) ₹ 1200 (d) ₹ 1000

4. The simple interest on a sum for 20 yr is 5/4 of the principal. What is the per annum rate of interest?
(a) 6.25% (b) 12.5% (c) 2.5% (d) 5%

5. At simple interest, a sum becomes 3 times in 20 yr. Find the time in which the sum will be double at the same rate of interest.
(a) 8 yr (b) 10 yr
(c) 12 yr (d) 14 yr

6. At 5% rate of simple interest, in how many years, interest of ₹ 2000 will be double of the principal?
(a) 4 yr (b) 40 yr
(c) 20 yr (d) 2 yr

7. Suresh borrowed ₹ 800 at 6% and Naresh borrowed ₹ 600 at 10% After how much time will they both have equal debts?
(a) $15\frac{1}{3}$ yr (b) $14\frac{1}{2}$ yr
(c) $18\frac{1}{3}$ yr (d) $16\frac{2}{3}$ yr

8. At 5% per annum rate of compound interest, what will become the amount ₹ 4000 after 24 months?
(a) ₹ 4100 (b) ₹ 4210
(c) ₹ 4400 (d) ₹ 4410

9. If at the rate of $12\frac{1}{2}\%$ per annum the compound interest is ₹ 510. What will be the simple interest on same amount for the same period at the same rate of interest?
(a) ₹ 480
(b) ₹ 400
(c) ₹ 450
(d) ₹ 460

10. The simple interest for certain sum in 2 yr at 4% per annum is ₹ 80. What will be the compound interest for the same sum, if conditions of rate and time period are same?
(a) ₹ 91.60 (b) ₹ 81.60
(c) ₹ 71.60 (d) ₹ 80

11. The sum for 2 yr gives a compound interest of ₹ 3225 at 15% rate. Then, sum is
(a) ₹ 10000 (b) ₹ 20000
(c) ₹ 15000 (d) ₹ 32250

12. A sum is invested for 3 yr at compound interest at 5%, 10% and 20% respectively. In three years, if the sum of amounts to ₹ 16632, then find the sum.
(a) ₹ 11000 (b) ₹ 12000
(c) ₹ 13000 (d) ₹ 14000

13. What amount will be received on a sum of ₹ 15000 in $1\frac{1}{4}$ yr at 12% per annum, if interest is compounded quarterly ?
(a) ₹ 16596.88 (b) ₹ 16789.08
(c) ₹ 17630.77 (d) ₹ 17389.10

14. A sum of ₹ 8400 was taken as a loan. This is to be paid in two equal instalments. If the rate of interest is 10% per annum, compounded annually, then the value of each instalment is
(a) ₹ 4200 (b) ₹ 4480
(c) ₹ 4840 (d) None of these

Answers

1. (c)	2. (a)	3. (d)	4. (a)	5. (b)
6. (b)	7. (d)	8. (d)	9. (a)	10. (b)
11. (a)	12. (b)	13. (d)	14. (c)	

Solutions

1. (c) Here, $P = ₹\,25000$, $T = 5\text{yr}$

$$SI = ₹\ 7500, R = ?$$

$$\therefore \quad SI = \frac{PRT}{100}$$

$$\Rightarrow \quad 7500 = \frac{25000 \times R \times 5}{100}$$

$$\Rightarrow \quad R \times 5 \times 250 = 7500 \Rightarrow R = \frac{7500}{5 \times 250} = 6$$

$$\Rightarrow \quad R = 6\%$$

2. (a) Let the sum be ₹ P.

Then, 50% of $P = \frac{P}{2} = SI$

$$SI = \frac{PRT}{100} \Rightarrow \frac{P}{2} = \frac{P \times 5 \times T}{100} \quad [\because R = 5\%]$$

$$\Rightarrow \quad \frac{P}{2} = \frac{5PT}{100} \Rightarrow \frac{1}{2} = \frac{T}{20} \quad \therefore \quad T = 10\,\text{yr}$$

3. (d) Let the principal be ₹ x

$$\therefore \quad 150 - 100 = \frac{x \times 5 \times 3}{100} - \frac{x \times 5 \times 2}{100}$$

$$\Rightarrow \quad 50 = \frac{x}{20} \Rightarrow x = ₹\ 1000$$

4. (a) Let principal $= x$ and then $SI = \frac{5}{4}x$

$$\therefore \quad SI = \frac{P \times R \times T}{100} \Rightarrow \frac{5}{4}x = \frac{x \times R \times 20}{100}$$

$$\therefore \quad R \text{ (rate)} = \frac{5 \times 100}{4 \times 20} = \frac{25}{4} = 6.25\%$$

5. (b) Let the sum $= ₹\,P$

Then, for 20 yr,

$$SI = (3P - P) = ₹\ 2P$$

$$\therefore \quad 2P = \frac{P \times R \times 20}{100} \quad \left[\because SI = \frac{P \times R \times T}{100}\right]$$

$$\Rightarrow \quad 2 = \frac{R}{5} \Rightarrow R = 10\%$$

Again, for another time (T)

$$SI = (2P - P) = P$$

$$\therefore \quad P = \frac{P \times 10 \times T}{100}$$

$$\therefore \quad T = 10\,\text{yr}$$

6. (b) Principal $= ₹\ 2000$

Required interest $= ₹\ (2 \times 2000) = ₹\ 4000$

Rate of simple interest (R) = 5% per annum

$$SI = \frac{2000 \times 5 \times T}{100} \quad \left[\because SI = \frac{PRT}{100}\right]$$

$$\Rightarrow \quad 4000 = \frac{2000 \times 5 \times T}{100} \Rightarrow T = 40\text{yr}$$

7. (d) Given, $R_1 = 6\%$, $R_2 = 10\%$

According to the question,

$$800 + \frac{800 \times 6 \times T}{100} = 600 + \frac{600 \times 10 \times T}{100}$$

$$800 + 48T = 600 + 60T$$

$$\Rightarrow \quad 12T = 200 \Rightarrow 3T = 50$$

$$\therefore \quad T = \frac{50}{3} = 16\frac{2}{3}\,\text{yr}$$

9. (a) Let the amount be ₹ x.

Compound interest $= ₹\ 510$

Rate of interest $= 12\frac{1}{2}\% = \frac{25}{2}\%$ per annum

$$\text{Then,} \quad x\left(1 + \frac{25}{2 \times 100}\right)^2 - x = 510$$

$$\left[\because CI = \left[P\left(1 + \frac{R}{100}\right)^n - P\right]\right]$$

$$\Rightarrow \quad \frac{81}{64}x - x = 510$$

$$\Rightarrow \quad \left(\frac{81 - 64}{64}\right)x = 510$$

$$\Rightarrow \quad x = \frac{510 \times 64}{17}$$

$$\Rightarrow \quad x = ₹\ 1920$$

$$\therefore \quad \text{Simple interest} = \frac{1920 \times 2 \times 25}{2 \times 100} = ₹\ 480$$

10. (b) Given, $n = 2$ yr, $R = 4\%$ and SI = 80

According to the formula,

$$CI = SI\left(1 + \frac{R}{100}\right)$$

$$= 80\left(1 + \frac{4}{200}\right) = \frac{80 \times 51}{50} = ₹\ 81.60$$

11. (a) Here, CI $= ₹\ 3225$, $r = 15\%$ and $n = 2$ yr

$$\therefore \quad CI = P\left[\left(1 + \frac{r}{100}\right)^n - 1\right]$$

$$\Rightarrow \quad 3225 = P\left[\left(1 + \frac{15}{100}\right)^2 - 1\right]$$

$$\Rightarrow \quad 3225 = P\left[\left(1 + \frac{3}{20}\right)^2 - 1\right]$$

$$\Rightarrow \quad 3225 = P\left[\left(\frac{23}{20}\right)^2 - 1\right]$$

$\Rightarrow \quad 3225 = P\left[\frac{529}{400} - 1\right]$

$\Rightarrow \quad 3225 = P \times \frac{129}{400}$

$\Rightarrow \quad P = \frac{3225 \times 400}{129}$

$\Rightarrow \quad P = 25 \times 400 = ₹\ 10000$

12. (b) Let P be the sum.

$\therefore 16632 = P\left(1+\frac{5}{100}\right)\left(1+\frac{10}{100}\right)\left(1+\frac{20}{100}\right)$

$\left[\because A = P\left(1+\frac{R_1}{100}\right)\left(1+\frac{R_2}{100}\right)\left(1+\frac{R_3}{100}\right)\right]$

$\Rightarrow \quad 16632 = P \times \frac{21}{20} \times \frac{11}{10} \times \frac{6}{5}$

$\Rightarrow \quad P = ₹\ 12000$

13. (d) Given, $P = ₹\ 15000$, $R = 12\%$

and $\quad n = 1\frac{1}{4} = \frac{5}{4}$ yr

According to the formula,

Amount $= P\left(1+\frac{R}{100 \times 4}\right)^{4n}$

$= 15000\left(1+\frac{12}{100 \times 4}\right)^{4 \times \frac{5}{4}}$

$= 15000\left(\frac{412}{400}\right)^5 = 15000\left(\frac{103}{100}\right)^5$

$= 15000 \times \frac{103}{100} \times \frac{103}{100} \times \frac{103}{100} \times \frac{103}{100} \times \frac{103}{100}$

$= \frac{15 \times 103 \times 103 \times 103 \times 103 \times 103}{10000000}$

$= ₹\ 17389.111$

$= ₹\ 17389.10$ (approx).

14. (c) Let each instalment be ₹ x.

Then, according to the question,

$\frac{x}{\left(1+\frac{10}{100}\right)} + \frac{x}{\left(1+\frac{10}{100}\right)^2} = 8400$

$\Rightarrow \quad \frac{10}{11}x + \frac{100}{121}x = 8400$

$\Rightarrow \quad \frac{10}{11}\left(\frac{21}{11}x\right) = 8400$

$\Rightarrow \quad x = \frac{8400 \times 121}{10 \times 21} = ₹\ 4840$

Chapter 11 Time and Work

Time and work are directly proportional to each other. More work more time and conversely less work less time if number of person or objects are equal.

Important Formulae and Facts

- If a person takes x days to complete a work, then the work done in 1 day will be $\frac{1}{x}$.
- If a person does $\frac{1}{x}$th part of a work in one day, then the person will finish the work in x days. If A is x % times more efficient than B to do a certain job, then A will take $\frac{1}{x}$ time of the time of B to do that work.

  Entire wages of one person = Total number of days × Wages of 1 day of that person
- If M_1 persons complete W_1 work in d_1 days by working h_1 hours per day earning R_1 and M_2 persons complete W_2 work in d_2 days by working h_2 hours per day earning R_2, then

$$\frac{M_1 \times d_1 \times h_1}{W_1 \times R_1} = \frac{M_2 \times d_2 \times h_2}{W_2 \times R_2}$$

- If A, B and C can do a piece of work in x, y and z days, respectively and they received ₹ k as wages by working together, then

$$\text{Share of } A = ₹\ \frac{yz}{xy + yz + xz} \times k$$

$$\text{Share of } B = ₹\ \frac{xz}{xy + yz + xz} \times k$$

$$\text{Share of } C = ₹\ \frac{xy}{xy + yz + xz} \times k$$

Exam Pattern Questions

1. Ram can complete a job alone in 36 days while Sunil takes 45 days to do it alone. How many days will it take the due to complete half of the job if they work together?

(a) 10 days (b) 9 days
(c) 12 days (d) 20 days

2. *A*, *B* and *C* can complete a piece of work in 24, 5 and 12 days respectively. Working together, they will complete the same work in

(a) $\frac{7}{24}$ days (b) $3\frac{1}{13}$ days
(c) 4 days (d) $\frac{1}{24}$ days

3. Shyama prepares the model of a shopping complex using cardboard, in 4 days, working 6 h per day at a stretch. But if she decided to finish it in 3 days, then how many more hours per day should she work?

(a) 2 h (b) 4 h (c) 6 h (d) 8 h

4. 36 men can complete a piece of work in 18 days. In how many days will 27 men complete the same work?

(a) 24 (b) 22 (c) 12 (d) 18

5. If 8 men can do a piece of work in 14 days, then in how much time will 7 men do the same piece of work?

(a) 16 days (b) 15 days
(c) 17 days (d) 18 days

6. If 90 men can do certain job in 16 days, working 12 h per day, then the part of that work which can be completed by 70 men in 24 days, working 8 h per day is

(a) $\frac{1}{3}$ (b) $\frac{2}{3}$ (c) $\frac{7}{9}$ (d) $\frac{5}{8}$

Answers

1. (a)	2. (b)	3. (a)	4. (a)	5. (a)
6. (c)				

Solutions

1. (a) One day work of Ram and Sunil

$= \frac{1}{36} + \frac{1}{45} = \frac{5+4}{180}$

$= \frac{9}{180} = \frac{1}{20}$

∴ To complete the job they both take = 20 days

∴ To complete half of the job they both take

$= 20 \times \frac{1}{2} = 10$ days

2. (b) $A + B + C$'s 1 day work

$= \frac{1}{24} + \frac{1}{5} + \frac{1}{12}$

$= \frac{5 + 24 + 10}{120}$

$= \frac{39}{120} = \frac{13}{40}$

∴ Required time $= \frac{40}{13}$

$= 3\frac{1}{13}$ days

3. (a) According to the question,

$D_1H_1 = D_2H_2$

$\Rightarrow \quad 4 \times 6 = 3 \times H_2$

$\therefore \quad H_2 = 8$

∴ Required more hours $= 8 - 6 = 2$ h

4. (a) $M_1D_1 = M_2 \times D_2$,

$36 \times 18 = 27 \times D_2$

$D_2 = \frac{36 \times 18}{27}$

$\Rightarrow \quad D_2 = 24$

Chapter 12 Speed, Time and Distance

Speed The rate at which a body travels to cover a certain distance is called speed of that body.

Distance The length of the path travelled by any object or a person between two places is known as distance.

Inportant Formulae and Facts

- Speed $= \frac{\text{Distance}}{\text{Time}}$

  The unit of speed is m/s or km/h.
- To convert a speed given in km/h → m/s, multiply it by $\frac{5}{18}$.
- To convert a speed given in m/sec → km/h, multiply it by $\frac{18}{5}$.
- If two objects/trains are moving in a same direction with speeds x km/h and y km/h respectively, then their relative speed will be $(x - y)$ km/h.
- If two objects/trains are moving in opposite directions, then their relative speed will be $(x + y)$ km/h.
- If an object / train covers same distance with speed of x km/h and y km/h respectively, then average speed of object will be $\frac{2xy}{x+y}$ km/h.
- If the ratio of speeds of A and B is a : b, then the ratio of times taken by them to cover the same distance is $\frac{1}{a} : \frac{1}{b}$.
- If a train passes a still object like tree, pole, etc, train has to travel a distance equal to its length.
- If a train passes a long object like platform, bridge, etc, train has to travel a distance equal to the sum of length of object and that of train.
- If speed of boat in still water is x km/h and speed of current is y km/h, then

  Speed of boat downstream, $u = (x + y)$ km/h

  Speed of boat upstream $v = (x - y)$ km/h

  Speed of boat in still water

  $$x = \frac{1}{2}(u + v) \text{ km/h}$$
- Speed of current, $y = \frac{1}{2}(u - v)$ km/h

Exam Pattern Questions

1. A person completes his journey in 6 h by a car at the speed of 45 km/h. To complete it in 5 h, the speed of car will be .... km/h.

(a) 55 (b) 54
(c) 53 (d) 52

2. A cyclist covers a distance of 750 m in 2 min 30 s. What is the speed of the cyclist?

(a) 12 km/h (b) 16 km/h
(c) 18 km/h (d) 22 km/h

3. Diljeet Singh, a policeman is 114 m behind a thief. Diljeet Singh runs 21 m and the thief 15 m in a minute. In what time will Diljeet Singh catch the thief ?

(a) 19 min (b) 16 min (c) 21 min (d) 23 min

4. A jeep is chasing a car which is 5 km ahead. Their respective speed are 90 km/h and 75 km/h. After how many minutes will the jeep catch the car?

(a) 18 min (b) 20 min (c) 24 min (d) 25 min

5. A train of 100 m long is running at the speed of 45 km/h. Find the time taken by it to pass a man standing near the railway track.
(a) 8 sec (b) 10 sec
(c) 12 sec (d) 2 sec

6. A train 300 m long is running with a speed of 54 km/h. In what time will it cross a telephone pole?
(a) 20 sec (b) 15 sec
(c) 17 sec (d) 18 sec

7. If a 80 m long train takes 15 min to cross a 70 m long platform, then how long will it take to cross another train, of 120 m, which is stationed on another parallel track?
(a) 20 min (b) 30 min
(c) 50 min (d) 40 min

8. A train of length 300 m is travelling with a speed of 54 km/h. It takes 40 sec to cross a bridge, then the length of the bridge will be
(a) 250 m
(b) 300 m
(c) 350 m
(d) None of these

9. Two trains of lengths 150 m and 180 m respectively are running in opposite directions on parallel tracks. If their speeds be 50 km/h and 58 km/h respectively, in what time will they cross each other?
(a) 11 sec (b) 30 sec
(c) 15 sec (d) 22 sec

10. If a train runs at 40 km/h, it reaches its destination late by 11 min. But if it runs at 50 km/h, it is late 5 min only. The correct time (in minutes) for the train to complete the journey is
(a) 13 (b) 15 (c) 19 (d) 21

11. The speed of a boat in still water is 22 km/h. If its speed in downstream is 24 km/h, the upstream speed will be
(a) 20 km/h (b) 22 km/h
(c) 24 km/h (d) 26 km/h

12. Speed of a boat in still water is 9 km/h. It goes 12 km downstream and comes back to the starting point in three hours. What is the speed of water in the stream?
(a) 3 km/h (b) 3.5 km/h
(c) 4 km/h (d) 5 km/h

13. If a sailer sails 12 km distance within 5 h against the flow of a river. If he sails 22 km distance in same time along the flow of the river. Then velocity of the river is
(a) 1 km/h (b) 2 km/h
(c) 1.5 km/h (d) 2.5 km/h

Answers

1. (b)	2. (c)	3. (a)	4. (b)	5. (a)
6. (a)	7. (a)	8. (b)	9. (a)	10. (c)
11. (a)	12. (a)	13. (a)		

Solutions

1. (b) Total distance
$= \text{Time} \times \text{Speed}$
$= 6 \times 45 = 270$ km
Now, Time = 5 h
$\therefore$ Speed needed $= \dfrac{\text{Distance}}{\text{Time}}$
$= \dfrac{270}{5} = 54$ km/h

2. (c) $\therefore$ Speed of cyclist
$= \dfrac{\text{Distance}}{\text{Time}}$
$= \dfrac{750}{2 \times 60 + 30} \times \dfrac{18}{5}$
$= \dfrac{150 \times 18}{150} = 18$ km/h

3. (a) In this case, (21 – 15) m or 6 m is covered by Diljeet Singh in 1 min.
$\therefore$ 114 m will be covered in
$\left(\dfrac{1}{6} \times 114\right)$ min = 19 min

4. (b) Relative speed
$= 90 - 75 = 15$ km/h
$\therefore$ Required time
$= \dfrac{\text{Distance}}{\text{Relative speed}}$
$= \dfrac{5}{15}\text{ h} = \dfrac{5}{15} \times 60$ min
= 20 min

5. (a) Here, cover distance to pass a man = 100 m and speed of train
$= 45 \times \dfrac{5}{18}$ m/s
$= \dfrac{25}{2}$ m/s

$\therefore$ Time taken to pass a man

$= \frac{\text{Distance}}{\text{Speed}}$

$= \frac{100}{\frac{25}{2}}$

$= \frac{100 \times 2}{25} = 8 \text{ sec}$

6. (a) Speed of train = 54 km/h

$= \left(\frac{54 \times 5}{18}\right) \text{m/s}$

$= 15 \text{ m/s}$

Required time $= \frac{\text{Length of train}}{\text{Speed of train}}$

$= \frac{300}{15} = 20 \text{ sec}$

7. (a) According to the question,

$\frac{80+70}{15} = \frac{80+120}{T}$

$\left[\because \text{Speed} = \frac{\text{Distance}}{\text{Time}}\right]$

$\Rightarrow \frac{150}{15} = \frac{200}{T}$

$\Rightarrow \frac{10}{1} = \frac{200}{T}$

$\Rightarrow T \times 10 = 200$

$\Rightarrow T = \frac{200}{10}$

$\Rightarrow T = 20 \text{ min}$

Hence, train will take 20 min to cross another train.

8. (b) Let the length of the bridge be x

Speed of train = 54 km/h

$= 54 \times \frac{5}{18} = 15 \text{ m/s}$

$\frac{\text{Distance}}{\text{Speed}} = \text{Time}$

$\Rightarrow \frac{(300+x)}{15} = 40$

$\Rightarrow x = 40 \times 15 - 300$

$x = 600 - 300$

$\Rightarrow x = 300 \text{ m}$

9. (a) $\therefore$ Required time

$= \frac{\text{Total length}}{\text{Respective speed}}$

$= \frac{150+180}{(58+50) \times \frac{5}{18}}$

$= \frac{330 \times 18}{108 \times 5} = 11 \text{ sec}$

10. (c) Let the distance be x km.

$\frac{x}{40} - \frac{11}{60} = \frac{x}{50} - \frac{5}{60}$

(Correct time is equal both conditions)

$\Rightarrow \frac{x}{40} - \frac{x}{50} = \frac{11}{60} - \frac{5}{60}$

$\Rightarrow \frac{(5-4)x}{200} = \frac{6}{60}$

$\Rightarrow x = \frac{6 \times 200}{60} = 20 \text{ km}$

$\therefore$ Required time

$= \frac{20}{40} - \frac{11}{60} = \frac{60-22}{120}$

$= \frac{38}{120} = \frac{19}{60} \text{h} = 19 \text{ min}$

11. (a) Speed of the boat in still water = 22 km/h

Speed of downstream

= 24 km/h

We know that,

Speed in still water $= \frac{1}{2}$ (Speed of upstream + Speed of downstream)

$\therefore$ Speed of upstream = (2 × Speed of still water – Speed of downstream)

= (2 × 22 km/h) – 24 km/h

= 44 km/h – 24 km/h

= 20 km/h

12. (a) Given,

Speed of boat in still water

= 9 km/h

Speed of water = x km/h

Speed of boat in downstream

$= (9 + x)$ km/h

Speed of boat in upstream

$= (9 - x)$ km/h

$\therefore \frac{12}{9+x} + \frac{12}{9-x} = 3 \text{ h}$

$\left[\because \text{Time} = \frac{\text{Distance}}{\text{Speed}}\right]$

$\Rightarrow \frac{108 - 12x + 108 + 12x}{81 - x^2} = 3$

$\Rightarrow \frac{216}{81 - x^2} = 3$

$\Rightarrow 243 - 216 = 3x^2$

$\Rightarrow x^2 = \frac{27}{3} = 9$

$\Rightarrow x = 3 \text{ km/h}$

13. (a) Let the speed of boat = B

Speed of river = S

$\therefore \frac{12}{B-S} = 5$

or $B - S = \frac{12}{5}$ ...(i)

and, $\frac{22}{B+S} = 5$

or $B + S = \frac{22}{5}$ ...(ii)

$\therefore$ Speed of river $= \frac{22}{5} - \frac{12}{5}$

$2s = \frac{10}{5} = 2 \text{ km/h}$

or $s = 1 \text{ km/h}$

Speed of river, $s = 1$ km/h

Chapter 13 Trigonometry

Trigonometry is a branch of mathematics in which we study measuring of angle and sides of a right angle triangles and to find relations between them.

System of Measurement of Angle

There are three system of measurement of angle.

(i) **Sexagesimal System**

$$1^\circ = 60' = 60 \text{ min}$$
$$1' = 60'' = 60 \text{ sec}$$

(ii) **Centesimal System**

$$1 \text{ Right Angle} = 100^g \text{ (100 grade)}$$
$$1^g = 100' = 100 \text{ min}$$
$$1' = 100'' = 100 \text{ sec}$$

(iii) **Circular System**

$\theta = \frac{l}{r}$ radian [here, l = length of arc, r = radius of circle, θ = angle subtended at the centre]

And $180^\circ = 200^g = \pi$ radians $= \pi^c$

Trigonometric Ratios and Their Relation

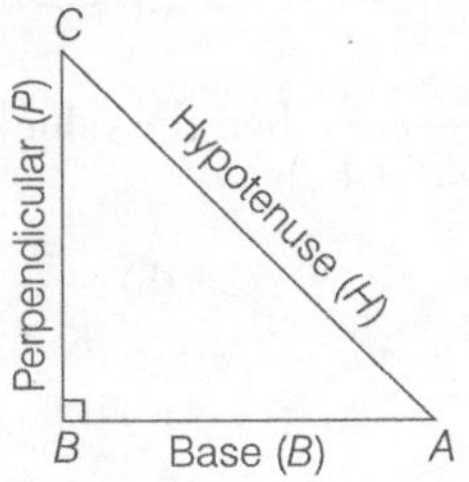

$\sin A = \frac{P}{H}$, $\cos A = \frac{B}{H}$,

$\tan A = \frac{P}{B}$

$\text{cosec } A = \frac{H}{P}$, $\sec A = \frac{H}{B}$, $\cot A = \frac{B}{P}$

$\sin A = \frac{1}{\text{cosec } A}$, $\cos A = \frac{1}{\sec A}$,

$\tan A = \frac{1}{\cot A}$

$\tan A = \frac{\sin A}{\cos A}$ or $\cot A = \frac{\cos A}{\sin A}$

Trigonometric Ratios of Some Angles

Trigonometric/ Angle Ratios	0°	30°	45°	60°	90°
sin A	0	1/2	$\frac{1}{\sqrt{2}}$	$\frac{\sqrt{3}}{2}$	1
cos A	1	$\frac{\sqrt{3}}{2}$	$\frac{1}{\sqrt{2}}$	$\frac{1}{2}$	0
tan A	0	$\frac{1}{\sqrt{3}}$	1	$\sqrt{3}$	∞ (Not defined)

Trigonometric Identities

$$\sin^2 A + \cos^2 A = 1;\ \sec^2 A = 1 + \tan^2 A;$$
$$\text{cosec}^2 A = 1 + \cot^2 A$$

Sign of Trigonometric Ratios

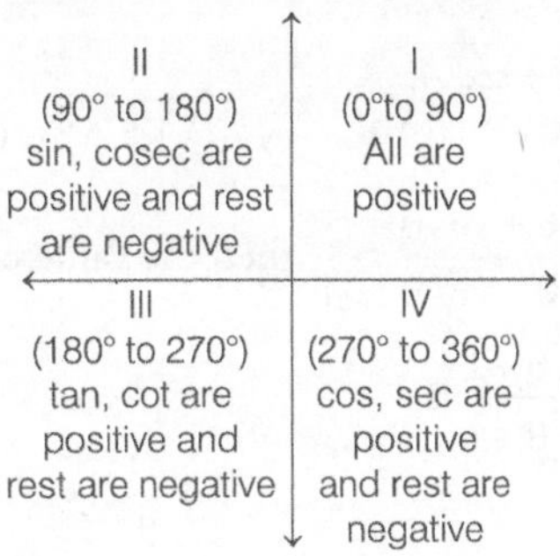

Trigonometric Ratios of Relative Angles

θ	$-\theta$	$90°-\theta$	$90°+\theta$	$180°-\theta$	$180°+\theta$
sin	$-\sin\theta$	$\cos\theta$	$\cos\theta$	$\sin\theta$	$-\sin\theta$
cos	$\cos\theta$	$\sin\theta$	$-\sin\theta$	$-\cos\theta$	$-\cos\theta$
tan	$-\tan\theta$	$\cot\theta$	$-\cot\theta$	$-\tan\theta$	$\tan\theta$
cot	$-\cot\theta$	$\tan\theta$	$-\tan\theta$	$-\cot\theta$	$\cot\theta$
sec	$\sec\theta$	$\mathrm{cosec}\,\theta$	$-\mathrm{cosec}\,\theta$	$-\sec\theta$	$-\sec\theta$
cosec	$-\mathrm{cosec}\,\theta$	$\sec\theta$	$\sec\theta$	$\mathrm{cosec}\,\theta$	$-\mathrm{cosec}\,\theta$

Angle of Elevation and Depression

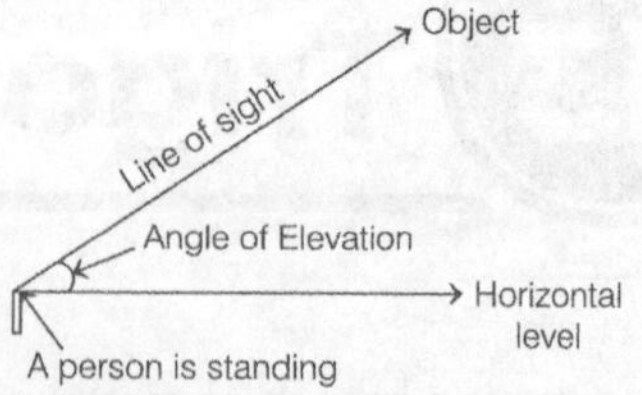

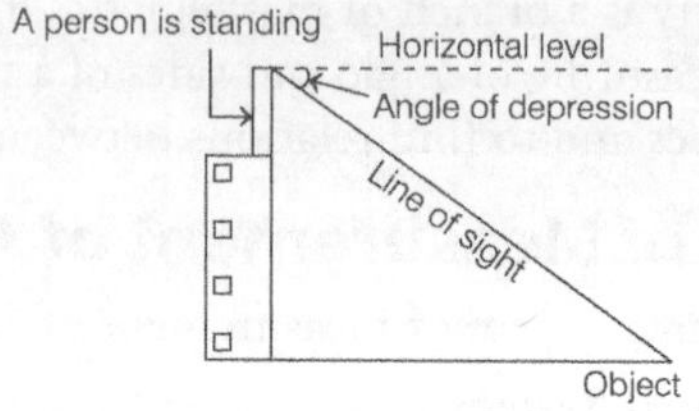

Exam Pattern Questions

1. If $\alpha+\beta=90°$ and $\alpha:\beta=2:1$, then the value of $\sin\alpha:\sin\beta$ is

(a) $\sqrt{3}:1$ (b) 2 : 1
(c) 1 : 1 (d) $\sqrt{2}:1$

2. If $\tan\left(\frac{\pi}{2}-\frac{\alpha}{2}\right)=\sqrt{3}$, then the value of $\cos\alpha$ is

(a) 0 (b) $1/\sqrt{2}$ (c) $\sqrt{3}/2$ (d) 1/2

3. If $\frac{\sin\theta+\cos\theta}{\sin\theta-\cos\theta}=3$, then the value of $\sin^4\theta-\cos^4\theta$ is

(a) $\frac{1}{5}$ (b) $\frac{2}{5}$ (c) $\frac{3}{5}$ (d) $\frac{4}{5}$

4. If $\sin A=\frac{5}{13}$, then what is the value of $\tan A+\sec A$?

(a) 1.8 (b) 1 (c) 1.5 (d) 2

5. If $\frac{\sin\theta+\cos\theta}{\sin\theta-\cos\theta}=\frac{5}{4}$, then the value of $\frac{\tan^2\theta+1}{\tan^2\theta-1}$ is

(a) $\frac{25}{16}$ (b) $\frac{41}{9}$
(c) $\frac{41}{40}$ (d) $\frac{40}{41}$

6. ΔPQR is right angled at Q. If $\mathrm{cosec}\,P=25/24$, then what is the value of $\cot R$?

(a) 25/7 (b) 24/25
(c) 7/24 (d) 24/7

7. If θ is an acute angle and $\cos\theta=\frac{3}{5}$, then the value of $\frac{\sin\theta\cdot\tan\theta-1}{2\tan^2\theta}$ is

(a) $\frac{16}{625}$ (b) $\frac{1}{36}$
(c) $\frac{3}{160}$ (d) $\frac{160}{3}$

8. If $\sin\theta=\frac{a^2-1}{a^2+1}$, then the value of $\sec\theta+\tan\theta$ will be

(a) $\frac{a}{\sqrt{2}}$ (b) $\frac{a}{a^2+1}$
(c) $\sqrt{2}a$ (d) a

9. If $\sec\theta-\mathrm{cosec}\,\theta=0$, then the value of $\tan\theta+\cot\theta$ is

(a) 0 (b) 1 (c) -1 (d) 2

10. The value of $[3\cos^2 60°+2\cot^2 30°-5\sin^2 45°]$ is

(a) 4 (b) 1
(c) $\frac{13}{6}$ (d) $\frac{17}{4}$

11. If $\sin(3x - 20°) = \cos(3y + 20°)$, then the value of $(x + y)$ is
(a) 20° (b) 30°
(c) 40° (d) 45°

12. The numerical value of
$\frac{5}{\sec^2\theta} + \frac{2}{1+\cot^2\theta} + 3\sin^2\theta$ is
(a) 5 (b) 2 (c) 3 (d) 4

13. If $\sec^2\theta + \tan^2\theta = \frac{7}{12}$, then $\sec^4\theta - \tan^4\theta$ is equal to
(a) $\frac{7}{12}$ (b) $\frac{1}{2}$ (c) $\frac{5}{12}$ (d) 1

14. The distance of the foot of a 20 m high tower from a point on the ground is $20\sqrt{3}$ m. What is the angle of elevation of the top of the tower from this point?
(a) 60° (b) 45° (c) 30° (d) 15°

15. If the length of the shadow of a tower is equal to its height, then what is the Sun's altitude at that time?
(a) 15° (b) 30° (c) 45° (d) 60°

Answers

1. (a)	2. (d)	3. (c)	4. (c)	5. (c)
6. (d)	7. (c)	8. (d)	9. (d)	10. (d)
11. (b)	12. (a)	13. (a)	14. (c)	15. (c)

Solutions

1. (a) Given, $\alpha + \beta = 90°$ and $\alpha : \beta = 2 : 1$

$\therefore \quad \alpha = \frac{2}{2+1} \times 90°$

$= \frac{2}{3} \times 90° = 60°$

Similarly, $\beta = \frac{1}{3} \times 90° = 30°$

$\therefore \sin\alpha : \sin\beta = \sin 60° : \sin 30°$

$= \frac{\sqrt{3}}{2} : \frac{1}{2} = \sqrt{3} : 1.$

2. (d) Given, $\tan\left(\frac{\pi}{2} - \frac{\alpha}{2}\right) = \sqrt{3}$

$\cot\frac{\alpha}{2} = \cot 30°$

On comparing,

$\frac{\alpha}{2} = 30°$

$\alpha = 60°$

$\therefore \quad \cos\alpha = \cos(60°) = \frac{1}{2}$

3. (c) Given, $\frac{\sin\theta + \cos\theta}{\sin\theta - \cos\theta} = 3$

$\Rightarrow \sin\theta + \cos\theta = 3\sin\theta - 3\cos\theta$

$\Rightarrow \quad 4\cos\theta = 2\sin\theta \Rightarrow \tan\theta = 2$

$\therefore$ Value of $\sin^4\theta - \cos^4\theta$

$= (\sin^2\theta + \cos^2\theta)(\sin^2\theta - \cos^2\theta)$

$[\because \sin^2\theta + \cos^2\theta = 1]$

$= \sin^2\theta - \cos^2\theta$

$= \cos^2\theta(\tan^2\theta - 1)$

$= \frac{\tan^2\theta - 1}{\sec^2\theta} = \frac{\tan^2\theta - 1}{1 + \tan^2\theta}$

$= \frac{4-1}{1+4} = \frac{3}{5}$

4. (c) Given, $\sin A = \frac{5}{13}$

$\therefore \ \cos A = \sqrt{1 - \sin^2 A} = \sqrt{1 - \frac{5^2}{13^2}}$

$= \sqrt{\frac{169-25}{169}} = \sqrt{\frac{144}{169}} = \frac{12}{13}$

$\therefore \quad \tan A = \frac{\sin A}{\cos A}$

$= \frac{5}{13} \times \frac{13}{12} = \frac{5}{12}$

and $\sec A = \frac{1}{\cos A}$

$= \frac{1}{12/13} = \frac{13}{12}$

$\therefore \quad \tan A + \sec A$

$= \frac{5}{12} + \frac{13}{12} = \frac{18}{12} = 1.5$

5. (c) Given, $\frac{\sin\theta + \cos\theta}{\sin\theta - \cos\theta} = \frac{5}{4}$

$\Rightarrow \quad \frac{\cos\theta\left(\frac{\sin\theta}{\cos\theta} + 1\right)}{\cos\theta\left(\frac{\sin\theta}{\cos\theta} - 1\right)} = \frac{5}{4}$

$\Rightarrow \quad \frac{\tan\theta + 1}{\tan\theta - 1} = \frac{5}{4}$

$\Rightarrow \quad 4\tan\theta + 4 = 5\tan\theta - 5$

$\Rightarrow \quad \tan\theta = 9.$

Now, $\frac{\tan^2\theta + 1}{\tan^2\theta - 1} = \frac{(9)^2 + 1}{(9)^2 - 1}$

$= \frac{81+1}{81-1} = \frac{82}{80} = \frac{41}{40}.$

6. (d) In ΔPQR,

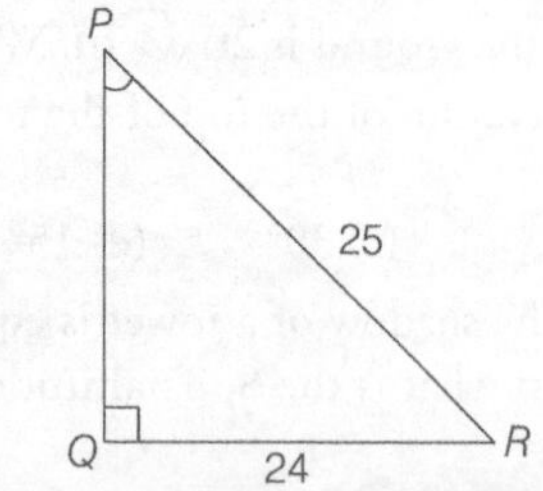

$PQ^2 = 25^2 - 24^2$

$= 625 - 576 = 49$

$\Rightarrow PQ = 7$

$\therefore \cot R = \dfrac{\text{Base}}{\text{Perpendicular}}$

$= \dfrac{QR}{PQ} = \dfrac{24}{7}$

10. (d) $3\cos^2 60° + 2\cot^2 30° - 5\sin^2 45°$

$= 3 \times \left(\dfrac{1}{2}\right)^2 + 2 \times (\sqrt{3})^2 - 5 \times \left(\dfrac{1}{\sqrt{2}}\right)^2$

$= \dfrac{3}{4} + 6 - \dfrac{5}{2} = \dfrac{3 + 24 - 10}{4} = \dfrac{17}{4}$

11. (b)

$\sin(3x - 20°) = \cos(3y + 20°)$

$\Rightarrow \sin(3x - 20°) = \sin[90° - (3y + 20°)]$

$\Rightarrow \sin(3x - 20°) = \sin(70° - 3y)$

$\therefore \quad 3x - 20° = 70° - 3y$

$\Rightarrow \quad 3x + 3y = 90°$

$\Rightarrow \quad 3(x + y) = 90°$

$\Rightarrow \quad x + y = 30°.$

12. (a) $\dfrac{5}{\sec^2\theta} + \dfrac{2}{1 + \cot^2\theta} + 3\sin^2\theta$

$= 5\cos^2\theta + \dfrac{2}{\text{cosec}^2\theta} + 3\sin^2\theta$

$[\because 1 + \cot^2\theta = \text{cosec}^2\theta]$

$= 5\cos^2\theta + 2\sin^2\theta + 3\sin^2\theta$

$= 5\cos^2\theta + 5\sin^2\theta$

$= 5(\sin^2\theta + \cos^2\theta)$

$[\because \sin^2\theta + \cos^2\theta = 1]$

$= 5 \times 1 = 5$

13. (a) $\because \sec^2\theta - \tan^2\theta = 1$ [identity]

Also, $\sec^2\theta + \tan^2\theta = \dfrac{7}{12}$ [given]

$\therefore \sec^4\theta - \tan^4\theta$

$= (\sec^2\theta - \tan^2\theta)(\sec^2\theta + \tan^2\theta)$

$= 1 \times \dfrac{7}{12} = \dfrac{7}{12}$

14. (c) Let, angle of elevation $= \theta$

In ΔABC, $\tan\theta = \dfrac{BC}{AB} = \dfrac{20}{20\sqrt{3}}$

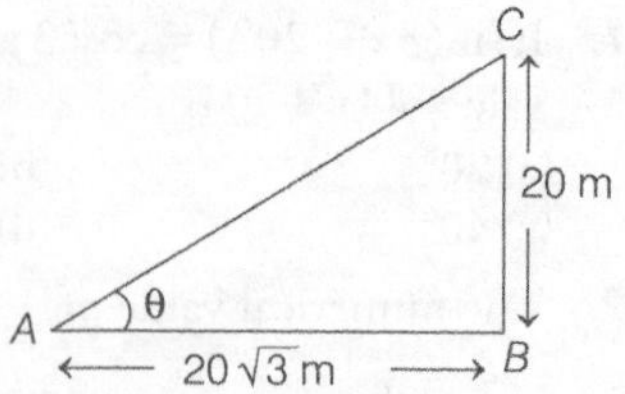

$\tan\theta = \dfrac{1}{\sqrt{3}} = \tan 30°$

$\tan\theta = \tan 30° \Rightarrow \theta = 30°$

15. (c) Let AB and BC be the height of tower and length of the shadow of a tower.

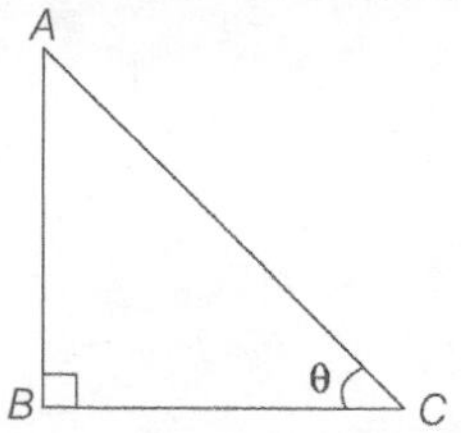

According to the question,

$AB = BC$ ... (i)

Now, in ΔABC,

$\tan\theta = \dfrac{AB}{BC} = \dfrac{AB}{AB}$ [from Eq. (i)]

$\Rightarrow \quad \tan\theta = 1$

$\Rightarrow \quad \tan\theta = \tan 45°$

$\Rightarrow \quad \theta = 45°$

Hence, the Sun's altitude is 45°.

Chapter 14 Geometry

Geometry is a branch of mathematics in which we study of shape, size of various figures.

Parallel Lines and Angles

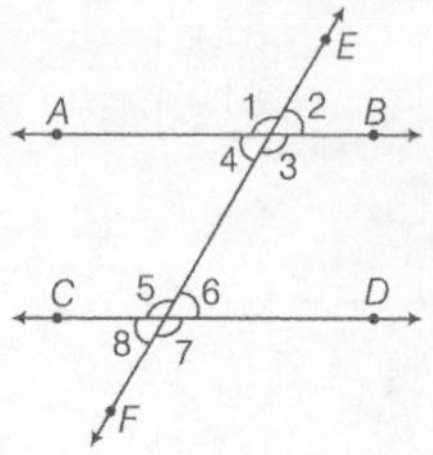

A line which cuts a pair of parallel line is called a transversal.

Here, two parallel lines AB and CD are cut by a transversal i.e. EF. Then,

- The corresponding angles are $\angle 1 = \angle 5$, $\angle 2 = \angle 6$, $\angle 4 = \angle 8$ and $\angle 3 = \angle 7$.
- The alternate angles are $\angle 1 = \angle 7$, $\angle 2 = \angle 8$, $\angle 3 = \angle 5$ and $\angle 4 = \angle 6$.
- The sum of the consecutive interior angles on the same side of a transversal is equal to 180°. i.e. $\angle 3 + \angle 6 = 180°$ and $\angle 4 + \angle 5 = 180°$

- The sum of the exterior angles on the same side of a transversal is equal to 180°.
  i.e. $\angle 1 + \angle 8 = 180°$ and $\angle 2 + \angle 7 = 180°$
- The vertically opposite angles are
  $\angle 1 = \angle 3, \angle 2 = \angle 4, \angle 8 = \angle 6$ and $\angle 5 = \angle 7$.

Triangle

Sum of interior angles of a triangle is 180° and sum of any two sides of a triangle is greater than third side.

Types of Triangles

(a) **Scalene Triangle** A triangle whose all sides are of different lengths is known as scalene triangle.

(b) **Isosceles Triangle** A triangle whose two sides are of equal length is known as isosceles triangle.

(c) **Equilateral Triangle** A triangle whose all sides are of equal length, is known as equilateral triangle.

Quadrilateral

It has four sides and four internal angles. The sum of the internal angles of a quadrilateral is equal to 360°.

Types of Quadrilateral

Parallelogram

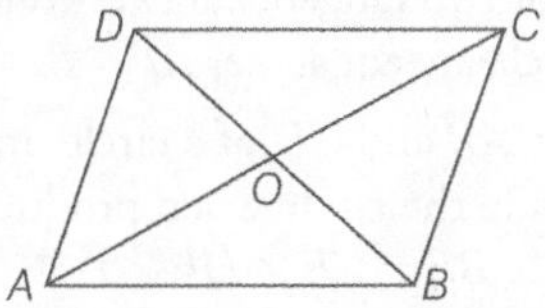

- The opposite sides are equal and parallel, i.e. $AB = DC$ and $AD = BC$.
- The sum of any two adjacent interior angles is equal to 180°.

$\angle A + \angle B = \angle B + \angle C$
$= \angle C + \angle D = \angle D + \angle A = 180°$

- The opposite angles are equal in magnitude, i.e. $\angle A = \angle C$ and $\angle B = \angle D$.
- The diagonals of a parallelogram are not equal in magnitudes but they bisect each other, i.e. $AC \neq BD$ but $AO = OC$ and $OB = OD$.
- Sum of the twice of squares of sides is equal to the sum of the squares of its diagonals
  $AC^2 + BD^2 = 2(AB^2 + BC^2)$

Rhombus

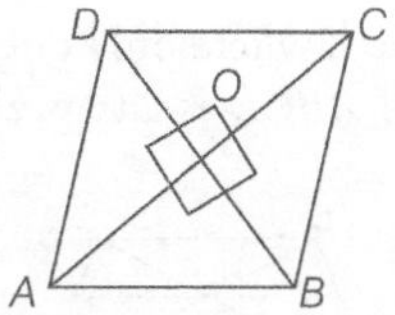

- The opposite sides are parallel and all the sides are of equal lengths, i.e. $AB = BC = CD = DA$.
- The sum of any two adjacent interior angles is equal to 180° i.e. $\angle A + \angle B = \angle B + \angle C = \angle C + \angle D = \angle D + \angle A = 180°$
- The opposite angles are equal in magnitude, i.e. $\angle A = \angle C$ and $\angle B = \angle D$.
- Sum of the squares of sides is equal to the sum of the squares of its diagonals.

Rectangle

- The opposite sides are parallel and are of equal lengths, i.e. $AB = CD$ and $AD = BC$.
- The adjacent sides are perpendicular i.e. $\angle A = \angle B = \angle C = \angle D = 90°$.

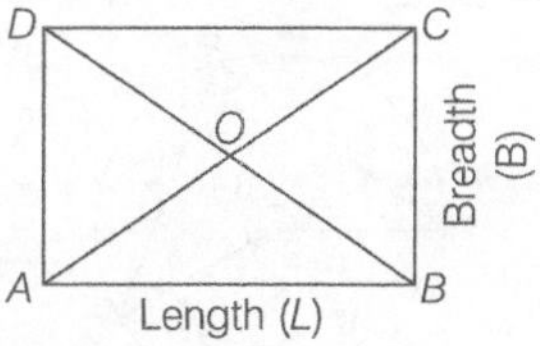

- The diagonals of a rectangle are of equal length and bisect each other, i.e. $AC = BD$ and $AO = OC = BO = OD$.

Square

- A parallelogram in which all the sides are equal and perpendicular to each other.
- The opposite sides are parallel and all the sides are of equal length i.e., $AB = BC = CD = DA$
- The diagonals of a square are of equal length, i.e. $AC = BD$.

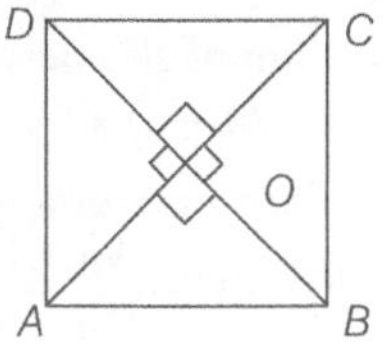

- The diagonals bisect each other at right angles and form four isosceles right angled triangles.
- The adjacent sides are perpendicular, i.e. $\angle A = \angle B = \angle C = \angle D = 90°$

Trapezium

- It is a quadrilateral, where only one pair of opposite sides are parallel. $ABCD$ is a trapezium with $AB || DC$.

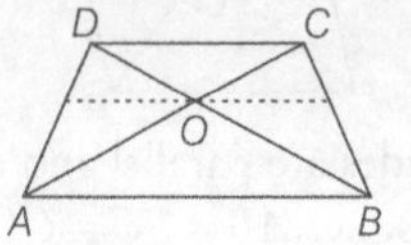

- In a trapezium $ABCD$,
$AC^2 + BD^2 = BC^2 + AD^2 + 2AB \cdot CD$

Also, $\frac{AO}{OC} = \frac{BO}{OD}$

- The line joining the mid-points of the non-parallel sides of a trapezium is half of the sum of the length of parallel sides.

Cyclic Quadrilateral

A quadrilateral whose vertices are on the circumference of a circle, is called a cyclic quadrilateral. The opposite angles of a cyclic quadrilateral are supplementary, i.e. $\alpha + \beta = 180°$. In a cyclic quadrilateral, exterior angle is equal to interior opposite angle.

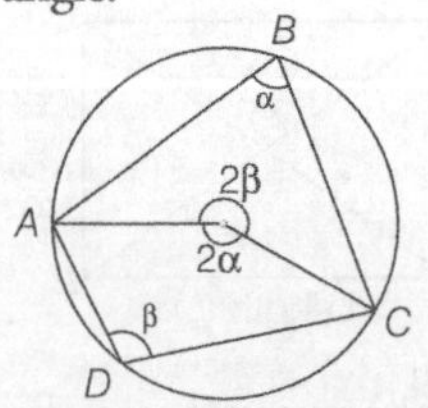

Polygon

A polygon in which all the sides are equal and also all interior angles are equal is called a regular polygon. They are named according to their number of sides as triangle, quadrilateral, pentagon, hexagon, for 3, 4, 5, 6 sides, respectively.

- Sum of all interior angles $= (n - 2) \times 180°$
$= (2n - 4) \times 90°$
- Each interior angle $= 180° -$ Exterior angle
$= 180° - \frac{360°}{n}$
- Each exterior angle $= \left(\frac{360°}{\text{Number of sides}}\right)$ (in degrees)
- Sum of all exterior angles = 360° (always constant)
- Number of diagonals of a polygon on n sides
$= \frac{n(n-3)}{2}$

Circle

- A collection of all points lie on a plane at a fixed distance from a fixed point, is known as circle. In given figure, O is known as centre of circle and distance OP is known as radius of circle and is denoted by r.

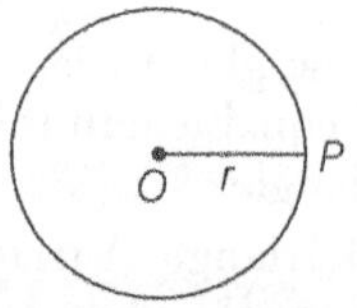

Important Theorems on Circle

- The perpendicular from the centre of a circle to a chord bisects the chord.
- Angle in a semi-circle is a right angle.
- Angles in the same segment of a circle are equal, i.e. $\angle ACB = \angle ADB$.

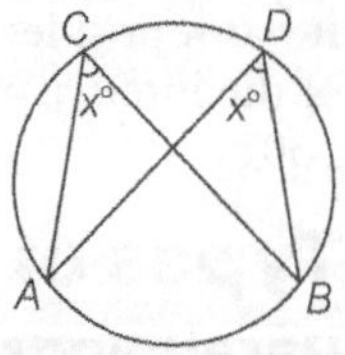

- The lengths of two tangents drawn from an external point to a circle are equal, i.e. $AP = BP$
- If two chords AB and CD of a circle, intersect inside a circle (outside the circle when produced at a point E), then $AE \times BE = CE \times DE$

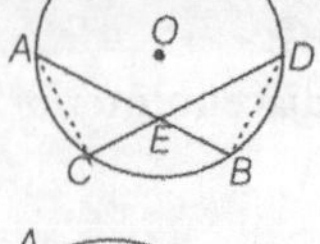

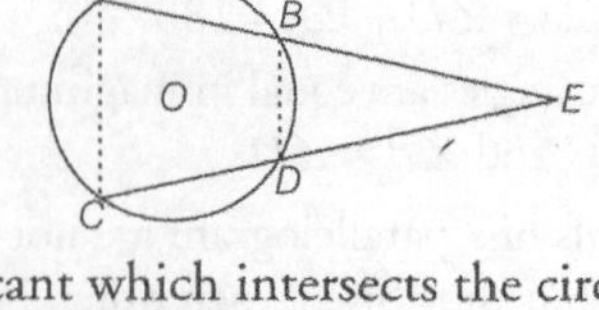

If PB be secant which intersects the circle at A and B and PT be a tangent at T, then $PA \cdot PB = (PT)^2$

Exam Pattern Questions

1. If the complement of an angle is one-fourth of its supplementary angle, then the angle, is

(a) 90° (b) 30°
(c) 60° (d) 120°

2. ABC is a triangle in which $DE \parallel BC$ and $AD : DB = 5 : 4$. Then, $DE : BC$ is

(a) $4 : 5$ (b) $4 : 9$
(c) $9 : 5$ (d) $5 : 9$

3. If the measure of three angles of a triangle are in the ratio $2 : 3 : 5$, then the triangle is

(a) right angled
(b) isosceles
(c) obtuse angled
(d) equilateral

4. If O is the orthocentre of a ΔABC and $\angle BOC = 100^\circ$, then measure of $\angle BAC$ is

(a) 100° (b) 180°
(c) 80° (d) 200°

5. One angle of a pentagon is 140°. If the remaining angles are in the ratio $1 : 2 : 3 : 4$, then what is the greatest angle?

(a) 144° (b) 150°
(c) 152° (d) 160°

6. In the given figure, straight lines AB and CD intersect at O. If $\angle \beta = 3\angle p$, then $\angle p$ is equal to

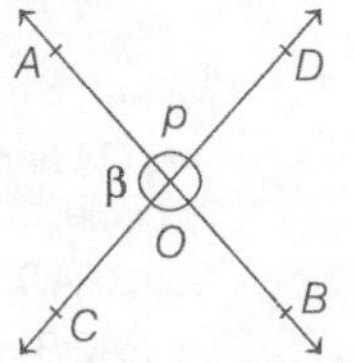

(a) 40° (b) 45°
(c) 50° (d) 55°

7. In the figure given below, EC is parallel to AB, $\angle ECD = 70^\circ$ and $\angle BDO = 20^\circ$. What is the value of $\angle OBD$?

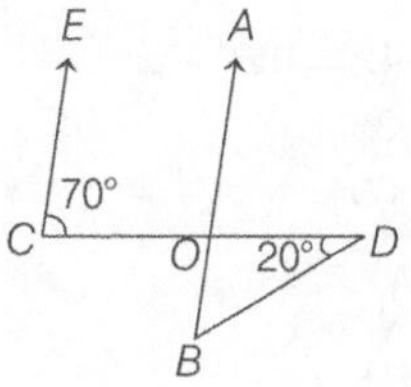

(a) 20° (b) 30° (c) 40° (d) 50°

8. In given figure, if QRS is an equilateral triangle TQS is an isosceles triangle and $X = 47^\circ$, then the value of y is

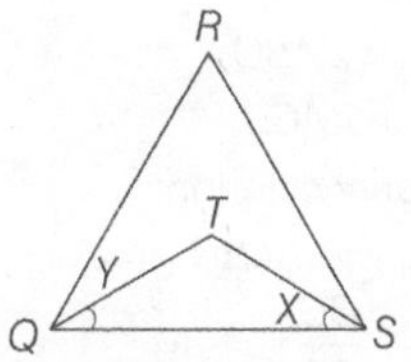

(a) 13° (b) 23° (c) 33° (d) 43°

9. Two triangles ABC and DEF are similar triangles. The ratio of their corresponding sides is $3 : 5$. What will be the ratio of their areas?

(a) $9 : 25$ (b) $5 : 3$ (c) $25 : 9$ (d) $6 : 4$

10. From a point P, two tangents PA and PB are drawn to a circle with centre O.
If $\angle AOB = 120^\circ$.

(a) 90° (b) 30° (c) 60° (d) 45°

Answers

1. (c)	2. (d)	3. (a)	4. (c)	5. (d)
6. (b)	7. (d)	8. (a)	9. (a)	10. (c)

Solutions

1. (c) Let the angle be $x°$.
According to the question,

$$90° - x = \frac{1}{4} \times (180° - x)$$

$\Rightarrow$ $360° - 4x = 180° - x$

$\Rightarrow$ $180° = 3x$

$\therefore$ $x = 60°$

2. (d)

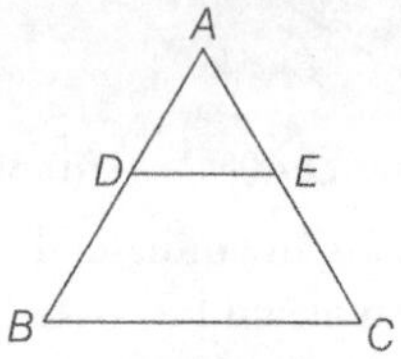

$DE || BC$

$\therefore$ $\angle ADE = \angle ABC$,

$\angle AED = \angle ACB$

By AA—similarity criterion,

$\Delta ADE \sim \Delta ABC$

$\therefore$ $\frac{AB}{AD} = \frac{BC}{DE}$

$\therefore$ $\frac{DB}{AD} = \frac{4}{5}$

$\Rightarrow$ $\frac{DB}{AD} + 1 = \frac{4}{5} + 1$

$\Rightarrow$ $\frac{DB + AD}{AD} = \frac{4+5}{5}$

$\Rightarrow$ $\frac{AB}{AD} = \frac{9}{5} = \frac{BC}{DE}$

$\therefore$ $\frac{DE}{BC} = \frac{5}{9} = 5:9$

3. (a) Angles of triangle $= 2x°, 3x°$ and $5x°$ (let)

$\therefore$ $2x° + 3x° + 5x° = 180°$

$\Rightarrow$ $10x° = 180°$

$\Rightarrow$ $x° = \frac{180}{10} = 18°$

Angles of triangle

$= 2x = 2 \times 18 = 36°$,

$3x = 3 \times 18 = 54°$,

$5x = 5 \times 18 = 90°$,

Hence, it is a right angled triangle.

4. (c) Here in ΔABC, AD, BE and CF are the altitudes at sides BC, AC and AB respectively and O is the orthocentre.

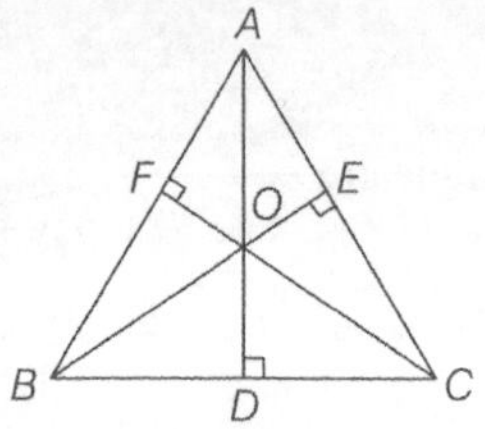

$\therefore$ $\angle BAC + \angle BOC = 180°$

$\Rightarrow$ $\angle BAC = 180° - 100°$

[$\because \angle BOC = 100°$, given]

$\therefore$ $\angle BAC = 80°$

6. (b) $\because \angle p + \angle \beta = 180°$ [linear pair]

$\Rightarrow$ $\angle p + 3\angle p = 180°$

$\Rightarrow$ $4\angle p = 180°$

$\therefore$ $\angle p = 45°$

7. (d) Given that, $EC || AB$

$\therefore$ $\angle ECO + \angle AOC = 180°$

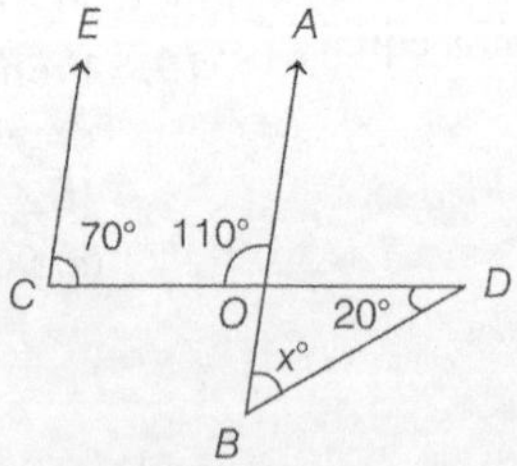

$\Rightarrow$ $\angle AOC = 180° - 70° = 110°$

$\therefore$ $\angle BOD = \angle AOC = 110°$

[vertically opposite angles]

Now, in ΔOBD,

$\angle BOD + \angle ODB + \angle DBO = 180°$

$\therefore$ $110° + 20° + x° = 180°$

$\Rightarrow$ $x° = 50°$

8. (a) $\because \Delta QRS$ is an equilateral triangle

$\therefore$ $\angle Q = \angle R = \angle S = 60°$

Again, ΔTQS is isosceles triangle

$\therefore$ $TQ = TS$

$\Rightarrow$ $\angle TQS = \angle TSQ$

$\therefore$ $\angle TQS = X = 47°$

from fig

$\angle Q = x + y$

$\Rightarrow$ $60° = 47° + y$

$\Rightarrow$ $y = 60° - 47° = 13°$

9. (a) We know that ratio of two similar triangles is equal to the ratio of squares of corresponding sides.

$\therefore$ $\frac{\text{area of } \Delta ABC}{\text{area of } \Delta DEF} = \left(\frac{3}{5}\right)^2$

$= \frac{9}{25} = 9:25$

10. (c) Given, $\angle AOB = 110°$

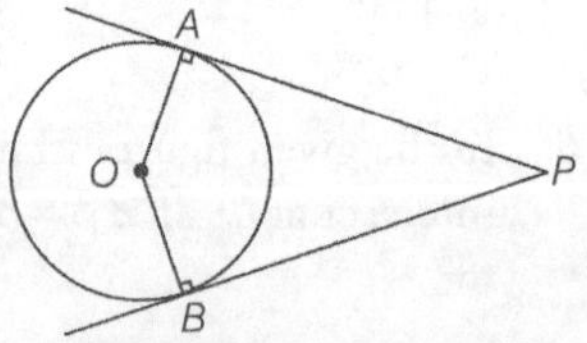

PA and PB are the tangents and OA and OB are the radius of circle.

So, $\angle PAO = \angle PBO = 90°$

$\because$ $PAOB$ is a quadrilateral

$\therefore$ $\angle PAO + \angle AOB + \angle PBO + \angle APB = 360°$

$\Rightarrow$ $90° + 120° + 90° + \angle APB = 360°$

$\Rightarrow$ $\angle APB = 360° - 300° = 60°$

Chapter 15

Mensuration

There are measured parameters, area, surface area and volume of various figures like triangle, rectangle, circle, cube, cuboid, cylinder, cone, sphere etc.

Triangle

Area $= \frac{1}{2} \times$ base $\times$ height $= \frac{1}{2} \times a \times h$

Scalene Triangle

(i) Perimeter $= a + b + c$

(ii) Area $= \sqrt{s(s-a)(s-b)(s-c)}$

where, $s = \frac{a+b+c}{2}$

This is also known as Heron's formula.

Right Angled Triangle

(i) Perimeter $= p + b + h$

(ii) Area $= \frac{1}{2} \times bp = \frac{1}{2} \times$ Base $\times$ Altitude

[$\because$ p = perpendicular,
b = base and h = hypotenuse]

Equilateral Triangle

(i) Perimeter $= 3a$

(ii) Area $= \frac{\sqrt{3}}{4} a^2 = \frac{\sqrt{3}}{4}$ (median)^2

(iii) Height $= \frac{\sqrt{3}}{2} a$

If two sides and angle between of them is known, then $\Delta = \frac{1}{2} bc \sin A = \frac{1}{2} ca \sin B$

$= \frac{1}{2} ab \sin C$

Rectangle

(i) Perimeter = 2 (length + breadth) $= 2(a+b)$

(ii) Area = length $\times$ breadth $= a \times b$

(iii) Diagonal $= \sqrt{a^2 + b^2}$

Square

(i) Perimeter $= 4a$

(ii) Area $= a^2 = \frac{1}{2}$ (diagonal)^2

(iii) Diagonal $= a\sqrt{2}$

Quadrilateral

Area $= \frac{1}{2} \times AC \times (DM + BN)$

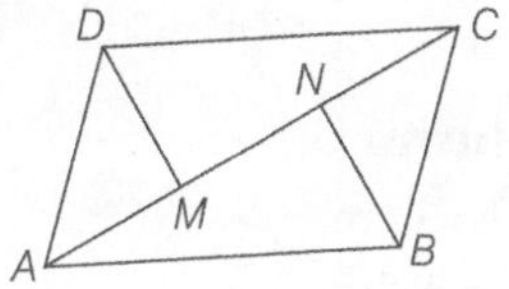

Parallelogram

(i) Perimeter $= 2(a+b)$

(ii) Area = base $\times$ height $= a \times h$

Rhombus

(i) Area $= \frac{1}{2} \times d_1 \times d_2$

(ii) Side $= \frac{1}{2} \sqrt{d_1^2 + d_2^2}$

(iii) Perimeter $= 4 \times$ side

(iv) $4a^2 = d_1^2 + d_2^2$

Trapezium

Area $= \frac{1}{2}(a+b) \times h$

Polygon

(i) Area of pentagon $= \frac{5a^2\sqrt{3}}{4}$

(ii) Area of hexagon $= \frac{6a^2\sqrt{3}}{4}$

Circle

(i) Area $= \pi r^2$

(ii) Circumference $= 2\pi r$

(iii) Diameter $= d = 2r$

(iv) Length of arc, $l = \frac{\pi r\theta}{180°}$

(v) Area of sector, $A = \frac{\pi r^2\theta}{360°}$

Circular Rings

(i) Area $= \pi(R^2 - r^2)$

(ii) Difference of the circumference of both rings $= 2\pi R - 2\pi r$

Units of Volume

$1000 \text{ mm}^3 = 1 \text{ cm}^3$

$1000 \text{ cm}^3 = 1 \text{ dm}^3$

$1000 \text{ dm}^3 = 1 \text{ m}^3$

$1 \text{ Litre} = 1 \text{ dm}^3 = 1000 \text{ cm}^3$

$1000 \text{ Litre} = 1 \text{ m}^3$

Cuboid

Let the length, width and height of a cuboid are l, b and h.

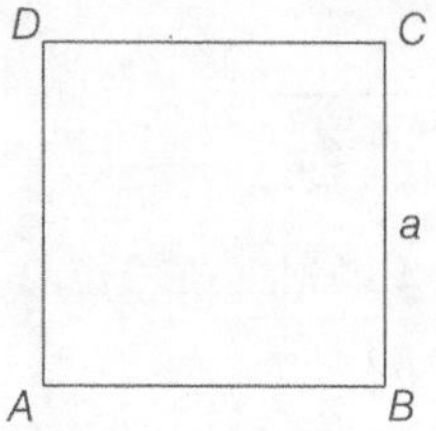

(i) Volume of cuboid, $V = \text{length} \times \text{width} \times \text{height} = lbh$

(ii) Surface area of the cuboid, $s = 2(lb + bh + hl)$

(iii) Diagonal $= \sqrt{l^2 + b^2 + h^2}$

Cube

Let the side of a cube is a.

(i) Volume, $V = (\text{side})^3 = a^3$

(ii) Surface area, $s = 6(\text{side})^2 = 6a^2$

(iii) Diagonal $= a\sqrt{3}$

(iv) Ratio of the total surface areas of two cubes = (side of the first cube)^2 : (side of the second cube)^2

Prism

(i) Volume = area of base × height

(ii) Surface area = perimeter of base × height

(iii) Total surface area = Surface area of prism + 2 × area of base

Cylinder

Let the radius of base is r and height is h.

(i) Volume $= \pi r^2 h$

(ii) Curved surface area $= 2\pi rh$

(iii) Total surface area $= 2\pi r(h + r)$

Hollow Cylinder

Let the internal and external radius are r_1 and r_2 and the height of cylinder is h.

(i) Volume $= \pi(r_2^2 - r_1^2)h$

(ii) Curved surface area $= 2\pi(r_2 + r_1)h$

(iii) Total surface area $= 2\pi h(r_2 + r_1) + 2\pi(r_2^2 - r_1^2)$

Pyramid

(i) Volume $= \frac{1}{3} \times$ area of base × height

(ii) Total surface area = area of base + area of all lateral faces

Cone

Let the radius of the base of cone is r and height of h.

(i) Volume $= \frac{1}{3}\pi r^2 h$

(ii) Curved surface area $= \pi rl$

(iii) Slant height, $l = \sqrt{h^2 + r^2}$

(iv) Total surface area $= \pi r (l + r)$

Sphere

Let r be the radius of the sphere.

(i) Volume $= \frac{4}{3}\pi r^3$

(ii) Curved surface area $= 4\pi r^2$

Hemisphere

Let r be the radius of the hemisphere.

(i) Volume $= \frac{2}{3}\pi r^3$

(ii) Curved surface area $= 2\pi r^2$

(iii) Total surface area $= 3\pi r^2$

Spherical Shell

Let r_1 and r_2 be internal and external radii of the shell.

$\therefore$ Volume $= \frac{4}{3}\pi (r_1^3 - r_2^3)$

Exam Pattern Questions

1. If the area of a square field is 196 sq cm, what will be the length of the fence to bind this field?

(a) 28 cm (b) 36 cm
(c) 56 cm (d) 196 cm

2. The diagonal of a square is $4\sqrt{2}$ cm. The diagonal of another square whose area is double that of the first square is

(a) 8 cm (b) $8\sqrt{2}$ cm
(c) $4\sqrt{2}$ cm (d) 6 cm

3. The perimeter and the breadth of a rectangle are 82 cm and 20 cm, respectively. Calculate the length of its diagonal.

(a) 58 cm (b) 21 cm (c) 42 cm (d) 29 cm

4. A rectangular field has an area of 1200 sq m. If its length is 40 m, then the ratio of the length to the breadth of the field is

(a) 3 : 4 (b) 4 : 3 (c) 2 : 1 (d) 5 : 2

5. The lengths of the two diagonals of a rhombus are 5 cm and 12 cm. Find its area.

(a) 30 cm^2 (b) 15 cm^2
(c) 60 cm^2 (d) 45 cm^2

6. The area of a trapezium is 384 cm^2. If its parallel sides are in the ratio 3 : 5 and the perpendicular distance between them is12 cm, the smaller of the parallel sides is

(a) 20 cm (b) 24 cm
(c) 30 cm (d) 36 cm

7. If area of a regular pentagon is $125\sqrt{3}$ sq cm, how long is its each side ?

(a) 10 cm (b) 15 cm
(c) 16 cm (d) 25 cm

8. A person travels 4.40 km distance by taking 10 rounds of his circular field. The area of his field is

(a) 1.34 hec (b) 1.54 hec
(c) 1.44 hec (d) 1.64 hec

9. The area of a circular field is 38.5 sq m. The cost per metre of a rope is ₹ 5. What is the total cost of rope to fence its boundary?

(a) ₹ 96.25
(b) ₹ 192.50
(c) ₹ 55
(d) ₹ 110

10. A railing of 288 m is required for fencing a semi-circular park. Find the area of the park. (take $\pi = 22/7$)

(a) 4928 m^2 (b) 9865 m^2
(c) 8956 m^2 (d) 9856 m^2

11. Find the area of circle with maximum radius that can be inscribed in the rectangle of length 16 cm and breadth 4 cm.

(a) 5π cm^2 (b) 6π cm^2 (c) 3π cm^2 (d) 4π cm^2

12. If the sides of a triangle are in the ratio of 3 : 4 : 5 and its area is 216 sq cm, then the perimeter of the triangle is

(a) 72 cm (b) 76 cm
(c) 84 cm (d) 80 cm

13. The area of a right angled triangle is 40 sq cm. If its base is equal to 28 cm, find its height.

(a) $3\frac{6}{7}$ cm (b) $4\frac{6}{7}$ cm
(c) $2\frac{6}{7}$ cm (d) $5\frac{6}{7}$ cm

14. A plate on square base made of brass is of length x cm and width 1 mm. The plate weighs 4725 gm. If 1 cubic cm of brass weighs 8.4 gm, then the value of x is

(a) 75 cm (b) 76 cm
(c) 72 cm (d) 74 cm

15. If the volume of a cube is 729 cm^3, what is the length of its diagonal?

(a) $9\sqrt{2}$ cm (b) $9\sqrt{3}$ cm
(c) 18 cm (d) $18\sqrt{3}$ cm

16. Find the surface area of a cuboid 10 m long, 5 m broad and 3 m high.

(a) 105 sq m (b) 104 sq m
(c) 170 sq m (d) 190 sq m

Answers

1. (c)	2. (a)	3. (d)	4. (b)	5. (a)
6. (b)	7. (a)	8. (b)	9. (d)	10. (a)
11. (d)	12. (a)	13. (c)	14. (a)	15. (b)
16. (d)				

Solutions

1. (c) Area = 196

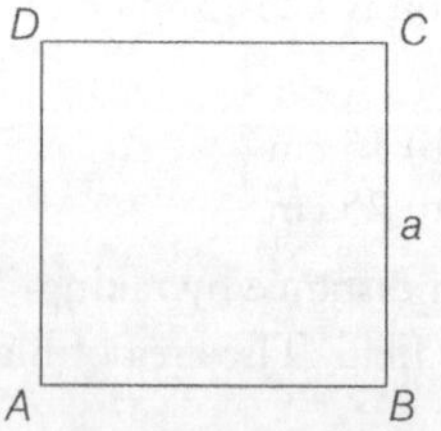

$\Rightarrow$ $a^2 = 196$

$\therefore$ $a = 14$ cm

$\therefore$ Length of the fence to bind the field

$= 4 \times 14$

$= 56$ cm

2. (a) Diagonal of square

$= \sqrt{2}a$ [$\because a =$ side]

$\Rightarrow 4\sqrt{2} = \sqrt{2}a$

$\Rightarrow$ $a = 4$ cm

Now, area of square

$= a^2 = (4)^2 = 16$

Side of a square whose area is 2×16.

$a_1^2 = 32 \Rightarrow a_1 = \sqrt{32} \Rightarrow a_1 = 4\sqrt{2}$

Now, diagonal of new square

$= \sqrt{2}a_1 = \sqrt{2} \times 4\sqrt{2} = 8$ cm

3. (d) Perimeter of rectangle

$= 2(l + b)$

$82 = 2(l + 20) \Rightarrow 41 = l + 20$

$\therefore$ $l = 21$ cm

$\therefore$ Length of diagonal

$= \sqrt{(21)^2 + (20)^2}$

$= \sqrt{441 + 400}$

$= \sqrt{841} = 29$ cm

4. (b) Given, area of rectangle

$= 1200\ m^2$

and length of rectangle = 40 m

$\therefore$ Area of rectangle

= Length × Breadth

$\Rightarrow 1200 = 40 \times$ Breadth

$\Rightarrow$ Breadth $= \frac{1200}{40} = 30$

Hence, the ratio of the length to the breadth = 40 : 30 = 4 : 3

5. (a) $\because$ Area of rhombus $= \frac{1}{2}$ product of diagonal

$= \frac{1}{2} \times 5 \times 12 = 30\ cm^2$

6. (b) Let the sides of trapezium be $5x$ and $3x$, respectively.

According to the question,

$\frac{1}{2} \times (5x + 3x) \times 12 = 384$

$\Rightarrow$ $8x = \frac{384 \times 2}{12}$

$\Rightarrow$ $x = \frac{64}{8} = 8$ cm

Length of smaller of the parallel sides = 3 × 8 = 24 cm

7. (a) We know that,

Area of regular pentagon

$= 5a^2 \frac{\sqrt{3}}{4}$

According to the question,

$\frac{5a^2\sqrt{3}}{4} = 125\sqrt{3}$

$\Rightarrow \quad a^2 = \frac{125\sqrt{3} \times 4}{5\sqrt{3}} = 100$

$\therefore \quad a = 10$ cm

8. (b) Distance covered by one round $= 2\pi r$

Distance covered by 10 rounds $= 20\pi r$

According to the question,

$20\ \pi r = 4.40$

$20 \times \frac{22}{7} \times r = 4.40$

$\Rightarrow \quad r = \frac{4.40 \times 7}{440}$

$\therefore \quad r = \frac{7}{100}$ km

Area of circular field $= \pi r^2$

$= \frac{22}{7} \times \frac{7}{100} \times \frac{7}{100}$ sq km

$= \frac{154}{10000}$ sq km

$= \frac{154}{10000} \times 100$ hectare

$= 1.54$ hec

9. (d) Given, area $= 38.5$

$\Rightarrow \quad \pi r^2 = 38.5$

$\Rightarrow \quad r^2 = \frac{38.5 \times 7}{22} = 12.25$

$\Rightarrow \quad r = \sqrt{12.25} = 3.5$ m

$\therefore$ Perimeter of field $= 2\pi r$

$= 2 \times \frac{22}{7} \times 3.5 = 22$ m

$\therefore$ Total cost of fencing

$= 22 \times 5 =$ ₹110

10. (a) Let the radius of the park be r, then

$\pi r + 2r = 288$

$\Rightarrow \quad (\pi + 2)\, r = 288$

$\Rightarrow \quad \left(\frac{22}{7} + 2\right) r = 288$

$\Rightarrow \quad r = \frac{288 \times 7}{36} = 56$

$\therefore$ Area of the park $= \frac{1}{2}\pi r^2$

$= \frac{1}{2} \times \frac{22}{7} \times 56 \times 56 = 4928\ m^2$

11. (d) Here, $b = 4$

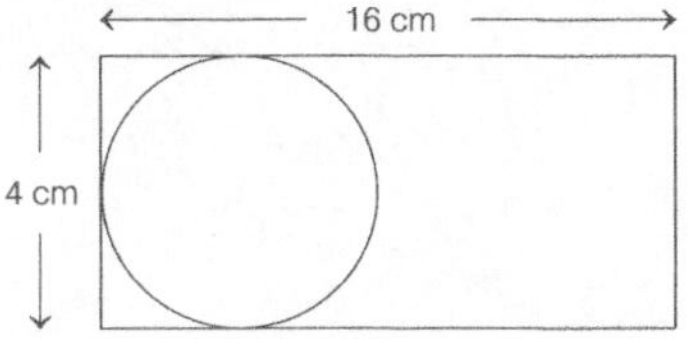

$\therefore$ Area of circle $= \frac{\pi b^2}{4}$

[by Technique 8]

$= \frac{\pi (4)^2}{4} = 4\pi\ cm^2$

12. (a) Let the sides of triangle are $3x$, $4x$ and $5x$.

$\because \quad (5x)^2 = (3x)^2 + (4x)^2$

$\therefore$ This triangle is a right-angled triangle.

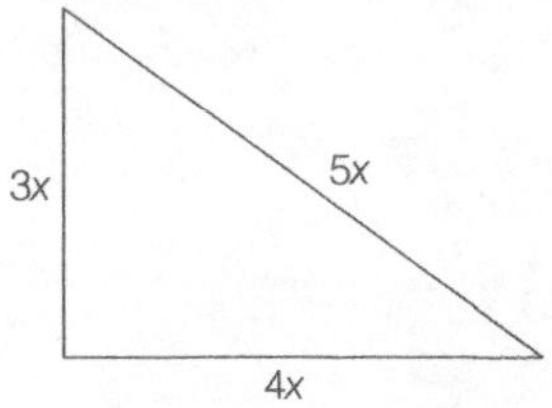

$\therefore \quad$ Area $= \frac{1}{2} \times$ base $\times$ height

$\Rightarrow \quad 216 = \frac{1}{2} \times 4x \times 3x$

$\Rightarrow \quad x = 6$ cm

Perimeter of triangle

$= 3x + 5x + 4x$

$= 3 \times 6 + 5 \times 6 + 4 \times 6$

$= 6(12) = 72$ cm

13. (c) Given that, area = 40 sq cm, base = 28 cm and height = perpendicular = ?

We know that,

Area $= \frac{1}{2} \times$ Base $\times$ Perpendicular

$\Rightarrow 40 = \frac{1}{2} \times 28 \times$ Perpendicular

$\therefore$ Perpendicular $= \frac{40}{14} = \frac{20}{7}$

$= 2\frac{6}{7}$ cm

14. (a)

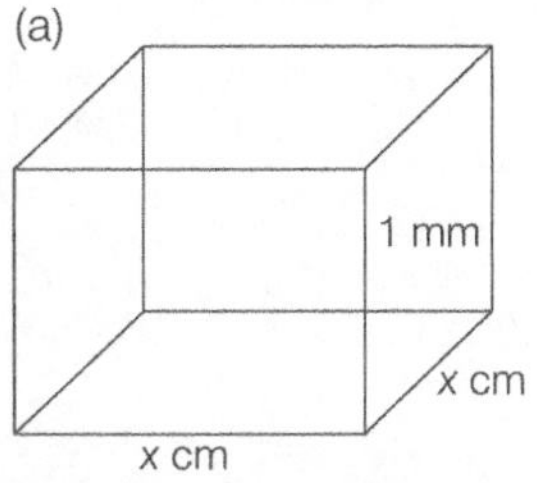

Given,

$\because$ 8. 4 gm weight of 1 cubic cm

$\therefore$ 4725 gm weight of

$\frac{1}{8 \cdot 4} \times 4725 = 562.5$ cubic cm

Volume of cuboid $= l \times b \times h$

$562.5 = x \times x \times \frac{1}{10}$

$\left[\because 1 \text{ mm} = \frac{1}{10} \text{ cm}\right]$

$x^2 = 5625 \Rightarrow x = 75$ cm

15. (b) Volume of cube $= (\text{Side})^3$

$\therefore \quad 729 = a^3 \Rightarrow a = 9$ cm

$\therefore$ Diagonal of cube $=$ Side $\times \sqrt{3}$

$= 9 \times \sqrt{3} = 9\sqrt{3}$ cm

16. (d) Given, $l = 10$ m, $b = 5$ m, $h = 3$ m

$\therefore \quad lb = 10 \times 5 = 50,$

$bh = 5 \times 3 = 15$

and $\quad lh = 10 \times 3 = 30$

$\therefore$ Surface area of a cuboid

$= 2(lb + bh + lh)$

$= 2(50 + 15 + 30)$

$= 2 \times 95 = 190$ sq m

PHYSICS

Chapter 01

Physical World and Measurement

Physical Quantities

The quantities which can be measured directly or indirectly are called physical quantities, e.g., distance, mass, time, length, electric current etc.

Units

A standard amount of a physical quantity chosen to measure the physical quantity of the same kind is called a physical unit. It should be easily reproducible, internationally accepted.

On the basis of magnitude and direction, all the physical quantities are classified into two groups.

- **Scalar Quantities** Physical quantities which have magnitude only. e.g., mass, speed, volume, work, time, power, energy etc are called scalar quantities.
- **Vector Quantities** Physical quantities which have magnitude and direction both. e.g., displacement, velocity, acceleration, force, momentum, torque etc are called vector quantities.

On the basis of units and measurement physical quantities are of the following two types

1. Fundamental Quantities and Their Units

- Those physical quantities which are independent of other physical quantities are called fundamental quantities. e.g., mass, temperature etc.
- The units which are used to measure the fundamental quantities are called fundamental units.

Fundamental Quantities and Their Units

Physical Quantities	Unit
Length	metre
Mass	kilogram
Time	second
Electric current	ampere
Thermodynamic temperature	kelvin
Amount of substance	mole
Luminous intensity	candela

2. Derived Quantities and Their Units

- Those quantities which can be derived from the fundamental quantities. e.g., velocity, volume, force.
- The units of dervied quantities are called derived units.

Important Formulae of Derived Units

Physical Quantities	Formulae	SI Units
Area of rectangle	Length × Breadth ($l \times b$)	m^2
Area of square	$(\text{Side})^2$	m^2
Area of triangle	$\frac{1}{2} \times$ Base × Height	m^2
Density	Mass/Volume	kg m^{-3}
Acceleration	Change in velocity /Time	ms^{-2}
Pressure	Force/Area	Nm^{-2} or pascal
Work or Energy	Mass × Acceleration due to Gravity × Height (PE = mgh)	N-m or J

Physical Quantities	Formulae	SI Units
Power	Work/Time	Js^{-1} or W
Torque	Force × Displacement	N-m
Impulse	Force × Time	N-s
Volume of cuboid	Length × Breadth × Height ($l \times b \times h$)	m^3
Velocity	$\frac{\text{Displacement}}{\text{Time}}$	ms^{-1}
Force	Mass × Acceleration	$kg\text{-}ms^{-2}$ or N
Linear momentum	Mass × Velocity	$kg\text{-}ms^{-1}$
Capacitance	$\frac{\text{Charge}}{\text{Potential difference}}$	F (farad)

Supplementary Quantities and Their Units

- Other than fundamental and derived quantities there are two more quantities called as supplementary quantities. e.g. Plane angle and solid angle.
- The units of supplementary quantities are called supplementary units.

Supplementary Quantities and Their Units

Physical Quantities	Unit
Plane angle	radian
Solid angle	steradian

System of Units

- **CGS System** It stands for centimetre, gram and second.
- **FPS System** It stands for foot, pound and second.
- **MKS System** It stands for metre, kilogram and seond.
- **SI System** This system contains seven fundamental units and two supplementary fundamental units.

Other Important Units

Some important units which is used frequently

1. $1\ \text{Å} = 10^{-10}$ m
2. 1 Nanometre (nm) $= 10^{-9}$ m
3. 1 Micrometre (μm) $= 10^{-6}$ m
4. 1 Light yearly $= 9.46 \times 10^{15}$ m
5. 1 Fermi $= 10^{-15}$ m
6. 1 Metric tonne = 1000 kg
7. 1 leap year = 366 day
8. 1 Parsec $= 3.083 \times 10^{16}$ m

Important Measuring Instruments

Measuring Instruments	Used to
Ammeter	measure strength of electric current
Audiometer	measure speed of sound
Odometer	measure distance covered by a vehicle
Barometer	measure atmospheric pressure
Actinometer	measure heating power of sunlight
Altimeter	measure height
Lactometer	check purity of milk
Periscope	to view object above sea-level
Hygrometer	measure the humidity of air
Galvanometer	measure small electric current
Pyrometer	measure temperature of a body by measuring the radiation by emitted body
Hydrometer	measure density or relative density of liquid
Fathometer	depth of ocean
Anemometer	wind speed
Luxmeter	intensity of light
Thermometer	temperature of body
Manometer	liquid pressure
Seismograph	intensity of earthquake
Phonometer	intensity of sound
Sphygmomanometer	blood pressure
Stethoscope	for listening heart beat
Cardiogram	a record of muscle activity within heart made by cardiograph
Potentiometer	internal resistance of a cell or to compare emf's of two cells

Exam Pattern Questions

1 Which among the following is the fundamental quantity?
(a) Mass (b) Volume (c) Velocity (d) Force

2 Kilowatt-hour is the unit of
(a) energy (b) power
(c) force (d) momentum

3 Radian is the SI unit of
(a) solid angle (b) plane angle
(c) acute angle (d) straight angle

4 SI unit of electric charge is
(a) ampere (b) esu
(c) kelvin (d) coulomb

5 What is the SI unit of speed?
(a) m (b) ms (c) ms^{-1} (d) m^{-1}

6 Ampere is the SI unit of
(a) electric charge (b) electric current
(c) electric potential (d) electric resistance

7 A light year is a unit of
(a) time (b) distance
(c) speed of light (d) intensity of light

8 Tesla is the unit of
(a) magnetic induction (b) magnetic field
(c) magnetic momentum (d) None of the above

9 Velocity is a .... quantity.
(a) practical (b) scalar
(c) fundamental (d) vector

10 Which of the following is not a vector quantity?
(a) Momentum (b) Displacement
(c) Torque (d) Speed

11 The quantity which has both magnitude and direction is known as
(a) scalar (b) variable (c) real (d) vector

12 Express 1 joule in terms of fundamental unit is
(a) 1 $kg^2m^2s^{-2}$ (b) 1 kg m^3s^{-2}
(c) 1 $kg^2m^2s^{-1}$ (d) 1 kg m^2s^{-2}

13 Which of the following is not matched?
(a) Decibel - Unit of sound
(b) Horse power - Unit of power
(c) Nautical mile - Unit of distance
(d) Celsius - Unit of heat

14 Match the List I with List II and select the correct answer using the codes given below.

	List I		List II
A.	Acceleration	1.	Joule
B.	Force	2.	Newton-second
C.	Work done	3.	Newton
D.	Impulse	4.	Metre per second^2

Codes

	A	B	C	D		A	B	C	D
(a)	1	2	3	4	(b)	2	3	4	1
(c)	4	3	1	2	(d)	3	4	1	2

15 Joule/Coulomb is equal to
(a) ohm (b) volt
(c) ampere (d) None of these

16 In domestic electric supply, we pay the bill for
(a) energy (kilowatt-hour)
(b) power (watt)
(c) current (coulomb/second)
(d) electric charge (coulomb)

17 Metric System or Decimal System is also known as
(a) MKS (b) CGS
(c) FPS (d) Both (a) and (b)

18 Noise is measured in
(a) watt (b) REM (c) centigrade (d) decibel

19 Liquid pressure measure by
(a) Manometer (b) Seismograph
(c) Hydrometer (d) None of these

20 Hydrometer is used to measure
(a) Density (b) Relative Density
(c) Both (a) and (b) (d) Wind speed

Answers

1 *(a)*	2 *(a)*	3 *(b)*	4 *(d)*	5 *(c)*	6 *(b)*	7 *(b)*	8 *(b)*	9 *(d)*	10 *(d)*
11 *(d)*	12 *(d)*	13 *(d)*	14 *(c)*	15 *(b)*	16 *(b)*	17 *(d)*	18 *(d)*	19 *(a)*	20 *(c)*

Chapter 02 Motion : Force and Laws of Motion

Rest and Motion

- If an object does not change its position with respect to its surroundings with time, then it is called at rest. e.g., a book lying on a desk is at rest, because its position with respect to the desk does not change with time.
- If an object changes its position with respect to its surroundings with time, then it is called in motion. e.g., a fish swims in water, car or bus moves on a road, train moves on the track, bird flying in air etc.

Important Definitions Related to Motion

Distance

The length of the actual path traversed by an object is called the distance. It is a scalar quantity and it can never be zero or negative during the motion of an object. Its unit is metre.

Displacement

The shortest distance between the initial and final positions of any object during motion is called displacement. It is a vector quantity. Its unit is metre. It may be positive, negative or zero.

Speed

The time rate of change of position of the object in any direction is called speed of the object.

$$\text{Speed } (v) = \frac{\text{Distance travelled } (s)}{\text{Time taken } (t)}$$

$$\text{Average speed} = \frac{\text{Total distance travelled}}{\text{Total time taken}}$$

Its unit is metre per second (m/s).

Instantaneous Speed The speed of a particle at any instant of time is known as its instantaneous speed.

$$\text{Instantaneous speed} = \lim_{\Delta t \to 0} \frac{\Delta s}{\Delta t} = \frac{ds}{dt}$$

Velocity

The rate of change of displacement of an object in a particular direction is called its velocity. Its unit is m/s.

$$\text{Velocity} = \frac{\text{Displacement}}{\text{Total time}}$$

It can be positive, zero and negative.

$$\text{Average velocity} = \frac{\text{Total displacement}}{\text{Total time}}$$

Instantaneous Velocity The velocity of a particle at any instant of time is known as its instantaneous velocity. Its unit is m/s.

Instantaneous velocity,

$$v = \lim_{\Delta t \to 0} \frac{\Delta r}{dt} = \frac{dr}{dt}$$

Acceleration

The time rate of change of velocity of a body is called acceleration. It is a vector quantity, denoted by a and its SI unit is m/s^2.

$$\therefore \text{Acceleration} = \frac{\text{Change in velocity } (\Delta v)}{\text{Time interval } (\Delta t)}$$

When velocity decreases due to acceleration, then it is called retardation.

Instantaneous Acceleration

Acceleration at any instant of time is known as instantaneous acceleration.

$$\text{Instantaneous acceleration } a = \lim_{\Delta t \to 0} \frac{\Delta v}{\Delta t} = \frac{dv}{dt}$$

Uniform and Non-Uniform Motion

- An object covers equal distances in equal intervals of time, then it is said to be in uniform motion. e.g., a car moving along a straight line path such that it covers equal distances in equal intervals of time, then it is said to be in **uniform motion.**
- On the other hand, if an object covers unequal distances in equal intervals of time then it is said to be in non-uniform motion. e.g., when a car is moving on a crowded street or a person is jogging in a park, these are said to be in **non-uniform motion.**

Equations of Motion

When a body is moving along a straight line with uniform acceleration, we can establish the relation between velocity of the body, acceleration of the body and the distance travelled by the body in a particular time interval by a set of equations. These equations are known as **equations of motion.**

The three equations of motion on a straight line are

- $v = u + at$
- $s = ut + (1/2)\, at^2$
- $v^2 - u^2 = 2as$

where u is the initial velocity of the body, a is the uniform acceleration of the body, v is the final velocity of the body after t second and s is the distance travelled in this time.

The three equations of free fall of an object near the surface of the earth are

- $v = u + gt$
- $h = ut + (1/2)\, gt^2$
- $v^2 = u^2 + 2gh$

where h is the height from which the object falls, t is the time of fall, u is the initial velocity and v is the final velocity when the body accelerates at g. Value of $g = 9.8$ m/s^2.

Uniform Circular Motion

If a body moves with uniform speed in a circular path, then its motion is called uniform circular motion. e.g., motion of an electric fan and motion of the moon and the earth.

Some basic terms related to circular motion are given below

- **Angular Displacement** It is defined as the angle through which an object moves on a circular path. It is the angle in radian, between the initial and final position.

  Displacement $\theta = \Delta s / r$

  where, Δs = length of arc and r = radius of circular path.
- **Angular Velocity** The time rate of change of angular displacement is called angular velocity. Its SI unit is rad s^{-1}.

  $$\text{Angular velocity, } \omega = \frac{\Delta\theta}{\Delta t}$$

  where, $\Delta\theta$ is the angular displacment and t is the time.

- **Angular Acceleration** Rate of change of angular velocity is called angular acceleration.

  Angular acceleration, $\alpha = \frac{d\omega}{dt} = \frac{d^2\theta}{dt^2}$

  Its unit is rad/s^2.

Force

- Force is an action which cause change is the state of motion of rest, its direction magnitude of speed, shape and size of a body.
- Force is a vector quantity, its SI unit is newton.

Inertia

The property of an object to rest any change in its state of motion along a straight line or rest is called inertia.

The mass of an object is a measure of its inertia.

Newton's Laws of Motion

- **First Law** Every body retains its state of rest or state of motion along a straight line until an external force is applied on it. This law is also known as **law of inertia.**

  e.g., the passengers in a bus falls backward, when it starts suddenly.
- **Second Law** The second law of motion states that the rate of change of momentum of an object is proportional to the applied unbalanced force in the direction of force.

  According to Newton's second law,

  Force, $F \propto$ Rate of change of momentum

  $$F \propto \frac{dp}{dt}$$

  where, dp = change in momentum

  and dt = change in time.

  On further calculation, Force, $F = ma$

  where, m = mass of the body

  and a = acceleration of the body.

  e.g., a cricket player (or fielder) moves his hands backward on catching a fast cricket ball.
- **Third Law** For every action, there is an equal and opposite reaction and both acts on two different bodies. So, this law is also known as **law of action and reaction.**

  e.g., recoiling of gun after firing a bullet and pushing of water backward by a swimmer.

Momentum

The momentum of a moving body is equal to the product of its mass and its velocity. It is a vector quantity having SI unit is kg-m/s.

If a body of mass (m) moves with a velocity (v), then momentum (p) is given by $p = mv$

Its dimensional formula is $[MLT^{-1}]$.

Law of Conservation of Momentum

If no external force acts upon a system of two (or more) bodies, then the total momentum of the system remains constant. This is called the law of conservation of momentum.

Consider a system of two bodies of masses m_1 and m_2 moving with initial velocities u_1 and u_2 respectively, in opposite direction. After collision, the bodies move with a common velocity of v, then according to law of conservation of momentum, $m_1 u_1 + m_2 u_2 = (m_1 + m_2)v$

Impulse

If a large force is acting on a body for a very short time, then the product of this large force (F) and time (Δt) is known as impulse and large force itself is called impulsive force.

Impulse = Change in momentum

= Force × Time

It is a vector quantity and its SI unit is N-s or kg-m/s.

Friction

When a body slides or rolls over another body or on a surface, then a force opposing the motion acts between those surfaces of the body which are in contact, this force is called force of friction.

e.g., whenever the surface of a body slides over the surface of another body, each body exerts a frictional force on the other which is parallel to the surface in contact.

Centripetal Force

A body performing circular motion is acted upon by a force directed along the radius towards the centre of the circle. This force is called the centripetal force.

∵ Centripetal force
= Mass × Centripetal acceleration

$$F = \frac{mv^2}{r}$$

$$\Rightarrow \quad F = mr\omega^2 \qquad [\because v = r\omega]$$

where, v = linear velocity of the body on circular track.

Centrifugal Force

- It is a force that arises when a body is moving actually along a circular path, by virtue of tendency of the body to regain its natural straight line path.
- It is regarded as reaction of centripetal force. It acts along the radius and away from the centre of the circle.
- It is a pseudo force.

Stability

Stability is the ability of an object to maintain its balance after being disturbed. The stability of object is extremely dependent upon its centre of gravity.

Centre of Gravity

- Centre of gravity of a rigid body is the point at which its whole weight can be supposed to act. Its position depends upon the distribution of mass of the body. It may be inside or outside the body.
- If the body is of symmetrical shape whose weight is distributed uniformly, then the centre of gravity of the body lies at its geometrical centre. e.g., the centre of gravity of a uniform straight wire is at its mid-point.

Equilibrium of an Object or Body

An object is said to be in equilibrium, if a number of forces acting on it produce no change in its state of rest or of uniform motion.

Types of Equilibrium

There are three types of equilibrium as given below

- **Static Equilibrium** A body is said to be in static (or stable) equilibrium, if it has a tendency to return to its original position, after being slightly disturbed from its equilibrium position.
- **Dynamic Equilibrium** A body is said to be in dynamic (unstable) equilibrium, if it has no tendency to come to its original position after being disturbed from its equilibrium position.
- **Neutral Equilibrium** A body is said to be in neutral equilibrium, if on being disturbed from its initial position, it stays in equilibrium in new position also.

Exam Pattern Questions

1 Which of the following is a scalar quantity?
(a) Velocity
(b) Acceleration
(c) Force
(d) Distance

2 What is called 'change in position in a particular direction of an object'?
(a) Velocity (b) Acceleration
(c) Displacement (d) None of these

3 Ahmed is driving his car with a velocity of 45 km/h. How much distance will be cover in one minute?
(a) 750 m (b) 900 m (c) 75 m (d) 450 m

4 A train covers the first half of the distance between two stations at a speed of 40 km/h and other half at 60 km/h, then its average speed is
(a) 100 km/h (b) 48 km/h
(c) 52 km/h (d) None of these

5 A body moving with uniform velocity. Its acceleration will be
(a) positive (b) negative
(c) zero (d) cannot determine

6 The rate of change of velocity is called
(a) acceleration (b) force
(c) momentum (d) impulse

7 Which equation is wrong in the following ?
(a) $s = ut + \frac{1}{2}at^2$
(b) $v = u + at$
(c) $v^2 - u^2 = 2\,as$
(d) $v = u + as$

8 A racing car is moving with an uniform acceleration of 4 ms^{-2}. How much distance will it cover in 10 s after it starts moving from rest?
(a) 200 m (b) 300 m
(c) 100 m (d) 2000 m

9 A particle falls freely from a height *h*, then find the height covered in 2 s.
(a) 9.8 m (b) 19.6 m (c) 4.9 m (d) 5 m

10 In which motion is the acceleration always directed normal to the direction of motion?
(a) Linear motion
(b) Circular motion
(c) Projectile motion
(d) Simple harmonic motion

11 In uniform circular motion of a body
(a) the velocity is constant but speed changes
(b) the speed is constant but velocity changes
(c) Both speed as well as velocity change
(d) Both speed as well as velocity is constant

12 When a body moves at a constant speed in a circular path, it has
(a) an acceleration directed tangentially
(b) an acceleration directed radially inward
(c) an acceleration away from the centre
(d) no acceleration is directed

13 Force can cause change in
(a) state of motion rest
(b) direction of motion
(c) shape and size of object
(d) All of the above

14 The property of a body by virtue of which it tends to remain in its state at motion or of rest is called
(a) force (b) momentum
(c) inertia (d) None of these

15 The inertia of a body depends on
(a) mass (b) velocity
(c) acceleration (d) length

16 The sole of shoes one made rough to increase
(a) sliding motion
(b) rolling motion
(c) frictional force
(d) momentum

17 Newton's first law is also called as
(a) law of conservation of momentum
(b) law of inertia
(c) law of energy conservation
(d) None of the above

18 Which of the following is a vector quantity?
(a) Time (b) Momentum
(c) Volume (d) Density

19 If the velocity of a moving body is doubled, then which of the following quantities is doubled?
(a) Acceleration (b) Weight
(c) Mass (d) Momentum

20 Momentum is the product of mass and
(a) distance
(b) velocity
(c) distance and velocity
(d) None of the above

21 Change in momentum will be equal to
(a) velocity (b) acceleration
(c) force (d) Impulse

22 Newton's second law also explains the law of
(a) velocity (b) acceleration
(c) momentum (d) speed

23 When a constant force is applied to a body, it moves with uniform
(a) speed (b) velocity
(c) acceleration (d) momentum

24 The rate of change of momentum is called
(a) acceleration
(b) kinetic energy
(c) force
(d) None of the above

25 A bullet of mass 0.01 kg is fired down a gun of mass 5 kg. If the velocity of bullet is 250 m/s, then the gun recoils at a velocity of

(a) 0.5 m/s (b) 0.25 m/s
(c) – 0.5 m/s (d) –0.25 m/s

26 The equation of relation between force, mass and acceleration is

(a) $a = mF$ (b) $m = aF$
(c) $ma = \frac{1}{F}$ (d) $ma = F$

27 A driver initially accelerates the car at 1.8 m/s^2 and subsequently at 1.2 m/s^2. The ratio of the forces exerted by the engine will be

(a) 3 : 2 (b) 2 : 3
(c) 2 : 1 (d) 7 : 2

28 The change in momentum for short time is called

(a) inertia
(b) momentum conservation
(c) impulse
(d) centripetal force

Answers

1 (d)	2 (c)	3 (a)	4 (b)	5 (c)	6 (a)	7 (d)	8 (a)	9 (b)	10 (b)
11 (b)	12 (c)	13 (d)	14 (c)	15 (a)	16 (c)	17 (b)	18 (b)	19 (d)	20 (b)
21 (d)	22 (c)	23 (c)	24 (c)	25 (c)	26 (d)	27 (a)	28 (c)		

Solutions

3 Velocity $= \frac{\text{Distance}}{\text{Time}} = \frac{45 \text{ km}}{1 \text{ h}}$

$= \frac{45000}{60} = 750$ m/min

∴ He travels 750m in one minute.

4 Average speed $= \frac{2(v_1 \times v_2)}{v_1 + v_2}$

$= \frac{2 \times 40 \times 60}{40 + 60} = 48$ km/h

8 Given, $u = 0$, $a = 4 \text{ ms}^{-2}$ and $t = 10$s

Using second equation of motion,

$s = ut + \frac{1}{2}at$

$= 0 + \frac{1}{2} \times 4 \times (10)^2 = 200$ m

9 Given, $t = 2, u = 0$

Using second equation of free fall,

$h = ut + \frac{1}{2}gt^2$

$= 0 + \frac{1}{2} \times 9.8 \times (2)^2$

$= 19.6$ m

25 Given, $m_1 = 0.01$ kg, $m_2 = 5$ kg,

$u_1 = 0, u_2 = 0$

$v_1 = 250$ m/s, $v_2 = ?$

Using conservation of momentum,

$m_1u_1 + m_2u_2 = m_1v_1 + m_2v_2$

$0 = 0.01 \times 250 + 5 \times v_2$

$\Rightarrow v_2 = -\frac{0.01 \times 250}{5}$

$= -0.5$ m/s

27 Given, $a_1 = 1.8 \text{ m/s}^2$, $a_2 = 1.2 \text{ m/s}^2$

Force, $F = ma = \frac{F_1}{F_2} = \frac{m a_1}{m a_2} = \frac{a_1}{a_2}$

$= \frac{1.8}{1.2} = \frac{3}{2}$ or 3:2

Chapter 03 Gravitation

Gravitation is defined as the non-contact force of attraction between any two bodies in the universe. The earth attracts all the bodies towards its centre. The force with which the earth pulls the bodies towards its centre is called the **gravitational force** of earth.

Universal law of Gravitation

Universal law of Gravitation was given by Issac Newton. According to this law, the attractive force between any two objects in the universe is directly proportional to the product of their masses and inversely proportional to the square of distance between them.

i.e. $$F \propto \frac{m_1 m_2}{r^2}$$

$$F = \frac{G\, m_1\, m_2}{r^2}$$

where, G is universal gravitational constant.

$$G = 6.67 \times 10^{-11}\ \text{N m}^2\ \text{kg}^{-2}$$

Free Fall

Whenever objects fall towards the earth under the earth's gravitational force alone, then this phenomena called freely falling objects and such a motion is called free fall.

Acceleration due to Gravity

- Whenever an object falls towards the earth, an acceleration is involved. This acceleration is due to the earth's gravitational pull and is called acceleration due to gravity (or acceleration due to the gravitational force of the earth).
- If mass of earth be M and an object falling freely towards it be m. The distance between centre of earth and the object is R. Then, acceleration due to gravity is

$$g = \frac{GM}{R^2}$$

- The acceleration due to gravity does not depend m, the mass of a falling object. The SI unit of g is m/s^2.
- As distance of an object from the centre of the celestial body increases, the value of g decreases.
- Earth is flattened at poles. Thus radius of earth is less at poles than at equator, hence the value of g is less at equator than at poles.

Mass

- Mass is the total content of the body which measures the inertia of a body. It is a scalar quantity and is measured in kilogram.
- Irrespective of the position of the body in the universe, mass always remains constant everywhere.
- The mass of the body cannot be zero.

Weight

The weight of an object is the force with which it is attracted towards the earth.

Weight of an object, $w = mg$

where, $m =$ mass and $g =$ acceleration due to gravity.

or $$w = \frac{GMm}{R^2}$$

Here, M = mass of the earth
and R = radius of the earth.

- Weight is a vector quantity, it acts in vertically downward direction and its SI unit is newton (N).
- Weight of an object is not constant, it changes from place to place.
- At the centre of earth, weight becomes zero.
- Spring balance is used to measure the weight of a body and pan balance is used to measure the mass of a body.
- The weight of an object on the moon is one-sixth of the weight on the earth.

$$w_m = \frac{1}{6} w_e$$

Planet

The heavenly body which revolves around the sun is called planet, e.g. the earth.

Kepler's Laws of Planetary Motion

- **Kepler's First Law** It states that the path of any planet in an orbit around the sun follows the shape of an ellipse with the sun at one of the foci.
- **Kepler's Second Law** It states that an imaginary line from the sun to the planet sweeps out equal areas in equal intervals of time.
- **Kepler's Third Law** It states that the cube of the mean distance of a planet from the sun is directly proportional to the square of time T to move around the sun. It is expressed as

$$r^3 \propto T^2, \Rightarrow r^3 = k \times T^2$$

$$k = \frac{r^3}{T^2}$$

where, T = time period of the planet (around the sun), r = radius as mean distance of the planet from the sun and k = Kepler's constant.

Satellite

A satellite is a body which is constantly revolving in an orbit around a comparatively much larger body. Satellite is of two types
- Natural satellite
- Artificial satellite

Orbital Velocity

Orbital velocity of a satellite is the maximum velocity required to put the satellite into a given orbit around the earth. It is denoted by v_o.

$$v_0 = \sqrt{\frac{GM}{R+h}}$$

where, M = mass of earth,
R = radius of earth,
h = height of satellite
and $R + h$ = orbital radius.

Escape Velocity

- The minimum velocity of the body that should be given to the body to enable it to escape away from earth's gravitational field is called escape velocity.
- Escape velocity,

$$v_e = \sqrt{2gR} = \sqrt{\frac{2GM}{R}}$$

where, g = gravitational acceleration
and R = radius of earth.

- Its value on the earth's surface is 11.2 km/s.
- Relation between orbital velocity of a satellite and escape velocity is $v_e = \sqrt{2}v_o$.

Exam Pattern Questions

1 Who defined the law of gravitation?
(a) Newton (b) Archimedes'
(c) Galileo (d) Faraday

2 For the relation $F = \frac{GMm}{r^2}$, the quantity G
(a) depends on the value of g at the place of observation
(b) is used only when the earth is one of the two masses
(c) is greatest at the surface of the earth
(d) is universal constant of nature

3 The value of universal gravitation constant G is
(a) 6.67×10^{-11} Nm^2/kg^2
(b) 5.67×10^{-11} Nm^2/kg^2
(c) 4.67×10^{-11} Nm^2/kg^2
(d) 3.67×10^{-11} Nm^2/kg^2

4 Two particles are placed at some distance. If the mass of each of the two particles is doubled keeping the distance between them unchanged, then the value of gravitational force between them will be
(a) 1/4 times (b) 4 times
(c) 1/2 times (d) unchanged

5 Intensity of gravitational field of the earth is maximum at
(a) poles (b) equator
(c) centre of earth (d) surface

6 Law of gravitation gives the gravitational force between
(a) the earth and a point mass only
(b) the earth and sun only
(c) any two bodies having some mass
(d) two charges bodies only

7 The value of quantity G is the law of gravitation
(a) depends on mass of earth only
(b) depends on radius of earth only
(c) depends on both mass and radius of earth
(d) is independent of mass and radius of the earth

8 The atmosphere is held to the earth by
(a) gravity
(b) wind
(c) clouds
(d) earth's magnetic field

9 The force of attraction between two unit point masses separated by a unit distance is called
(a) gravitational potential
(b) acceleration due to gravity
(c) gravitational field
(d) universal gravitational constant

10 Which of the following statement is true?
(a) g is the same at all places on the surface of the earth.
(b) g is less at the earth's surface then at a height above or at a depth below it.
(c) g has its maximum value at the equator.
(d) g is the greater at the poles than at the equator.

11 When a body falls freely towards the earth, then its total energy
(a) increases
(b) decreases
(c) remains constant
(d) first increases and then decreases

12 A body is falling from a height h after it has fallen a height $\frac{h}{2}$. It will possess
(a) only potential energy
(b) only kinetic energy
(c) half potential and half kinetic energy
(d) more kinetic and less potential energy

13 The value of acceleration due to gravity
(a) is same on equator and poles
(b) is least on poles
(c) is least on equator
(d) increases from pole to equator

14 Two objects of different masses falling freely near the surface of moon would
(a) have same velocities at any instant
(b) have different acceleration
(c) experience force of same magnitude
(d) undergo a change in their inertia

15 An apple falls from a tree because of gravitational attraction between the earth and apple. If F_1 is the magnitude of force exerted by the earth on the apple and F_2 is the magnitude of force exerted by apple on earth, then

(a) F_1 is very much greater than F_2
(b) F_2 is very much greater than F_1
(c) F_1 is only a little greater than F_2
(d) F_1 and F_2 are equal

16 Astronauts in space cannot stand erect, this is because in space
(a) pressure is very high (b) pressure is very low
(c) there is no gravity (d) there is high gravity

17 The weight of an object at the centre of the earth of radius R is
(a) zero
(b) infinite
(c) R times the weight at the surface of the earth
(d) $1/R^2$ times the weight at the surface of the earth

18 What is weight in newtons of a 10kg object on the moon?
(a) 15 N (b) 15.33 N (c) 16 N (d) 16. 33N

19 If one moves from the surface of earth to moon, what will be the effect on its weight?
(a) Weight of a person decreases continuously with height from the surface of earth
(b) Weight of a person increases with height from the surface of earth
(c) Weight of a person first decreases with height and then increases with height from the surface of earth
(d) Weight of a person first increases with height and then decreases with height from the surface of earth

20 If m_e is the mass of a body on the surface of the earth and m_m is the mass of the same body on the moon, then
(a) $m_e = 6m_m$ (b) $m_e < m_m$
(c) $m_e > m_m$ (d) $m_e = m_m$

21 If w_e is the weight of a body on the surface of the earth and w_m is the weight of the same body on the moon, then
(a) $w_e = 6w_m$ (b) $w_e = w_m$
(c) $w_e < w_m$ (d) $w_e = w_m = 0$

22 One goes from the centre of the earth to a distance two-third the radius of the earth, where will the acceleration due to gravity be the greatest?
(a) At the centre of the earth
(b) At a depth half the radius of the earth
(c) At a depth one-third the radius of the earth
(d) At a depth two-third the radius of the earth

23 Spring balance is used to measure the …… of a body.
(a) mass (b) weight
(c) force (d) acceleration

24 Pan balance is used to measure the …… of a body.
(a) mass (b) weight
(c) velocity (d) speed

25 Who gave laws of planetary motion?
(a) Newton (b) Lenz
(c) Kepler (d) Galileo

Answers

1 (a)	2 (d)	3 (a)	4 (b)	5 (a)	6 (c)	7 (d)	8 (a)	9 (d)	10 (d)
11 (c)	12 (c)	13 (c)	14 (a)	15 (d)	16 (c)	17 (a)	18 (d)	19 (c)	20 (d)
21 (c)	22 (c)	23 (b)	24 (a)	25 (c)					

Solutions

4 $F = \frac{G\,m_1 m_2}{r^2}$

$$F' = G\frac{(2m_1)(2m_2)}{r^2} = 4\frac{G\,m_1 m_2}{r^2} = 4F$$

9 We have, $F = \frac{GMm}{r^2} = G\frac{1\times 1}{(1)^2}$

$$F = G$$

18 Mass of an object, $m = 10$ kg

Weight on the earth, $w = mg = 10 \times 9.8 = 98$ N

Weight on the moon $= \frac{1}{6}$ of the weight on the earth

$$= \frac{1}{6} \times 98 = 16.33 \text{ N}$$

Chapter 04 Work, Energy and Power

Work

When a body is displaced by applying a force on it in the direction of applied force, then work is said to be done.

Work done by a Constant Force

If a constant force F acts on an objects and object is displaced through a distance s in the direction of force.

Then, work $W =$ force $\times$ displacement in the direction of force

$$W = F \times s$$

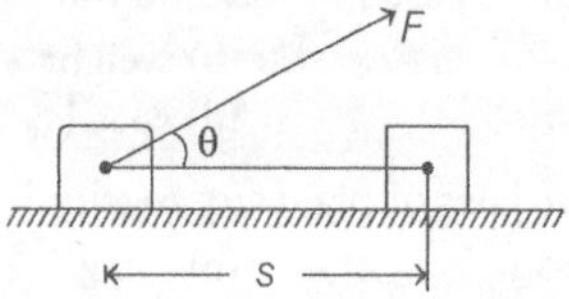

- Work is scalar quantity and its unit is joule.
- If there is an angle θ between the direction of force and direction of displacement, then

$$W = Fs \cos\theta$$

Value of work will be maximum at $\theta° = 0$ and minimum at $\theta = 90°$.

Types of Work

- **Positive Work** When the force and displacement are in the same direction, then work done will be positive. e.g., a boy pulls an object towards himself.
- **Negative Work** When the force and displacement are in opposite direction, then work done will be negative.
- **Zero Work** When the force and displacement are in perpendicular direction, then work done will be zero. e.g., if a body in moving on circle, then after completing one circle work done is zero because of zero displacement.

Energy

The ability of a body to do some work is called energy. It is a scalar quantity and its unit is joule in SI and erg in CGS. Larger unit of energy is kilojoule (kJ).

Mechanical Energy

The energy that is possessed by an object due to its motion or due to its position is called mechanical energy.

It is of two types

- **Kinetic Energy** The energy possessed by a body due to its motion is called its kinetic energy.

$$\text{KE} = \frac{1}{2} mv^2$$

where, $v =$ velocity of a body at any time,
and $m =$ mass of the body.

e.g., when a fast moving cricket ball hits a stationary wicket, the wicket is thrown away.

- **Potential Energy** The energy possessed by a body due to change in its position of shape is called potential energy.

$$\text{PE} = mgh$$

where, $g =$ acceleration due to gravity,
$h =$ height above the surface
and $m =$ mass of the body.

e.g., water stored in dam, a stone placed on the roof of building has potential energy due to their height.

Relation between Kinetic Energy and Linear Momentum

$$KE = \frac{p^2}{2m}$$

From above relation, it is clear that an object cannot have kinetic energy without having momentum and *vice-versa.*

Law of Conservation of Energy

According to law of conservation of energy, energy can only be transformed from one form to another, it can neither be created nor be destroyed. The total energy before and after transformation always remains constant.

$$KE + PE = \text{constant}$$

e.g., when an athlete runs, the body's internal energy is converted into kinetic energy.

Work-Energy Theorem

The kinetic energy of an object in measured by the amound of work, $W = \frac{1}{2}m(v^2 - u^2)$

This is known as work-energy theorem.

If initial velocity $u = 0$, then $W = \frac{1}{2}mv^2$

This work done is equal to the kinetic energy of the object.

Commercial Unit of Energy

The commercial unit of electric energy is kilowatt-hour (kWh).

It is the amount of electric energy consumed by an appliance of power 1000 W in one hour.

$$1 \text{ kWh} = 1 \text{ kW} \times 1 \text{h} = 1000 \text{ W} \times 3600 \text{ s}$$
$$= 1000 \text{ Js}^{-1} \times 3600 \text{ s}$$
$$1 \text{ kWh} = 3.6 \times 10^6 \text{ J}$$

Power

Power is defined as the rate of doing work or the rate of transfer of energy. The unit of power is watt (W).

$$\text{Power } (P) = \frac{\text{Work } (W)}{\text{Time } (t)} = \frac{F \cdot s}{t} \quad [\because W = F \cdot s]$$

$$P = F \cdot v \left[\because \frac{s}{t} = v\right]$$

We express larger rate of energy transfer in kilowatt (kW).

$$1 \text{ W} = 1 \text{ J/s}$$

or
$$1 \text{ kW} = 1000 \text{ W}$$
$$= 1000 \text{ Js}^{-1}$$
$$1 \text{ MW} = 10^6 \text{ W}$$
$$1 \text{ horse power (HP)} = 746 \text{ W}$$

Exam Pattern Questions

1 The earth moving around the sun in a circular orbit is acted upon by a force and hence work done on the earth by the force is
(a) zero (b) positive
(c) negative (d) None of these

2 If F force is applied on a body and body get displaced by s displacement, then work done on the body will be
(a) work = force/displacement
(b) work = displacement/force
(c) work = force × displacement
(d) None of the above

3 In case of negative work, the angle between the force and displacement is
(a) 0° (b) 45°
(c) 90° (d) 180°

4 The work done on an object does not depend upon the
(a) displacement
(b) force applied
(c) angle between force and displacement
(d) initial velocity of the object

5 Work has the same unit as
(a) power (b) energy
(c) momentum (d) impulse

6 Work done is zero by
(a) a weight lifter while holding a weight of 100 kg on his shoulders for 1 min
(b) a locomotive against gravity when it is running on a level plane with a speed of 60km/h
(c) a person holding a suitcase on his head and standing at a bus terminal
(d) All of the above

7 What is the angle between force and displacement for maximum work?
(a) 0° (b) 30°
(c) 45° (d) 90°

8 A pair of bullocks exerts a force of 140 N on a plough. The field being ploughed is 15m long, how much work is done in ploughing the length of field?
(a) 1100 J (b) 2100 J
(c) 550 J (d) 4200 J

9 Water stored in an dam possesses
(a) kinetic energy
(b) potential energy
(c) electrical energy
(d) no energy

10 A body is moving up with a velocity *v*. If the velocity of this body is suddenly tripled, then its kinetic energy will be
(a) triple
(b) double
(c) one-third
(d) nine times

11 The potential energy of a system increases, if work is done
(a) by the system against a conservative force
(b) by the system against a non-conservative force
(c) upon the system by a conservative force
(d) upon the system by a non-conservative force

12 A body is thrown upward with some initial velocity, then at top position
(a) total energy is in the form of kinetic energy
(b) total energy is in the form of potential energy
(c) kinetic energy and potential energy is same
(d) potential energy is zero

13 When a body falls freely towards the earth, then its total energy
(a) decreases
(b) increases
(c) remains same
(d) first decreases and then increases

14 The mass of the body is halved and its speed is doubled. What happens to the kinetic energy of the body?
(a) Halved (b) Four times
(c) Doubled (d) Remains same

15 The energy possessed by a body due to its position is called
(a) kinetic energy (b) potential energy
(c) mechanical energy (d) total energy

16 The energy stored in a watch spring is
(a) kinetic energy (b) potential energy
(c) electrical energy (d) chemical energy

17 When velocity of a moving body increases by a applying force, then which of the following is true?
(a) Work done on the body is equal to change in its kinetic energy.
(b) Work done on the body is greater than change in kinetic energy.
(c) Work done on the body is less than change in kinetic energy.
(d) Change in potential energy is equal to work done on the body

18 If momentum of a body is increased to doubled, then its kinetic energy will be
(a) doubled
(b) half
(c) four times
(d) remains same

19 The example of conservative energy is
(a) gravitational energy
(b) magnetic energy
(c) electrostatic energy
(d) All of the above

20 A body of mass 4 kg is throwing upward with a speed of 4 m/s. The maximum height attained by the body is [given $g = 10\ \text{m/s}^2$]
(a) 0.4 m (b) 0.6 m
(c) 0.8 m (d) 1 m

Answers

1 (a)	2 (c)	3 (d)	4 (d)	5 (b)	6 (d)	7 (a)	8 (b)	9 (b)	10 (d)
11 (a)	12 (b)	13 (c)	14 (c)	15 (b)	16 (b)	17 (a)	18 (c)	19 (d)	20 (c)

Solutions

3 $W = F \cdot s \cos\theta$

$\because \cos 180° = -1$

$\therefore \quad W = -F \cdot d$

For negative work, the angle between the force and displacement should be 180°.

7 Work done will be maximum, if

$\cos\theta = 1$ or° $\theta = 0°$

$W = Fs\cos\theta = Fs$

8 $F = 140$ N,

$s = 15$m

$W = Fs = Fs\cos\theta \quad [\because \theta = 0°]$

$= 140 \times 15 \times \cos\theta$

$= 140 \times 15 \times \cos 0°$

$= 140 \times 15 \times 1 \quad [\because \cos 0° = 1]$

$= 2100$ J

10 (d) Kinetic energy $K \propto v^2$

$$\frac{K_2}{K_1} = \left(\frac{v_2}{v_1}\right)^2 = \left(\frac{3v_1}{v_1}\right)^2 = 9$$

$K_2 = 9K_1 \quad [v_2 = 3v_1]$

14 $(m') = \frac{m}{2}$,

Speed $\quad v' = 2v, K_1 = \frac{1}{2}mv^2$

Kinetic energy, $K' = \frac{1}{2}m'v'^2$

$= \frac{1}{2}\frac{m}{2}(2v)^2$

$= mv^2$

$= 2.\frac{1}{2}mv^2$

$= 2K_1$

18 (c) Kinetic energy, $K = \frac{p^2}{2m}$ [where, p = momeutum]

$$\therefore \quad \frac{K_2}{K_1} = \left(\frac{p_2}{p_1}\right)^2 = \left[\frac{2p_1}{p_1}\right]^2 = 4$$

$[p_2 = 2p_1]$

$\therefore \quad K_2 = 4K_1$

20 (c) If h be the maximum height attained by the body then at top position, kinetic energy converted into potential energy.

$\therefore \quad mgh = \frac{1}{2}mv^2$

$h = \frac{v^2}{2g}$

$= \frac{4^2}{2 \times 10} = 0.8$ m

Chapter 05

Physical Properties and States of Matter

Matter

Matter is anything that has mass and volume or we can say that anything that has mass occupies space and can be felt by our one or more sense organ is called matter.

Important characteristics of matter are as follows

(i) Matter is made up of very small particles (atoms or molecules) that are beyond our imagination.

(ii) The particles have space in between them, called the **intermolecular space.**

(iii) They are continuously moving, i.e. they possess kinetic energy.
As the temperature rises, speed of the particles increases. Due to which the kinetic energy of the particles increases.

(iv) They attract each other. The force of attraction responsible for keeping them together is called **intermolecular force.**

States of Matter

Almost all substances exist in three states under appropriate conditions of temperature and pressure.

1. Solids

In this state of matter, the substances have definite mass, volume and shape, e.g., wood, table, pen, book, etc.

- Solids have a definite shape and a definite volume.
- Intermolecular forces operating between the molecules are very strong due to which their positions are fixed. Molecules can only vibrate to and fro about their mean positions.
- Molecules are closely packed and associated with minimum energy.

Note The melting point of a solid is an indication of strength of intermolecular forces of attraction.

Solids can be of following two types

- **Crystalline solids** Constituent particles are arranged in an orderly arrangement over the long range. e.g., graphite, diamond, NaCl etc.
- **Amorphous solids** Constituent particles do not possess the orderly arrangement over the long range. e.g., glass, rubber and plastic etc. Glass is a supercooled liquid.

2. Liquids

In this state, the substances have no fixed shape but have a fixed volume. They take up the shape of the container in which they are kept. e.g., water, oil, milk, etc.

- Liquids have no definite shape but have a definite volume.
- Intermolecular forces operating between the molecules are weak due to which they can slide over one another but cannot escape the boundary in normal conditions.
- Molecules are closely packed and associated with intermediate energy due to motion.

3. Gases

In this state, matter have no fixed shape and volume. They only occupy the shape and size of the container in which they are kept. e.g., air, H_2, O_2, N_2, etc.

- Gases have neither definite shape nor volume.
- Intermolecular forces operating between the molecules are very weak due to which their positions are not fixed and thus they can move freely.

- Molecules are wide apart and are associated with maximum energy.
- Gases exert pressure on the walls of the container due to collision of molecules with the walls of the container.

Note Compressibility depends upon the intermolecular spaces between the particles of matter.

Compressibility $\propto$ Intermolecular spaces

Solid < Liquid < Gas

Physical Properties of Matter

Elasticity

- It is the property of material of a body by virtue of which the body acquires its original shape and size after the removal of deforming force.
- A force which changes the configuration of a body is called a **deforming force**. Steel is more elastic than rubber.
- **Perfect Elastic Body** If a body completely regains its original configuration on removal of external deforming forces, it is called a perfectly elastic body.
- **Plastic Body** If a body has no tendency to regain its original configuration and tends to maintain its deformed state even after the removal of the deforming force, then the body is called a plastic (or non-elastic) body.

Stress

- The internal restoring force acting per unit area of cross-section of the deformed body is called stress. Its SI unit is N/m^2 or pascal.

Strain

- The change in length, volume and shape of the body per unit of the original value under the application of the deforming force is called strain. Strain is unitless quantity.

$$\text{i.e., strain} = \frac{\text{change in length}}{\text{original length}}$$

Hooke's Law

According to this law within the elastic limit, the stress developed in a body is directly proportional to the strain produced in the body.

i.e., stress $\propto$ strain

$\Rightarrow$ Stress $= E \times$ Strain

where, E is the modulus of elasticity

There are three types of modulus of elasticity

- **Young's modulus of elasticity** (Y) Within the elastic limit, it is defined as the ratio of normal stress to the longitudinal strain.

$$\text{Thus, } Y = \frac{\text{normal stress}}{\text{longitudinal strain}}$$

$$= \frac{F/A}{\Delta L/L} = \frac{F \cdot L}{\pi r^2 \Delta L} = \frac{MgL}{\pi r^2 \Delta L}$$

- **Bulk modulus of elasticity** (K) Within the elastic limit, it is defined as the ratio of normal stress to the volumetric strain.

$$\text{Thus, } K = \frac{\text{normal stress}}{\text{volumetric strain}} = -\frac{F/A}{\Delta V/V} = \frac{pV}{\Delta V}$$

$$[\because F/A = p]$$

- **Modulus of rigidity or shear modulus of elasticity** (η) With in the elastic limit, it is defined as the ratio of tangential stress to the shearing strain.

$$\text{Thus, } \eta = \frac{\text{tangential stress}}{\text{shearing strain}} = \frac{F/A}{\theta} = \frac{FL}{Ax}.$$

Pressure

It is the force acting perpendicularly on a unit area of an object.

$$\text{Pressure } (p) = \frac{\text{Force } (F)}{\text{Area } (A)} = \frac{\text{Thrust}}{\text{Area}}$$

The SI unit of prssure is Nm^{-2}, which is also called pascal (Pa) named after the scientist Blaise Pascal. It is a scalar quantity.

$$1 \text{ Pa} = 1 \text{ Nm}^{-2}$$

Atmospheric Pressure

- The gaseous envelope surrounding the earth is called atmosphere and the pressure exerted by atmosphere is called atmospheric pressure.
- It is maximum at the surface of earth and goes on decreasing as we move up into earth's atmosphere.
- The value of atmospheric pressure on the surface of earth at sea level is called one atmosphere (1 atm) and is nearly equal to 1.013×10^5 Nm^{-2}.

- SI unit of atmospheric pressure is Nm^{-2} or pascal and CGS unit is dyne/cm^2.
- Atmospheric pressure is also measured in mm or in cm of mercury column. It is also measured in torr.

1 torr = 1 mm of mercury

- The unit of atmospheric pressure used for metreological purpose is called bar.

1 bar = 10 Pa

and 1 millibar $= 10^{-3}$ bar $= 100$ Pa

Mercury Barometer

An Italian scientist **Evangelista Torricelli** (1608-1647), first devised an instrument to measure atmospheric pressure. It is known as **barometer**. A long glass tube closed at one end and filled with mercury is inverted into a trough of mercury.

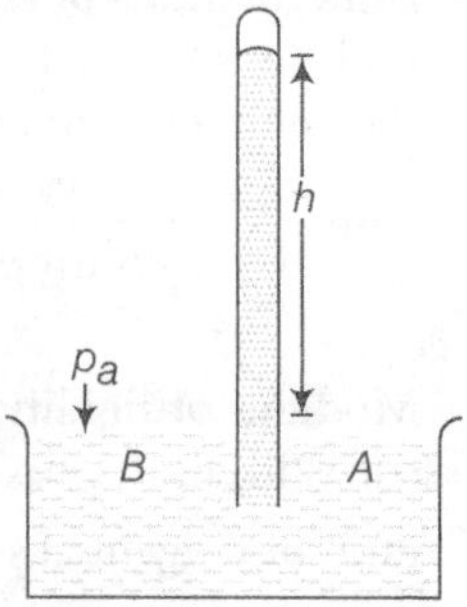

We find that mercury column in the tube has height of about 76 cm above the mercury level in the trough.

The space above mercury in the tube contains mercury vapour and its pressure can be neglected.

Let us consider points *B* and *A* as shown in the figure.

Let *h* is the height of mercury column and ρ is the density of mercury so

$$p_A = p_B = p_a = h\rho g$$

Volume

The space occupied by an object (solid, liquid and gas) is called the value of that object. Its SI unit is cubic metre.

Density

Mass (m) per unit volume (V) is known as density (d). i.e., $d = \dfrac{m}{V}$

It is a scalar quantity having SI unit kg/m^3.

Relative Density (Specific Gravity)

The relative density (specific gravity) of a substance is the ratio of its density to that of water at 4° C.

$$\text{Relative density} = \frac{\text{Density of substance}}{\text{Density of water at } 4°\text{C}}$$

Note Density of water at 4°C is 1×10^3 kg/m^3 and density of ice is 0.9 g/cm^3.

Pressure of Liquid

The normal force exerted by a liquid per unit area of the surface in contact is called pressure of liquid or hydrostatic pressure.

Pressure exerted by a liquid column $p = h\rho g$

where, h = height of liquid column,

ρ = density of liquid

and g = acceleration due to gravity.

Pascal's Law

It states that a pressure applied to fluid in a closed container is transmitted equally to every point of the fluid and the walls of the container.

Buoyancy

The upward force exerted by the liquid on the objects immersed in it, is called upthrust or buoyant force and this phenomena is called buoyancy.

Archimedes' Principle

When an object is fully or partially immersed in a liquid, it experiences an upward force that is equal to the weight of the fluid displaced by it.

Weight of displaced fluid =

Weight of object in air − Weight of object in fluid

Viscosity

It is the property of liquid by virtue of which it opposes the relative motion between its adjacent layers viscosity of an ideal fluid is zero.

Surface Tension

- It is the tendency of liquid surfaces to shrink into the minimum surface area possible.
- Its SI unit is N/m or J/m^2 and it is a scalar quantity.

- It is measured as the force acting per unit length of imaginary line drawn on the free surface of liquid.

$$\text{Surface tension} = \frac{\text{Force}}{\text{Length}}$$

- Small liquid drops are spherical due to the property of surface tension.

Gaseous Laws

Mass (m), volume (V), pressure (p) and temperature (T) of a gas are the measurable properties. The laws which inter-relate these properties, are called gas laws.

Let's discuss the various gas laws which give the relationship between measurable properties of gases.

- **Boyle's Law** At constant temperature, the volume of the given mass of a gas is inversely proportional to its pressure.

$$V \propto \frac{1}{p} \quad \text{[at constant temperature]}$$

$$pV = \text{constant or } p_1V_1 = p_2V_2$$

- **Charles' Law** At constant pressure, the volume of given mass of the gas is directly proportional to its absolute temperature.

$$V \propto T \quad \text{[at constant pressure]}$$

or $$\frac{V_1}{T_1} = \frac{V_2}{T_2}$$

Absolute zero is that temperature at which all molecular motion ceases.

Exam Pattern Questions

1 Out of solid, liquid and gas which has maximum elasticity?
(a) Solid (b) Gas
(c) Liquid (d) Cannot be compared

2 A body floats in a liquid, if the buoyant force is
(a) zero (b) greater than its weight
(c) less than its weight (d) equal to its weight

3 A deep sea diver may hurt his ear drum during diving because of
(a) lack of oxygen
(b) high atmospheric pressure
(c) high water pressure
(d) All of the above

4 For a steel boat floating on a lake, the weight of the water displaced by the boat is
(a) less than the weight of the boat
(b) more than the weight of the boat
(c) equal to the weight of the part of the boat which is below the water level of the lake
(d) equal to the weight of the boat

5 Density of water is
(a) maximum at 0°C
(b) minimum at 0°C
(c) maximum at 4°C
(d) minimum at 4°C

6 A stone weighing 750 g appears to weighs only 500g when it is submerged in water of density 1 $g(cc)^{-1}$. The volume of the stone is
(a) 250 cc (b) 500 cc
(c) 750 cc (d) 1000 cc

7 The fraction of the total volume of an iceberg of density 0.93 g cm^{-3} floating in North sea with density of 1.03 g cm^{-3} is
(a) 1% (b) 11% (c) 21% (d) 75%

8 Suppose, we have an iron nail and an iron ball of same mass. When submerged in water, then the iron ball may float but the nail always sinks. This is because
(a) buoyant force on the ball is larger than that of the nail due to their shapes
(b) viscous force on the ball is higher
(c) viscous force on the nail is higher
(d) gravitational force affects the ball differently from the nail

9 Which of the most elastic?
(a) Iron (b) Copper
(c) Quartz (d) Wood

10 Hooke's law defines
(a) stress (b) strain
(c) modulus of elasticity (d) elastic limit

11 Write copper, steel, glass and rubber in order of increasing coefficient of elasticity.
(a) Steel, Rubber, Copper, Glass
(b) Rubber, Copper, Glass, Steel
(c) Rubber, Glass, Steel, Copper
(d) Rubber, Glass, Copper, Steel

12 Under elastic limit, the stress is
(a) inversely proportional to strain
(b) directly proportional to strain
(c) square root of strain
(d) independent of strain

13 The common name for all liquids and gases is
(a) solid (b) fluid
(c) matter (d) None of these

14 Unit of pressure is
(a) newton (b) pascal
(c) volt (d) watt

15 Pins and nails are made to have pointed end because
(a) it transmits very small pressure
(b) it transmits a large pressure
(c) it provide a large area
(d) None of the above

16 Which one of the following is correct relation for density (d) and volume (V)?
(a) $d \propto V$ (b) $d \propto \frac{1}{V}$
(c) $d \propto V^2$ (d) $d \propto \frac{1}{V^2}$

17 Increase in pressure at one point of the enclosed liquid in equilibrium at rest is transmitted equally to all other points. This is as per
(a) impulse
(b) conservation of momentum
(c) Ohm's law
(d) Pascal's law

18 Which of the following is unit of atmospheric pressure?
(a) Bar (b) Torr (c) Nm^{-2} (d) All of these

19 Buoyancy depends on
(a) density (b) volume (c) weight (d) force

20 An object weighs 10 N in air and when immersed fully in water, it weighs only 8N. The weight of the liquid displaced by the object will be
(a) 2N (b) 8N (c) 10N (d) 12 N

21 When a piece of ice floating on surface of water in a glass melts completely, then the level of water
(a) increases (b) decreases
(c) remains the same (d) None of these

22 A boat floating in a water tank is carrying a number of stones, if the stones were unloaded into water, then the water level
(a) increases (b) decreases
(c) remains same (d) Data is insufficient

23 Small liquid drops are spherical due to
(a) pressure (b) density
(c) surface tension (d) force

Answers

1 (a)	2 (d)	3 (c)	4 (c)	5 (c)	6 (a)	7 (b)	8 (a)	9 (c)	10 (c)
11 (d)	12 (b)	13 (b)	14 (b)	15 (b)	16 (b)	17 (d)	18 (d)	19 (a)	20 (a)
21 (c)	22 (b)	23 (c)							

Solutions

6 $\because$ Density of stone $= \frac{750}{750 - 500} = 3$

We know that, volume $= \frac{\text{mass}}{\text{density}} = \frac{750}{3} = 250$ cc

7 Given, density of ice $= 0.93$ g cm^{-3},
Density of water $= 1.03$ g cm^{-3}
$\therefore$ Immersed part of ice berg

$$= \frac{\text{Density of ice}}{\text{Density of water}} = \frac{0.93}{1.03} = \frac{93}{103}$$

The volume of a piece of ice will be above water

$$= 1 - \frac{93}{103} = \frac{10}{103}$$

$$\because \text{Percentage fraction} = \frac{\frac{10}{103} \times 100}{\frac{93}{100}} \simeq 11\%$$

Chapter 06

Heat and Temperature

Temperature

Temperature is a quantity that expresses the degree of hotness or coldness of a body. Temperature is the state or condition which would determine the direction of flow of heat.

Measurement of Temperature

The device which measures the temperature of the body is called **thermometer.**

Different Scales to Measure the Temperature

Scale	Freezing point	Boiling point	No. of Divisions
Celsius	0°C	100°C	100
Fahrenheit	32°F	212°F	180
Reaumur	0°R	80°R	80
Kelvin	273 K	373 K	100
Rankine	460	672° Ra	180

Relation between various temperature scales is given below

$$\frac{C}{100} = \frac{F-32}{180} = \frac{K-273}{100} = \frac{R}{80} = \frac{Ra-492}{180}$$

where, C, F, K, R, Ra are the readings of different scales.

Important Points about Temperature

- The normal temperature of human body is 98.6° F or 37°C.
- The highest possible temperature achieved in laboratory is about 10^8 K.
- – 40° is the temperature at which celsius and fahrenheit thermometers read same.
- At 574.25°, the fahrenheit and kelvin scales read the same.
- Alcohol thermometers are better than mercury thermometer because alcohol expands more than water.
- Gas thermometers are superior to mercury thermometers as the variation of pressure (or volume) with temperature is uniform and the range is also high.

Heat

Heat is a form of energy which always flows from hotter body to colder body by virtue of temperature difference and produces a sensation of warmth. It is responsible for the change in thermal condition of the body.

The SI unit of heat is joules another widely used unit for the heat is calorie.

$$1 \text{ cal} = 4.18 \text{ J}.$$

Specific Heat

The amount of heat required to raise the temperature of unit mass of the substance through 1°C is called the specific heat of gas. It is denoted by s.

i.e., specific heat, $s = \dfrac{Q}{m \times \Delta t}$

where, Q = amount of heat given to the substance,
m = mass of the substance
and Δt = rise in temperature.

- Its SI unit is J/kg°C and CGS units is cal/g°C.
- The specific heat of water at 15°C is 4200 J $kg^{-1}\,°C^{-1}$, which is high as compared with most other substances.

Heat Capacity or Thermal Capacity

Thermal capacity is the amount of heat required to raise the temperature of a given amount of a substance through 1°C or 1K.

Thus, thermal capacity

$$= \text{mass} \times \text{specific heat} = \frac{Q}{\Delta t},$$

where, $Q =$ heat absorbed or rejected by body

and $\Delta t =$ change in temperature.

Its unit is JK^{-1} or cal $°C^{-1}$.

The value of heat capacity of a body depends upon the nature of body and its mass.

Principle of Calorimetry

According to this principle, "if two substances of different temperatures are brought in contact with each other, then heat flows from the substance at higher temperature to lower temperature, till their temperatures become same (equilibrium state)."

Latent Heat

The amount of heat transferred per unit mass during the change of phase of a substance without any change in its temperature is called latent heat of the substance for particular change.

$$Q = mL$$

$$\Rightarrow \quad L = \frac{Q}{m}$$

where, $m =$ mass of substance

and $Q =$ quantity of heat required.

Its SI unit is J-kg^{-1}.

Transmission of Heat

As we know that heat flows from the body at higher temperature to the body at lower temperature, this flow of heat is known as transfer of heat from one place to another.

There are three processes of heat transmission

1. **Conduction** In solids, heat is transmitted from higher temperature to lower temperature without actual movements of the particles. This mode of transmission of heat is called conduction.
2. **Convection** The mode of transfer of heat from one part of the medium to the another part by the actual movement of the heated particles of the medium is called convection. In liquid and gases, transmission of heat takes place by convection process.
3. **Radiation** The mode of transfer of heat from one body to another without any actual movement the particles involved and without heating the intervening medium is called radiation. For radiation, there is no need of any medium because it is of electromagnetic nature. e.g., sitting near the fire during winter.

Heat Engine

Heat engine is a device which converts heat into mechanical work. A heat engine essentially consists of three parts

1. Source of heat at higher temperature.
2. Working substance (steam in steam engine, fuel vapors and air in diesel engine).
3. Sink of heat at lower temperature.

Types of Heat Engines

There are two types of heat engines

1. **External Combustion** Engine in which heat is produced by burning the fuel in a chamber outside the main body of the engine is called external combustion. e.g., steam engine is an external combustion engine.
2. **Internal Combustion** Engine in which heat is produced by burning the fuel inside the main body of the engine is called internal combustion. These are also called **four stroke engines.**

   e.g., petrol engine and diesel engine are internal combustion engines.

Thermal Efficiency of Heat Engine (η)

It is defined as the ratio of net work done per cycle by the engine to the total amount of heat absorbed per cycle by the working substance from the source.

$$\eta = \frac{\text{Net work done per cycle}}{\text{Total amount of heat absorbed per cycle}}$$

Efficiency of heat engine is given by

$$\eta = \left(1 - \frac{T_2}{T_1}\right) \times 100\%$$

where, T_1 = temperature of source

and T_2 = temperature of sink.

The thermal efficiency of a heat engine is always less than 100%, i.e., it is always less than 1.

Exam Pattern Questions

1 Which of the following is a measure of hotness of a body?
(a) Temperature (b) Heat
(c) Specific heat (d) Latent heat

2 A glass of ice-cold water left on a table on a hot summer day eventually warms up whereas a cup of hot tea on the same table cools down because
(a) its surrounding media are different
(b) the direction of heat flow depends on the surrounding temperature with respect to the object
(c) heating or cooling does not depend on surrounding temperature
(d) Both (a) and (b)

3 The common physical property which is to be used as the basis for constructing thermometer is
(a) the variation of the volume of a liquid with temperature
(b) the variation of the pressure of a gas with temperature
(c) the variation of the resistance of a wire with temperature
(d) All of the above

4 Gas thermometers are more sensitive than the liquid thermometers because the gases
(a) are lighter
(b) have low specific heat
(c) have high specific heat
(d) have large coefficient of expansion

5 The normal temperature of a healthy person is 37° on
(a) kelvin scale (b) reaumur scale
(c) fahrenheit scale (d) celsius scale

6 An iron ball at 40° C is dropped in a mug containing water at 40°C. The heat will
(a) flow from iron ball to water
(b) not flow from iron ball to water or from water to iron ball
(c) flow from water to iron ball
(d) increase the temperature of both

7 On a hilly region, water boils at 95° C. The temperature expressed in fahrenheit is
(a) 100°F (b) 20.3°F (c) 150°F (d) 203°F

8 Temperature of a body in celsius scale is 60°C. In kelvin scale, its temperature will be
(a) 373 K (b) 333 K (c) 363 K (d) 337 K

9 The temperature at which centigrade and fahrenheit scales give the same reading is
(a) − 40° (b) 40° (c) − 30° (d) 30°

10 The ice point and the steam point of water are two convenient fixed points and are known as the
(a) cooling point and heating point, respectively
(b) heating point and cooling point, respectively
(c) freezing point and boiling point, respectively
(d) boiling point and freezing point, respectively

11 On centigrade scale °C, the temperature of a body increases by 30°. The increase in temperature on fahrenheit scale (°F) is
(a) 50° (b) 40° (c) 30° (d) 54°

12 Which one among the following denotes the smallest temperature?
(a) 1° on the celsius scale
(b) 1° on the kelvin scale
(c) 1° on the fahrenheit scale
(d) 1° on the reaumur scale

13 In the winter season, if we touch two blocks one of iron and another of wood in the early morning, then the block of iron appears to be more cold because
(a) the temperature of the iron block is less than that of the wooden block
(b) iron is a bad conductor of heat in comparison of the wood
(c) iron has high specific heat capacity
(d) the block of iron is heavier than the wooden block

14 The temperature of a body is an indicator of
(a) average kinetic energy of the molecules of body
(b) the total velocity of the molecules of body
(c) the total potential energy of the molecules of body
(d) average total energy of the molecules of body

15 Which one of the following has the highest value of specific heat?
(a) Glass (b) Copper
(c) Lead (d) Water

16 A electric heater kept in vacuum, is heated continuously by passing electric current. Its temperature
(a) will go on rising with time
(b) will stop rising after sometime as it will lose heat to the surrounding by conduction
(c) will become constant after sometime because of loss of heat due to radiation
(d) None of the above

17 Water is used in hot water bags because
(a) it is easily obtained
(b) it is cheaper and not harmful
(c) it has high specific heat
(d) it is easy to heat water

18 Heat stored in water vapour is
(a) specific heat (b) latent heat
(c) absolute heat (d) relative heat

19 What changes will happen to a bowl of ice and water kept at exactly zero degree celsius?
(a) All ice will melt
(b) All water will become ice
(c) No change will happen
(d) Only some ice will melt

20 Which of the following produces more severe burns?
(a) Boiling water (b) Hot water
(c) Steam (d) Melting icebergs

Answers

1 (a)	2 (b)	3 (d)	4 (d)	5 (d)	6 (b)	7 (d)	8 (b)	9 (a)	10 (c)
11 (d)	12 (b)	13 (a)	14 (a)	15 (d)	16 (c)	17 (c)	18 (b)	19 (c)	20 (c)

Solutions

7 Using relation, $\frac{C}{100} = \frac{F - 32}{180}$

Given, C = 95° C, $\frac{95}{100} = \frac{F - 32}{180}$

$\Rightarrow \quad F = 171 + 32 = 203° F$

8 Using the relation, $\frac{C - 0}{100} = \frac{K - 273}{100}$

$\Rightarrow \quad C = K - 273 \Rightarrow K = 60 + 273 = 333\,K$

9 Using the relation, $\frac{F - 32}{180} = \frac{C}{100}$

If $F = C = x$, then substituting $\frac{x - 32}{9} = \frac{C}{5}$

$\Rightarrow x = -40°$

11 From the relation, $\frac{F - 32}{180} = \frac{C}{100}$

$$\frac{F_1 - 32}{180} = \frac{C_1}{100} \quad \text{...(i)}$$

$$\frac{F_2 - 32}{180} = \frac{C_2}{100} \quad \text{...(ii)}$$

[initial temperatures $F_1 = C_1$ and final temperatures $= F_2, C_2$]

Subtracting Eq. (i) from Eq. (ii), we get

$$\frac{F_2 - F_1}{180} = \frac{C_2 - C_1}{100}$$

Given, $C_2 - C_1 = 30°$ C,

$\Rightarrow \quad F_2 - F_1 = 180 \times \frac{30}{100} = 54° F$

Chapter 07 Light

Light is a form of energy that makes us to see. An object reflects the light that falls on it. This reflected light, when received by our eyes, enables us to see. The speed of light in vacuum or in air is 3×10^8 m/s.

Reflection of Light

The phenomenon of rebouncing back of light rays in same medium on striking a smooth surface is called reflection of light.

- Silver metal is one of the best reflectors of light.
- Laws of reflection is applied to all kinds of reflecting surface.

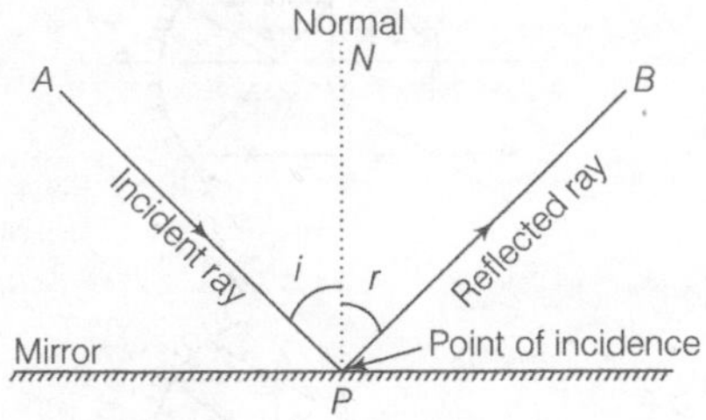

The laws of reflection are

- The incident ray, the reflected ray and the normal to the reflecting surface at the point of incidence all lie in the same plane.
- Angle of incidence ($\angle i$) is always equal to the angle of reflection ($\angle r$).

Mirror

Mirror is a polished surface like glass, which reflects almost all the light that is incident on it.

Types of Mirror

There are two types of mirror

1. **Plane Mirror** If the reflecting surface of a mirror is plane, then the mirror is called a plane mirror.
   Image formed by a plane mirror is always virtual, erect and equal in size to the object.
2. **Spherical Mirror** A highly polished curved surface whose reflecting surface is a cut part of a hollow glass sphere is called a spherical mirror.

There are two types of spherical mirror

1. **Concave Mirror** The spherical mirror whose reflecting surface is inwards and outer surface is polished is called concave mirror. It is also called converging mirror because it is generally used to converge the beam of light after reflection.
2. **Convex Mirror** A spherical mirror whose outer surface is reflecting the inner surface is polished is called convex mirror. It is also called diverging mirror because it generally diverges beam of light after reflection.

Image Formation by a Concave Mirror

Position of object	Position of image	Size of image	Nature of image	Ray Diagram
At infinity	At F	Highly diminished	Real and inverted	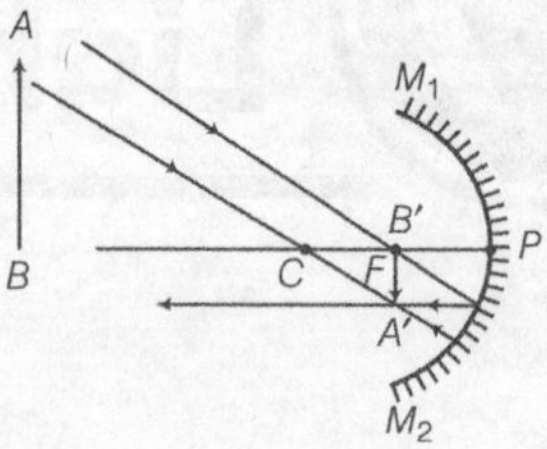
Between infinity and C	Between F and C	Diminished	-do-	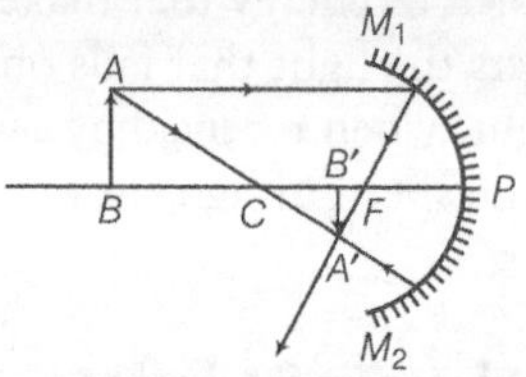
At C	At C	Same size	-do-	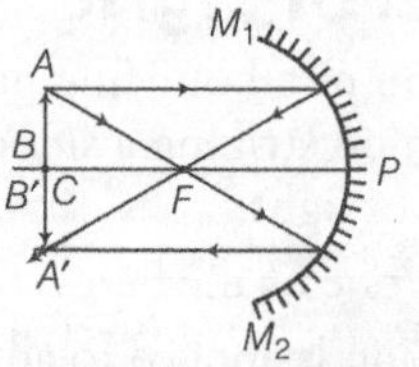
Between F and C	Between infinity and C	Enlarged	-do-	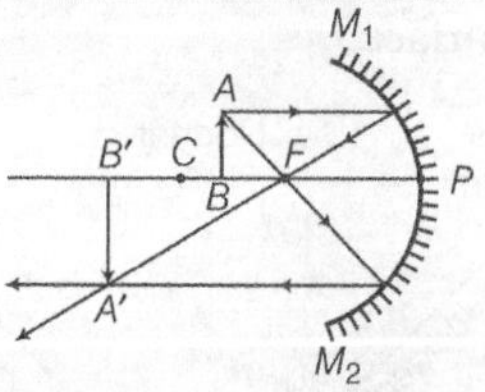
At F	At infinity	Highly enlarged	-do-	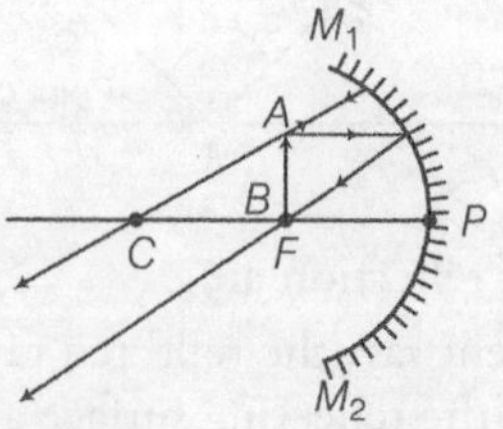
Between F and P	Behind the pole	Enlarged	Virtual and erect	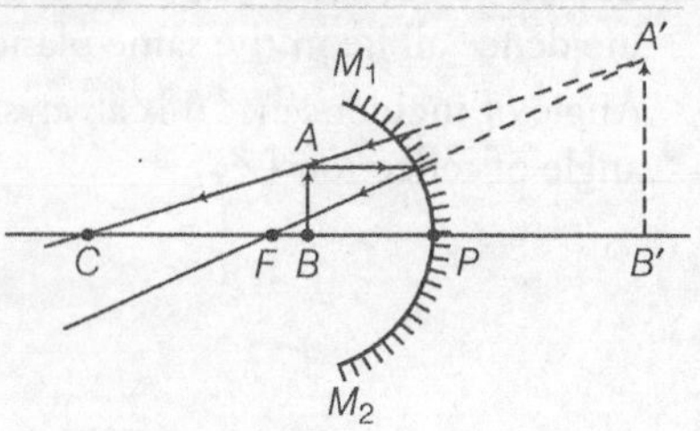

Image Formation by a Convex Mirror

Position of object	Position of image	Size of image	Nature of image	Ray Diagram
At infinity	At F	Highly diminished	Erect and virtual	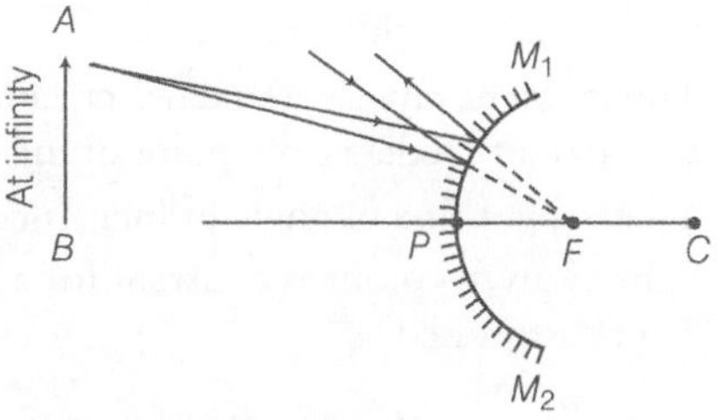
Between infinity and pole	Between F and P	Diminished in size	Erect and virtual	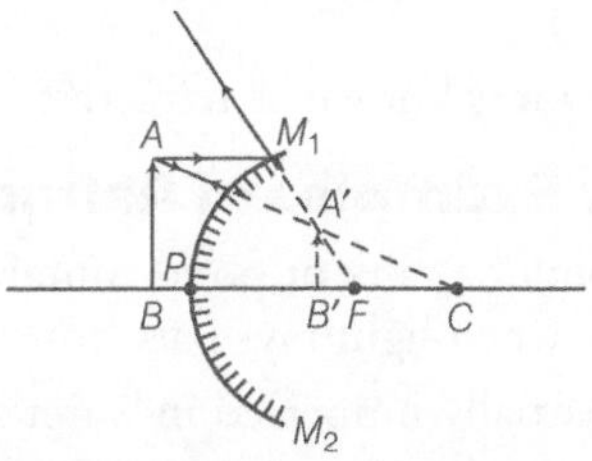

Mirror Formula

- The relation between quantities u, v and f is called mirror formula.

  It is expressed as $\frac{1}{v}+\frac{1}{u}=\frac{1}{f}$

  where u, v and f are to be used according to their new cartesian sign convention and R is the radius of curvatures, $R=2f$.
- This formula is valid in all situations for all spherical mirrors and for all positions of the object.

Linear Magnification

- It is expressed as the ratio of height of image to the height of object. It is represented by m.

  i.e. $\text{Magnification, } m=\frac{\text{Height of image } (h_i)}{\text{Height of object } (h_o)}$
- Magnification is also related to the object distance (u) and image distance (v). It can be expressed as

$$m=\frac{\text{Image distance }(v)}{\text{Object distance }(u)}=\frac{-v}{u}$$

where, u and v are to be used with their appropriate sign.

Uses of Concave Mirrors

- Concave mirrors are commonly used in torches, search lights and vehicles headlights to get powerful parallel beams of light.
- Concave mirrors are used as shaving mirrors to see larger image of the face.
- Dentists use concave mirrors to see large images of the teeth.
- Large concave mirrors are used to concentrate sunlight to produce heat in solar furnaces.

Uses of Convex Mirrors

- Convex mirrors are commonly used as rear view mirrors in vehicles because they always give an erect image and have wider field of view as they are curved outwards.
- Big convex mirrors are used as shop security mirrors, the shop owner can keep an eye on the customers to look for thieves and shoplifters among them.

Refraction of Light

"Change in path of a light ray as it passes from one medium to another medium is called refraction of light."

The laws of refraction are

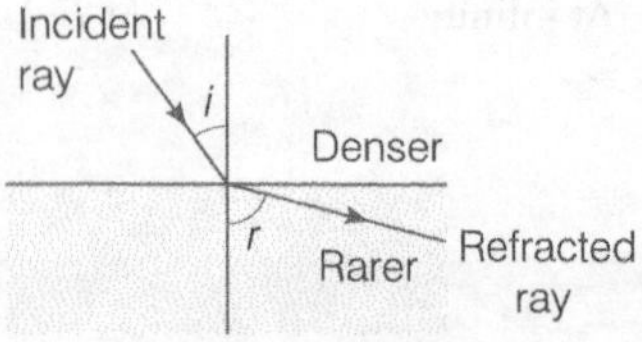

- The incident ray, the refracted ray and the normal to the interface of two transparent media at the point of incidence, all lie in the same plane.
- The ratio of sine of angle of incidence to the sine of angle of refraction for light of given colour is constant for a given pair of media (Snell's law). It can be expressed as

$$\frac{\sin i}{\sin r} = \mu = \text{constant } (\mu \text{ or } \eta)$$

This constant is known as refractive index (μ).

Everyday Examples of Refraction of Light

- The bottom of a tank or pond containing water appears to be raised due to refraction of light which takes place when light rays pass from the pool of water into the air.
- A pencil partially immersed in water appears to be broken because of the refraction of light coming from the part of pencil that is under water.

Lens

Lens is a transparent medium bounded by two surfaces of which one or both surfaces are spherical.

Spherical Lenses

There are two types of lenses

1. **Convex lens (converging lens) A lens which is thicker at the centre and thinner at its ends.**
2. **Concave lens (diverging lens)** A lens which is thinner at the centre and thicker at its ends.

Image Formation by a Convex Lens

Position of Object	Position of Image	Size of Image	Nature of Image	Ray Diagram
At infinity	at F_2	extremely diminished	real and inverted	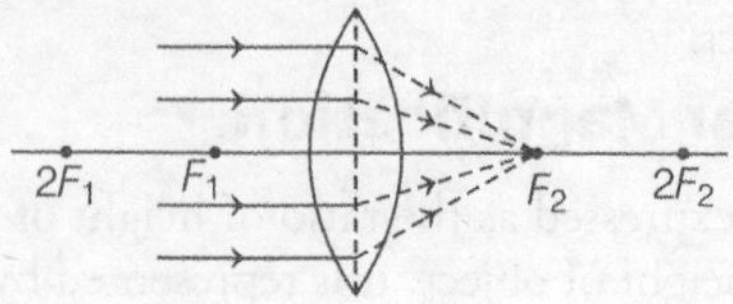
Beyond $2F_1$ (at finite distance)	between F_2 and $2F_2$	diminished	real and inverted	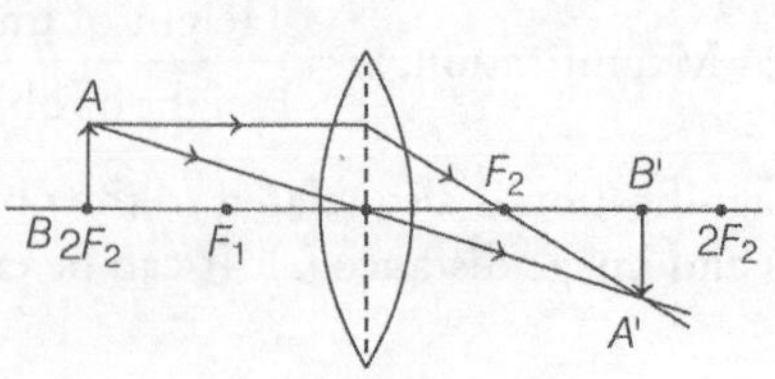

Position of Object	Position of Image	Size of Image	Nature of Image	Ray Diagram
At $2F_1$	at $2F_2$	same size	real and inverted	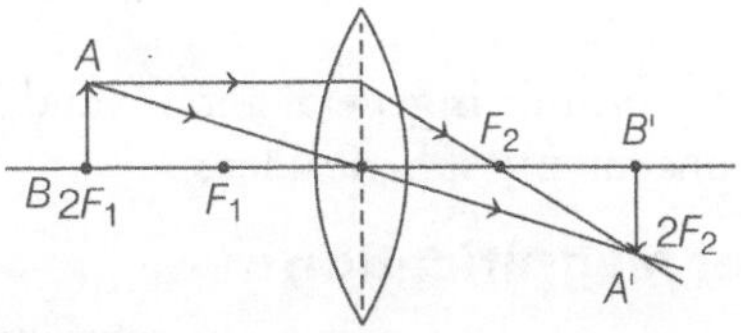
Between F_1 and $2F_1$	beyond $2F_2$	magnified	real and inverted	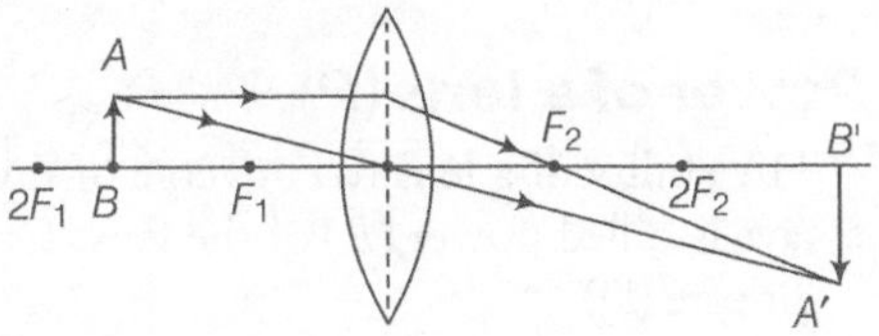
At F_1	at infinity	highly magnified	real and inverted	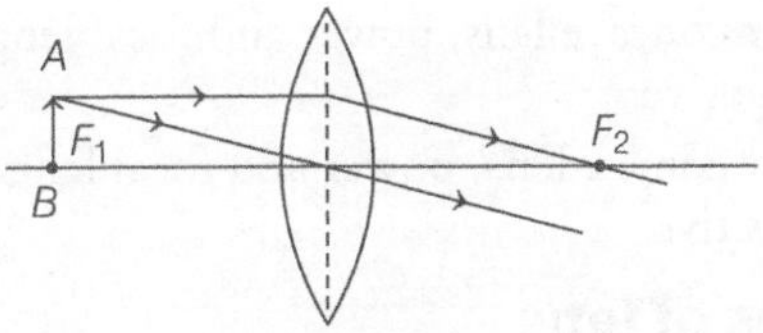
Between lens and F_1	on same side of the lens as the object	magnified	virtual and erect	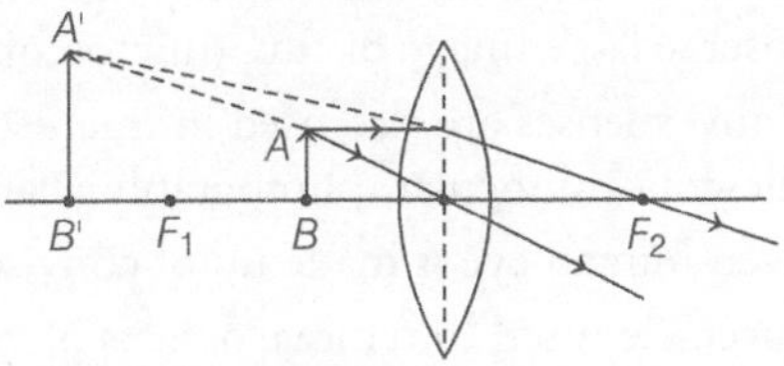

Image Formation by a Concave Lens

Position of Object	Position of Image	Size of Image	Nature of Image	Ray Diagram
At infinity	at focus on same side of lens as object	highly diminished	virtual and erect	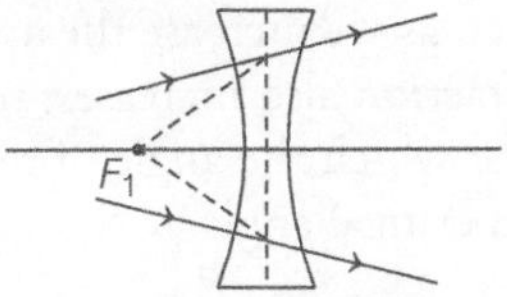
At finite distance	between focus and optical centre on the same side of lens as object	diminished	virtual and erect	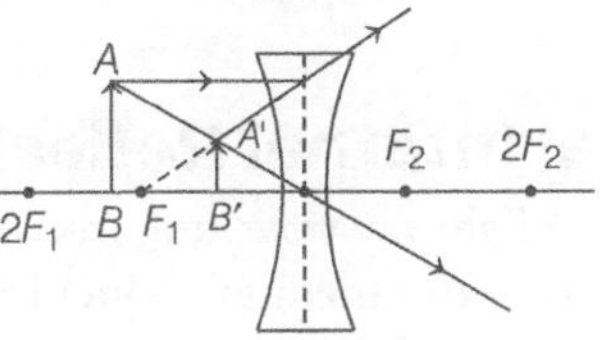

Lens formula

The lens formula is expressed as $\frac{1}{v} - \frac{1}{u} = \frac{1}{f}$

The lens formula is general and is valid in all situations for any spherical lens.

Linear Magnification

Magnification, $m = \frac{v}{u} = \frac{I}{O} = \frac{\text{Size of image}}{\text{Size of object}}$

Power of a lens (*P*)

- The ability of a lens to converge or diverge light rays is called power (P) of the lens. Its SI unit is dioptre (D).

  Power, $P = \frac{100}{\text{Focal length } (f)(\text{in cm})}$

- For concave lens, power and focal length are negative.
- For convex lens, power and focal length are positive.

Uses of lens

- Convex lens is used as magnifying glass to observe large image of tiny (microscopic) objects.
- Convex lenses are also used in microscope, telescope, binocular, photographic camera etc.
- Even human eye is made up of convex lens.
- Spectacles used to remove defects of vision are also made up of both the lenses.

Critical Angle

When a light ray goes to rarer medium from denser medium then as we increase the angle of incidence, angle of refraction also increases, so the angle of incidence for which the angle of refraction becomes 90° is called critical angle.

$$\mu = \frac{1}{\sin C}$$

Total Internal Reflection (TIR)

When a light ray travelling from a denser medium towards a rarer medium is incident at the interface at an angle of incidence greater than critical angle, then light rays are reflected back into the denser medium (i.e., same medium). This phenomenon is called total internal reflection.

Necessary conditions for total internal reflection to takes place are

- The ray incident on the interface of two media should travel from denser medium to rarer medium.
- The angle of incidence should be greater than critical angle for the two media.

Dispersion of Light

When a narrow beam of light is incident on a prism, the emergent beam is not only deviated but at the same time splits up into a coloured band of seven colours. This phenomenon is called dispersion of light, e.g. Rainbow formation.

The seven colours of band are Violet, Indigo, Blue, Green, Yellow, Orange and Red (can be memorised as VIBGYOR).

Scattering of Light

- The reflection of light from an comparably smaller sized particle in all directions is called scattering of light.
- The colour of scattered light depends on the size of scattering particles. Very fine particles scatter mainly blue light while particles of larger size scatter light of longer wavelength (red light).
- If the size of the scattering particles is large enough, then the scattered light may even appear white.
- Some phenomena based on scattering of light are
  - During the day time sky appears blue.
  - Reddish appearance of sun at sunrise and sunset.

Human Eye

Human eye is an optical instrument which forms real image of the objects.

- Least distance of distinct vision is 25 cm.
- Far point of normal eye is at infinity.

Defects of Vision	Symptom	Cause	Remedy
Myopia	a person can see nearby objects clearly but cannot see distance objects	decrease in focal length of lens due to excessive curvature of lens elongation of eyeball	concave lens
Hypermetropia	a person cannot see near by objects clearly but can see distant objects	focal length of eye lens becomes large or shorting of eye-ball	convex lens
Presbyopia	Old aged people cannot read comfortably near point gradually recedes away sometimes they cannot see far objects also	weakness of ciliary muscles, hardening of eyelens or loss of elasticity	bifocal lens
Astigmatism	eye cannot focus objects both in horizontal and vertical lines clearly	imperfact shape of cornea or lens or of both	cylindrical lens
Colourblindness	the person cannot distinguish between certain colours	absence of cones with some specific colours	Not curable

Optical Magnifying Instruments Microscope

It is an optical instrument which forms a magnified image of a small nearby object and thus increases the visual angle subtended by the image at the eye, so that the object is seen to be bigger and distinct.

Simple Microscope A simple microscope is a convex lens of short focal length which is fixed in a frame provided with handle.

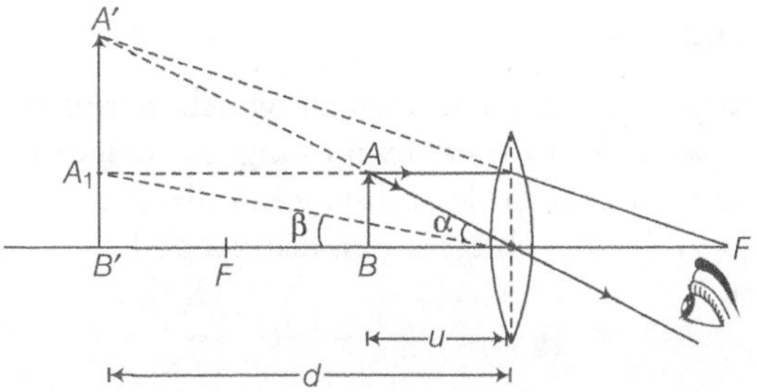

Magnification of Simple Microscope

- When final image is formed at least distance of distinct vision, $M = 1 + \frac{D}{f}$
- For relaxed eye, $M = \frac{D}{f}$

where, D = least distance of distinct vision

Compound Microscope It consists of two converging lenses arranged coaxially. The one facing the object is called **objective** and the one close to eye is called **eye piece.** The objective has a smaller aperture and smaller focal length than those of the eyepiece.

Magnification of Compound Microscope

- For relaxed eye, $M_\infty = -\frac{v_o}{u_o}\left(\frac{D}{f_e}\right)$

  In this position, length of microscope,

  $$L_\infty = v_o + f_e$$

- When final image is formed at least distance of distinct vision,

  $$M_D = -\frac{v_o}{u_o}\left(1 + \frac{D}{f_e}\right)$$

  Length of microscope, $L_D = v_o + u_e$

  where,

  v_o = distance of first image from object lens,

  u_o = distance of object from objective lens

  and f_e = focal length of eyepiece $L = f_o + f_e$.

Telescope

Telescope is an optical instrument which increases, the visual angle at the eye by forming the image of a distant object at the least distance of distinct vision, so that the object is seen distinct and bigger.

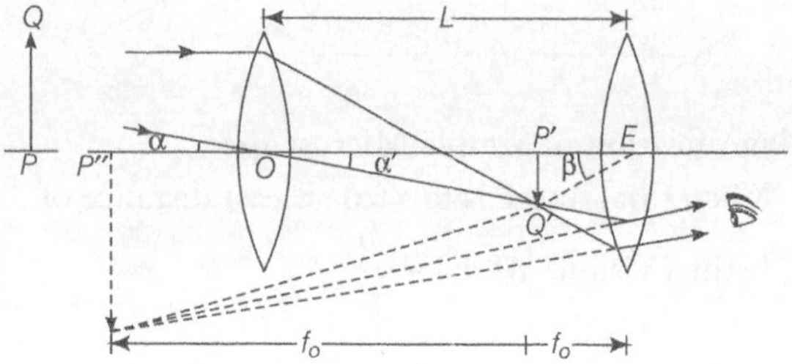

Magnification of Astronomical Telescope

- For relaxed eye, $M_{\infty} = -\frac{f_o}{f_e}$

In this position, length of telescope,

$$L_{\infty} = f_o + f_e$$

- When final image is formed at least distance of distinct vision, $M_D = -\frac{f_o}{f_e}\left(1 + \frac{f_e}{D}\right)$
- Length of telescope, $L_D = f_o + f_e$

where, f_o = focal length of objective lens and

f_e = focal length of eyepiece

It is used for observing distinct images of heavenly bodies like stars, planets, etc.

Exam Pattern Questions

1 A beam of light is
(a) a ray of light
(b) a bundle of rays
(c) few rays moving in different directions
(d) more than one ray

2 Speed of light in vacuum is
(a) highest attainable speed
(b) attainable by small particles in vacuum
(c) attainable by dust particles in interstellar space
(d) None of the above

3 Which type of mirror is used in the headlights of vehicles?
(a) Plane mirror
(b) Concave mirror
(c) Convex mirror
(d) Parabolic mirror

4 Shaving mirror is
(a) convex (b) concave
(c) plane (d) parabolic

5 A person standing in front of a mirror finds his image thinner but with normal height. The mirror in question is
(a) concave and spherical
(b) convex and spherical
(c) convex and cylindrical with vertical axis
(d) convex and cylindrical with horizontal axis

6 A point object is placed at a distance 30 cm from a convex mirror of focal length 30 cm. The image will be formed at
(a) infinity
(b) pole
(c) focus
(d) 15 cm behind the mirror

7 In reflection over a spherical mirror, ray parallel to principal axis after reflection from mirror pass through
(a) focus
(b) centre of curvature
(c) pole of mirror
(d) any point

8 Incident ray always lies in a plane
(a) perpendicular to plane containing normal and reflected ray
(b) perpendicular to normal
(c) perpendicular to plane containing reflected ray
(d) containing reflected ray and normal

9 A ray of light gets reflected from the plane mirror. The incident ray and the reflected ray are perpendicular to each other. The angle of incidence is
(a) 60° (b) 30° (c) 45° (d) 0°

10 An object is placed at 10 cm from a concave mirror of radius of curvature 15 cm, then
(a) it forms an erect image
(b) it forms a small and inverted image
(c) it forms a point image
(d) if forms a magnified, real and inverted image

11 Incident ray, normal at the point of incidence and refracted ray are always
(a) mutually perpendicular
(b) inclined at acute angles
(c) parallel
(d) coplanar

12 Quantity which does not changes during refraction is
(a) direction
(b) speed
(c) frequency
(d) wavelength

13 Which of the following is not caused by atmospheric refraction of light?
(a) Twinkling of starts at night
(b) Sun appearing higher in the sky than its actually is
(c) Sun becoming visible two or three minutes before actual sunrise
(d) Sun appearing red at sunset

14 The position, relative size and nature of the image formed by a concave lens for an object placed at infinity are respectively
(a) at focus, diminished and virtual
(b) at focus, diminished and real
(c) between focus and optical centre, diminished and virtual
(d) between focus and optical centre, magnified and real

15 While looking at an image formed by a convex lens (one-half of the lens is covered with a black paper), which one of the following will happen to the image?
(a) Half of the image will be visible
(b) Intensity of the image will be diminished
(c) Image will be inverted now
(d) One can see an image of smaller size

16 The focal length of a convex lens which forms real and inverted image of a needle at a distance of 50 cm from it will be provided size of image size of object
(a) 20 cm (b) 100 cm
(c) 25 cm (d) 45 cm

17 What is the reason for formation of mirage in desert?
(a) Refraction of light
(b) Reflection of light
(c) Total internal reflection of light
(d) Dispersion of light

18 Rainbow is produced when sunlight falls on drops of rain. Which of the following physical phenomena are responsible for this?
(a) Dispersion
(b) Refraction
(c) Total internal reflection
(d) All of the above

19 The blue colour of water in the sea is due to
(a) absorption of other colours except blue by water molecules
(b) scattering of blue light by water molecules
(c) reflection of blue light by impurities in sea water
(d) reflection of blue sky by sea water

20 The power of concave lens of focal length 2 m will be
(a) +0.5 D (b) +0.25 D
(c) +5 D (d) – 0.5 D

21 The nature and focal length of a lens whose power is +2D will be
(a) 25 cm
(b) – 25 cm
(c) + 50 cm
(d) –100 cm

22 Light travels slower in glass than in air because
(a) refractive index of air is less than that of glass
(b) refractive index of air is greater than that of glass
(c) density of glass is greater than that of air
(d) density of glass is less than that of air

23 Which of the following is correct?
(a) Clear sky appears blue due to poor scattering of blue wavelength of visible light
(b) Red part of light shows more scattering than blue light in the atmosphere
(c) In the absence of atmosphere, there would be no scattering of light and sky will be black
(d) None of the abvoe

24 The human eye is like a camera and hence, it contains a system of lens. The eye lens forms
(a) a straight or upright, real image of the object on the retina
(b) an inverted, virtual image of the object on the retina
(c) an inverted, real image of object on the retina
(d) a straight or upright, real image of the object on the iris

25 Red colour is used for danger singnals because
(a) it causes fear
(b) it undergoes least scattering
(c) it undergoes maximum scattering
(d) None of the above

Answers

1 (b)	2 (a)	3 (b)	4 (b)	5 (c)	6 (a)	7 (a)	8 (d)	9 (c)	10 (d)
11 (d)	12 (c)	13 (d)	14 (a)	15 (b)	16 (c)	17 (c)	18 (d)	19 (a)	20 (d)
21 (c)	22 (a)	23 (c)	24 (c).	25 (b)					

Solutions

9 From law of reflection, $\angle i = \angle r = \theta$

$\Rightarrow \quad i + r = 2\theta = 90^\circ$

As, incident ray perpendicular to reflected ray

$\Rightarrow \quad 2\theta = 90^\circ$ or $\theta = 45^\circ$

10 $f = \frac{-15}{2} = -7.5$ cm ($\because$ $R = -15$ cm)

The object distance, $u = -10$ cm

Hence, using mirror formula, $\frac{1}{v} + \frac{1}{u} = \frac{1}{f}$

$\frac{1}{v} + \frac{1}{(-10)} = \frac{1}{-75}$

$\Rightarrow v = \frac{10 \times 7.5}{-2.5} = -30$ cm

$m = -\frac{v}{u} = -\frac{-30}{-10} = -3$, image is magnified, real and inverted.

20 Given, $f = +2$ m

As, per formula, $P = \frac{1}{-f} = -\frac{1}{2} = -0.50$ D

21 Given, $P = +2$ D, hence lens is convex lens.

Focal length, $f = \frac{1}{P} = \frac{1}{2} = 0.5$ m $= 50$ cm

Chapter 08 Wave Motion and Sound

Wave

A wave is a disturbance which propagates energy from one place to the other without the transport of matter.

Types of Waves

Waves are of two types, i.e., mechanical waves and electromagnetic waves.

1. **Mechanical Waves** The waves which require material medium (solid, liquid or gas) for their propagation are called mechanical waves or elastic waves. e.g., sound wave, water wave, jump rope wave etc.

Mechanical waves are of following two types

(i) **Longitudinal waves** The individual particles of medium move in a parallel to the direction of propagation of the disturbance.

(ii) **Transverse waves** The individual particles of medium move about its mean position in a direction perpendicular to the direction of wave propagation.

2. **Electromagnetic waves** The waves which do not require medium for their propagation, i.e., which can propagate even through the vacuum are called electromagnetic wave. e.g., radio waves, light waves, X-rays, gamma (γ) rays etc.

Wave velocity

The distance covered by a wave per unit time in its directions of propagation is called its wave velocity or phase velocity. It is denoted by v.

Relation between wave velocity, frequency and wavelength is

$$\text{Wave velocity} = \frac{\text{Distance}}{\text{Time}}$$

$$v = \frac{\lambda}{T} \text{ or } v = n\lambda \qquad \left\{\because n = \frac{1}{\lambda}\right\}$$

i.e. Wave velocity = Frequency × Wavelength

Sound

- Sound is a form of energy which produces the sensation of hearing in our ears.It is a mechanical wave. It is measured in decibel (dB).
- The speed of sound is maximum in solids and minimum in gases.
- A sound is produced by vibrating objects.
- The sound of human voice in produced due to vibrations in the vocal cords.

Characteristics of Sound

- **Pitch** Pitch is the characteristic of a sound that depends on the frequency received by a human ear. A sound wave of high frequency has high pitch and sound wave of low frequency has two pitch.
- **Loudness** Loudness of a sound depends on the amplitude of the vibrating body that producing sound.It depends on the sensitivity of human ear.
- **Intensity** In the amount of sound energy passing each second through unit area is known as the intensity of sound. The unit of intensity is watt per square metre (W/m^2).
- **Quality** The quality of sound is that characteristic of sound which enables us to distinguish one sound from another having the same pitch and loudness. A sound of single frequency is called a tone.

Propagation of Sound

- Sound wave propagates through compressible media such as air or water.
- The source of sound creates a disturbance in the medium which travels through the medium.
- The particles of the medium do not move forward but the disturbance is carried forward.

Speed of Sound

- Sound propagates through a medium at a finite speed. The medium can be a solid substance, a liquid or a gas.
- The speed of sound depends on the properties of medium through which it travels.
- The speed of sound in a medium depends on temperature of the medium (as temperature increases, speed of sound also increases).
- The speed of sound decreases when we go from solid to gaseous state.
- The speed of sound in aim is about 344 ms^{-1} at 22°C and 331 ms^{-1} at 0°C.

Range of Hearing

- The average frequency range over which the human ear is sensitive is called **audible range.** The audible range is from 20 Hz to 20000 Hz.
- The sound of frequencies lower than 20 Hz are known like as **infrasonic sound.** Earthquake's and some animals whales, elephants and rhinoceroses produce infrasonic sound of frequency 5 Hz.
- The sound of frequencies higher than 20000 Hz are called **ultrasonic sound.** Dog can hear ultrasonic sound of frequency up to 50000 Hz, monkey, bats, cats and dolphins can also hear ultrasonic sound.

Echo

Echo is a repetation of sound due to the reflection of original sound by a large obstacle. The minimum distance between the source and obstacle for echo is 17.2 m.

Resonance

Resonance is the tendency of a system to vibrate with increasing amplitudes at some frequencies of excitation. These are known as the system's resonant frequencies.

SONAR

- SONAR stands for Sound Navigation and Ranging.
- It is a device using ultrasonic waves to measure the distance, direction and speed of under water objects.

Doppler Effect in Sound

- Whenever there is a relative motion between a source of sound and listener, the apparent frequency of sound heard by the listener is different from the actual frequency of sound. This phenomenon is called doppler's effect.
- It is observed both in mechanical and electromagnetic waves.

Exam Pattern Questions

1 Which of the following is/are type/types of wave?
(a) Mechanical wave
(b) Electromagnetic wave
(c) Both (a) and (b)
(d) None of the above

2 The waves which require material medium for their propagation are called
(a) microwaves (b) electromagnetic waves
(c) mechanical waves (d) None of the above

3 Longitudinal waves cannot travel through
(a) vacuum (b) solid (c) liquid (d) gas

4 Which of the following statement(s) is/are false your mechanical waves?
(a) These waves require a medium for propagation, they cannot propagate through vacuum.
(b) They involve oscillation of particles.
(c) They depend on the elastic properties of the medium.
(d) They have the same speed in all the mediums.

5 Matter waves are associated with

(a) electrons and protons (b) neutrons
(c) atoms and molecules (d) All of these

6 Longitudinal wave is one in which the component of medium oscillate
(a) perpendicular to the direction of propagation of wave
(b) along the direction of the propagation of wave
(c) opposite to the direction of propagation of wave
(d) None of the above

7 A light spring is suspended from a hook which is attached to a 200 g weight at its lower end. The weight is pulled down and then released. The disturbance produced in the spring is
(a) pulse (b) longitudinal wave
(c) transverse wave (d) None of these

8 Sound wave is a
(a) transverse wave (b) longitudinal wave
(c) electromagnetic wave (d) radio wave

9 Sound cannot pass through
(a) water (b) steel
(c) air (d) vacuum

10 Among the following materials sound travel fastest in
(a) steel (b) air
(c) vacuum (d) water

11 In which medium velocity of sound is maximum?
(a) Metals (b) Air
(c) Water (d) Polymere

12 The speed of sound in air is
(a) 231 m/s (b) 331 m/s
(c) 142 m/s (d) 0 m/s

13 On which scale loudness of sound is measured?
(a) Decibel (b) Hertz (c) Volt (d) Watt

14 Note is a sound
(a) of a single frequency
(b) of mixture of two frequencies only
(c) of mixture of several frequencies
(d) always unpleasant to listen

15 A key of a mechanical piano struck gently and then struck again but much harder this time. In the second case
(a) sound will be louder but pitch will not be different
(b) sound will be louder and pitch will also be higher
(c) sound will be louder but pitch will be lower
(d) Both loudness and pitch will remain unaffected

16 Loudness of sound is depend on
(a) frequency (b) amplitude
(c) velocity (d) wavelength

17 Ultrasound can be heard by
(a) dog (b) bat
(c) rhinoceros (d) human beings

18 Earthquake produces which kind of sound before the main shock wave begin?
(a) Ultrasound (b) Infrasound
(c) Audible sound (d) None of these

19 The frequency of sound wave is measured in
(a) metre (b) second (c) hertz (d) mega

20 In SONAR, we use
(a) audible wave (b) infrasonic wave
(c) ultrasonic wave (d) radio wave

Answers

1 (c)	2 (c)	3 (a)	4 (d)	5 (d)	6 (b)	7 (b)	8 (b)	9 (d)	10 (a)
11 (a)	12 (b)	13 (a)	14 (c)	15 (c)	16 (b)	17 (b)	18 (b)	19 (c)	20 (c)

Chapter 09 Electricity

Electric Charge

- A charge is a physical quantity which is defined by excess or deficiency of electrons on a body.
- It is represented by q and the SI unit of electric charge is **coulomb** (C).

  i.e., $q = ne$

  where, n = number of electrons in substance and e = electron charge $= 1.6 \times 10^{-19}$ C
- A body is said to be **negatively charged**, if it **gains** electrons. e.g., an ebonite rod rubbed with fur acquires negative charge.
- A body is said to be **positively charged**, if it **loses** electrons. e.g., a glass rod rubbed with a silk cloth acquires positive charge.

Coulomb's Law

The force of attraction or repulsion between two stationary point charge is directly proportional to the product of their charges and inversely proportional to the square of distance between them.

i.e., $$F = \frac{kq_1 q_2}{r^2}$$

Conductors

- Conductors are those materials in which charge carriers flow easily.
- Conductors have large number of free electrons. e.g., aluminium, copper, silver, iron etc.

Insulator

- The materials which have no free charge carriers (electrons) and hence no current flows through them, are called insulators.

  e.g., paper, glass, rubber etc.

Semiconductor

- The materials which conductivity lies between insulator and conductor are called semiconductor. e.g., germanium, silicon etc.

Electric Field

The space in the surrounding of any charge in which its influence can be experienced by other charge is called electric field.

Electric Current

- It is defined as the rate of flow of electric charge through any cross-section of a conductor in unit time.
- If q amount of charges flows through a conductor in t time, then

  $$\text{Electric current } (I) = \frac{\text{Charge } (q)}{\text{Time } (t)} = \frac{ne}{t} \quad [\because q = ne]$$

  where, n = number of electrons flowing through the conductor.

  The SI unit of electric current is **ampere** (A).
- The direction of electric current is taken as opposite to the direction of the flow of electrons (negative charges).

Electric Potential

- It is defined as the amount of work done when a unit positive charge is moved from infinity to a point.
- If work done in moving a positive charge q from infinity to a point is W, then electric potential V of that point is

  $$V = \frac{W}{q}$$

- The SI unit of electric potential is volt (V) and is named after Italian physicist Alessandro Volta (1745-1827). It is a scalar quantity.

Electric Potential Difference (ΔV)

- It is defined as the work done per unit charge in moving a unit positive charge from one point to other point.
- The electric potential difference between two points is said to be **1 volt**, if 1 joule of work is done in moving 1 coulomb of electric charge from one point to other point.

  Potential difference,

$$\Delta V = V_2 - V_1 = \frac{W}{q} \text{V.}$$

where, W = work done and q = charge.

Ohm's Law

According to Ohm's law, the electric current flowing through a conductor is directly proportional to the potential difference applied across its ends, providing the physical conditions (such as temperature) remain unchanged.

If V is the potential difference applied across the ends of a conductor through which current I flows, then according to Ohm's law,

$$V \propto I \quad \text{[at constant temperature]}$$

or $$V = IR$$

or $$I = \frac{V}{R}$$

where, R is the constant of proportionality called **resistance of the conductor** at a given temperature.

Resistance

It is that property of a conductor by virtue of which it opposes/resists the flow of charges through it. Its SI unit is **ohm** and is represented by the Greek letter Ω.

Resistivity

- It is defined as the resistance of a conductor of unit length and unit area of cross-section. Its SI unit is **ohm-metre** (Ω-m).

$$\text{Resistivity, } \rho = R.\frac{A}{l} \ \Omega\text{-m}$$

where, ρ = resistivity of conductor,
l = length of conductor
and A = area of cross-section of conductor.

- The resistivity of a material does not depend on its length or thickness but depends on the nature of the substance and temperature.
- It is a characteristic property of the material of the conductor and varies only, if its temperature changes.

Combinations of Resistors

- **Series Combination of Resistors** When two or more resistors are connected end to end, then they are said to be **connected in series**.

  Equivalent resistance $R = R_1 + R_2 + R_3$

  In series combination, current through each resistor is same while potential difference across each resistor is different.

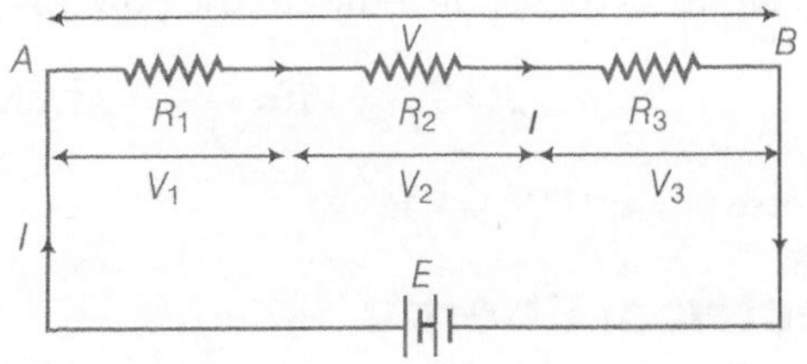

- **Parallel Combination of Resistors** In this combination, first ends of all the resistances is connected to one point and second ends of all the resistances is connected to other point.

  In parallel combination of resistors, potential difference across each resistor is same while current flowing through each resistor is different. If R be the equivalent resistance, then

$$\frac{1}{R} = \frac{1}{R_1} + \frac{1}{R_2} + \frac{1}{R_3}$$

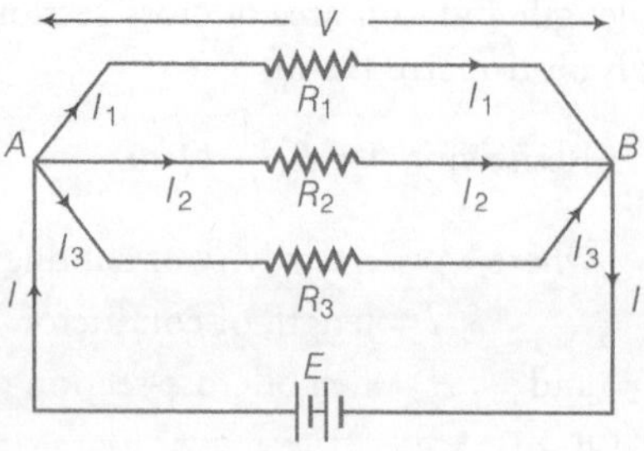

Heating Effect of Electric Current

- When an electric current is passed through a high resistance wire like nichrome wire, then the wire becomes very hot and produces heat. In purely resistive circuits, the source of energy continuously gets dissipated entirely in the form of heat. This is called the heating effect of current.

$$H = \frac{VIt}{4.2} = \frac{V^2 t}{4.2R} = \frac{I^2 Rt}{4.2} \text{ cal}$$

Electric Power

- It is defined as the amount of electric energy consumed in a circuit per unit time.
- If W be the amount of electric energy consumed in a circuit in t seconds, then the electric power is given by

$$P = \frac{W}{t} = VI = \frac{V^2}{R} = I^2 R \text{ W}$$

1 Horse power (HP) = 746 W

Electrical Energy

- The total work done by the source of emf is maintaining the electric current in the circuit for a given time is called electrical energy consumed in the circuit.
- The SI unit of electric energy is joule, but another unit is watt-hour.

Kilowatt-hour (kWh)

It is bigger unit of electric energy. It is known as Board of Trade unit (BOT).

$$1 \text{ kWh} = P \text{ (in kW)} \times t \text{ (in hour)}$$
$$1 \text{ kWh} = 1000 \times 3600$$
$$1 \text{ kWh} = 3.6 \times 10^6 \text{ joule}$$

The electric energy consumed in kWh is given by

$$W = \frac{V \text{ (in volt)} \times I \text{ (in amp)} \times t \text{ (in hour)}}{1000}$$

Electric Hazards and Safety Measures

Due to fault in electrical circuit, there is a possibility to catchup fire in connected electrical appliances. We suffer with high electric shock if we hold circuit without precautions.

Live wire has high value of current, therefore we should touch live wire with the help of using insulator.

Electric Fuse Fuse is used as a safety device in household circuits and is based on heating effect of current. It is connected in series with the mains supply.

A fuse consists of an alloy of lead and tin which has appropriate melting point.

Fuse helps to protect the electric elements (appliances) from hazards caused by heavy circuit.

Electric Bulb It is an electric device based on heating effect of electric current. An electric bulb has a filament made of tungsten. Tungsten has a high resistivity and a high melting point (3380°C).

Exam Pattern Questions

1 The property acquired by the material body when it is rubbed with another body is
(a) mass (b) capacitance
(c) charge (d) All of these

2 Electric charge on a body at rest produces
(a) magnetic field (b) electric field
(c) Both (a) and (b) (d) None of these

3 Charge can take only those values, which are integral multiples of charge on
(a) deuteron (b) positron (c) α-particle (d) electron

4 If a metallic conductor has positive charge, then its mass
(a) remains same (b) decreases
(c) increases (d) becomes double

5 A soap bubble is given positive charge, then its radius
(a) decreases (b) increases
(c) remains same
(d) decreased to half of its initial radius

6 The rate of flow of electric charge through a circuit is called
(a) electric current (b) electric power
(c) electromotive force (d) None of these

7 A piece of wire of resistance R is cut into five equal parts. These parts are connected in parallel. If equivalent resistance of this combination is R', then the ratio of R/R' is
(a) $\frac{1}{25}$ (b) $\frac{1}{5}$ (c) 5 (d) 25

8 The lowest total resistance which can secured by combinations of four resistances 4Ω, 8 Ω, 12 Ω and 24Ω is
(a) 8 Ω (b) 6 Ω (c) 4 Ω (d) 2 Ω

9 The energy which is given to each coulomb of charge passing through 4 V battery is
(a) 2 J (b) 4 J (c) 16 J (d) 8 J

10 The number of electrons constituting one coulomb of charge is [given, charge on one electron $= 1.6 \times 10^{-19}$ C]
(a) 1.6×10^{-19} electrons (b) 1.6×10^{19} electrons
(c) 3.2×10^{19} electrons (d) 6.25×10^{18} electrons

11 The factor on which resistance of a conductor depends is/are
(a) length of conductor
(b) area of cross-section of conductor
(c) nature of material of conductor
(d) All of the above

12 The coils of electric toaster are made of alloy rather than a pure metal because alloy has
(a) higher resistivity than their constituent metals
(b) lower resistivity than their constituent metals
(c) low melting point than their constituent metals
(d) None of the above

13 If length of a conductor is increased to double by drawing it, then its resistivity becomes
(a) double (b) half
(c) four times (d) remains same

14 An electric iron of resistance 20 Ω takes a current of 5 A, the heat developed in 30 s is
(a) 10 kJ (b) 15 kJ (c) 5 kJ (d) 20 kJ

15 Nichrome wire is used to make the element of electric heater because it has
(a) high melting point (b) low melting point
(c) high resistivity (d) Both (a) and (c)

16 In how much time will a bulb of 100 W consume an energy of 3 kWh?
(a) 10 h (b) 20 h (c) 30 h (d) 33.33 h

17 In the following diagram, what will be the value of the current reading in the ammeter?

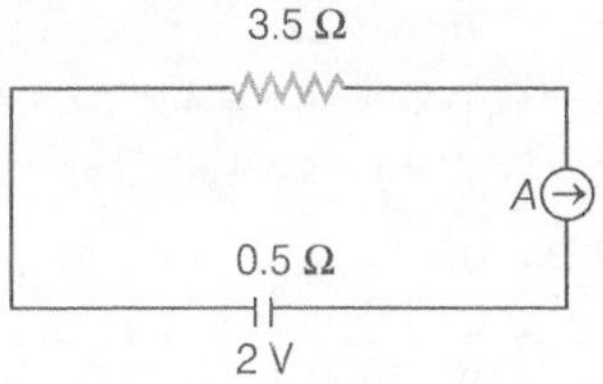

(a) 4 A (b) 2 A
(c) 3 A (d) 0.5 A

18 When temperature of a conductor increases, then its resistance
(a) decreases
(b) increases
(c) remains same
(d) may increases or decreases

19 The work done on moving a charge of 5C from a point 40 V to 80 V, is
(a) 200 J (b) 50 J
(c) 150 J (d) 100 J

20 Electric appliances in household circuit are connected in parallel because
(a) this way they require high current
(b) it one appliance fails then other remains working
(c) same voltage gets each appliance
(d) Both (b) and (c)

21 Which of the following does not represent electrical power in a circuit?
(a) VI (b) I^2R
(c) IR^2 (d) $\frac{V^2}{R}$

22 An electric fuse works on the
(a) magnetic effect of current
(b) heating effect of current
(c) chemical effect of current
(d) All of the above

23 A fuse wire has
(a) high melting point (b) low melting point
(c) highly elastic (d) highly fatigue

24 In a filament type light bulb, most of the electric power consumed appears as
(a) infrared rays (b) visible rays
(c) microwave rays (d) fluorescent rays

25 If the current flowing through a fined resistor is double, the heat produced in it will become
(a) double (b) four times
(c) half (d) remains same

Answers

1 (c)	2 (b)	3 (d)	4 (b)	5 (a)	6 (a)	7 (d)	8 (d)	9 (b)	10 (d)
11 (d)	12 (a)	13 (d)	14 (b)	15 (d)	16 (c)	17 (d)	18 (b)	19 (a)	20 (d)
21 (c)	22 (b)	23 (b)	24 (a)	25 (b)					

Solutions

8 Resistance is minimum, when all resistors are connected in parallel.

$$\therefore \quad \frac{1}{R_{eq}} = \frac{1}{4} + \frac{1}{8} + \frac{1}{12} + \frac{1}{24}$$

$$\frac{1}{R_{eq}} = \frac{1}{2}$$

$$R_{eq} = 2\,\Omega$$

9 Given, $q = 1\,C$, potential, $V = 4\,V$

$\therefore$ Energy, $W = qV = 1 \times 4 = 4\,J$

10 We know that, $q = ne$

$$\therefore \quad n = \frac{q}{e} = \frac{1}{1.6 \times 10^{-19}} \quad [q = 1\,C, e = 1.6 \times 10^{-19}\,C]$$

$$= 6.25 \times 10^{18} \text{ electrons}$$

14 Given, resistance, $R = 20\,\Omega$,
Current, $I = 5\,A$, time, $t = 30\,s$
We know that,
Heat developed, $H = I^2Rt = (5)^2 \times 20 \times 30$
$= 5 \times 5 \times 20 \times 30 = 15000\,J = 15\,kJ$
15 kJ heat is developed in 30 s.

16 Time, $t = \frac{\text{Energy}}{\text{Power}} = \frac{3\text{ kWh}}{100\text{ W}}$

$$= \frac{3000}{100} = 30\,h$$

17 Total resistance,

$$R = 3.5 + 0.5 = 4\,\Omega$$

Current, $I = \frac{V}{R} = \frac{2}{4} = 0.5\,A$

19 Work done, W = Charge (q) × Potential difference (ΔV)

$$= 5 \times (80 - 40)$$
$$= 5 \times 40 = 200\,J$$

25 Heat $\propto$ (Current)^2

$$H \propto I^2$$

$$\frac{H^2}{H_1} = \left(\frac{I_2}{I_1}\right)^2 = \left(\frac{2I_1}{I_1}\right)^2$$

$$\frac{H_2}{H_1} = 4$$

$$H_2 = 4H_1$$

Chapter 10

Magnet and Magnetism

Magnet and Magnetism

A **magnet** is a material or an object that produces a magnetic field. The magnetic field is invisible but is responsible for most notable property of a magnet.

A naturally occurring ore of iron, magnetite attracts small pieces of iron towards it. The phenomenon of attraction of small bits of iron, steel, cobalt, nickel, etc. towards the ore is called **magnetism**.

Types of Magnet

Magnets are of two types

1. **Natural magnets** are generally irregular in shape and weak in strength.
2. **Artificial magnets** have desired shape and desired strength. A bar magnet, a horse shoe magnet, compass needle etc., all are the examples of artificial magnets.

Properties of Magnet

- When a bar magnet is suspended freely, it points in the North-South direction. The tip of the magnet which points to the geographic North is called the **North pole** and the tip which points to the geographic South is called the **South pole** of the magnet.
- There is a **repulsive force,** when North poles (or South poles) of two magnets are brought close together.
- Conversely, there is an **attractive force** between the North pole of one magnet and the South pole of the other.
- We cannot isolate the North or South pole of a magnet, i.e. magnetic poles exist in pairs. If a bar magnet is broken into two halves, we get two similar bar magnets with somewhat weaker properties. Unlike electric charges, isolated magnetic North and South poles are known as magnetic monopoles which do not exist.
- It is possible to make magnets out of iron and its alloys. When a piece of a substance, such as soft iron, steel, cobalt, nickel etc., is placed near a magnet, it acquires magnetism.

Magnetic Field

The space around a magnet in which its effect can be experienced i.e., its force can be detected is called magnetic field.

Magnetic field is a **vector** quantity. The SI unit of magnetic field is **tesla** named after an American engineer Nikola Tesla. The smaller unit of magnetic field is **gauss.** Its SI unit is Tesla or N/A-m.

Magnetic Field Lines

The magnetic field lines in a magnetic field are those imaginary lines which continuously represent the direction of the magnetic field.

The tangent drawn at any point on a line shows the direction of magnetic field at the point.

Properties of Magnetic Field Lines

The magnetic field lines have the following properties

- The magnetic field lines originate from North pole of a magnet and end at its South pole, by convention.

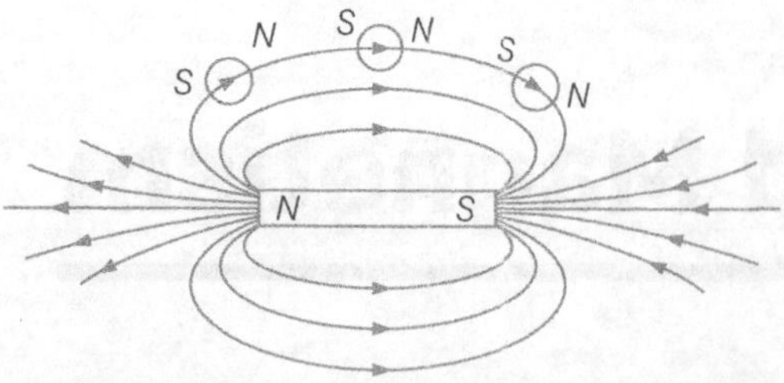

- The magnetic field lines are closed and continuous curves.
- The magnetic field lines are crowded near the poles, where the magnetic field is strong and separated far from the poles, where the magnetic field is weak.
- The magnetic field lines never intersect each other. If they do, so that would mean there are two directions of the magnetic field at the point of intersection, which is impossible.
- When magnetic compass is placed at different points on magnetic field lines, then it comes to rest along the direction of magnetic field at that point.
- The direction of the magnetic field is indicated by the arrow of the lines at any point.

Magnetic Field due to a Current through a Straight Conductor

The magnetic field lines around a current carrying straight conductor are concentric circles whose centres lie on the wire.

The magnitude of magnetic field B produced by a straight current carrying wire at a given point is

- Directly proportional to the current I passing through the wire

  i.e., $B \propto I$ ...(i)

  If current is increased, then the magnetic field produced is stronger and *vice-versa*.
- Inversely proportional to the distance r from the wire

  i.e., $B \propto \frac{1}{r}$ ...(ii)

  The magnetic field is stronger at the point which is nearer to the conductor and goes on decreasing for the far away point.

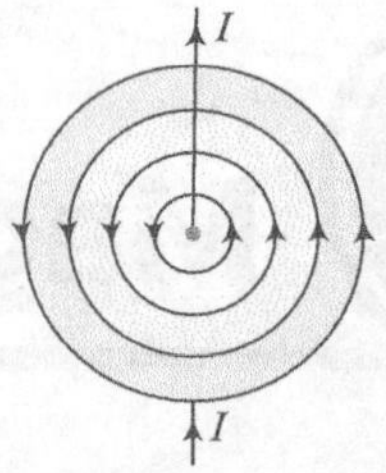

By using Eqs. (i) and (ii), we get

$$B \propto \frac{I}{r}$$

Maxwell's Right Hand Thumb Rule

The direction of the magnetic field produced by a current carrying conductor is given by Maxwell's right hand thumb rule.

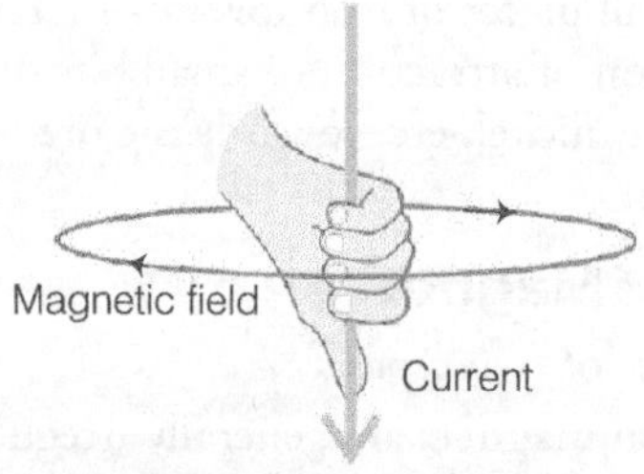

It states that, if you hold the current carrying straight wire in the grip of your right hand in such a way that the stretch thumb points in the direction of current, then the direction of the curl of the fingers will give the direction of the magnetic field. This rule is also called Maxwell's corkscrew rule.

Magnetic Field due to a Current through a Circular Loop

The magnetic field produced by current carrying circular wire at a given point depends on the following factors

- **Amount of current flowing through a wire** The strength of magnetic field (B) due to a current carrying circular wire is directly proportional to the amount of current (I) flowing through it.

  i.e., $B \propto I$ ... (i)
- **Number of turns of the circular wire** The strength of the magnetic field due to a current carrying circular wire is directly proportional to the number of turns (N) of the wire.

  i.e., $B \propto N$ ... (ii)

Thus, the strength of magnetic field produced by a current carrying circular coil can be increased by

- increasing the number of turns of wire in the coil.
- increasing the current flowing through the coil.
- decreasing the radius of the coil.

Magnetic Field due to a Current in a Solenoid

A solenoid is defined as a coil consisting a large number of circular turns of insulated copper wire. These turns are wound closely to form a cylinder.

The strength of magnetic field produced by a current carrying solenoid depends on the following factors

- The number of turns of solenoid ($B \propto N$).
- The strength of current ($B \propto I$).
- The nature of core material used to make solenoid.

The field lines inside the solenoid are parallel to each other. Thus, the strength of magnetic field is the same at all points inside a solenoid.

Electromagnet

An electromagnet is a solenoid coil that gets magnetised, i.e., it becomes a magnet due to flow of current. It works on the **principle of magnetic effect of current.**

It consists of a long insulated copper wire wound around a soft iron core. The magnetic effect remains only till the current is flowing through the solenoid.

Soft iron is used for making electromagnet or temporary magnet.

Fleming's Left Hand Rule

The direction of force which acts on a current carrying conductor placed in a magnetic field is given by Fleming's left hand rule. It states that, if the forefinger, thumb and middle finger of left hand are stretched mutually perpendicular and the forefinger points along the direction of external magnetic field, middle finger indicates the direction of current, then thumb points the direction of force acting on the conductor.

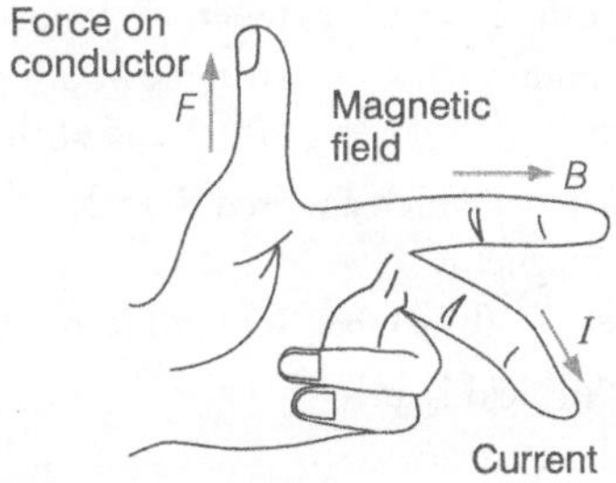

Electric Motor

An electric motor is a rotating device used for converting electric energy into mechanical energy.

An electric motor is based on the principle that when a rectangular coil is placed in a magnetic field and current is passed through it, two equal and opposite forces act on the coil which rotates it continuously.

DC Motor A DC motor is an electrical machine which converts direct current, electrical energy into mechanical energy.

AC Motor An AC motor is an electrical device which converts alternating current, electrical energy into mechanical energy.

Exam Pattern Questions

1 Which type of magnet is used in electric bell?
(a) Bar magnet (b) Electrical magnet
(c) Horse shoe magnet (d) Natural magnet

2 Repulsion , on bringing nearer the same poles of two magnets will
(a) increase (b) decrease
(c) remains same (d) no repulsion

3 At the centre of a bar magnet, magnetism is
(a) minimum (b) maximum
(c) zero (d) None of these

4 The material which are used to make electromagnet is
(a) steel (b) copper (c) hard iron (d) soft iron

5 Magnetic field is a
(a) scalar quantity
(b) vector quantity
(c) scalar as well as vector
(d) Neither scalar nor vector

6 The magnetic lines of forces
(a) intersect at infinity
(b) intersect at neutral point
(c) do not intersect
(d) intersect within the magnet

7 A bar made of soft iron is inserted inside a current carrying solenoid. The magnetic field inside the solenoid will
(a) increase (b) decrease
(c) remains same (d) None of these

8 The magnetic field lines in the solenoid near the axis are
(a) circular about the axis of solenoid
(b) perpendicular to the axis of solenoid
(c) parallel to the axis of solenoid
(d) None of the above

9 If the front face of a circular wire carrying current behaves like a South pole. The direction of current in this face of the circular wire is
(a) clockwise (b) anti-clockwise
(c) upwards (d) downwards

10 The force experienced by a current carrying conductor placed in a magnetic field is zero, when the angle between the conductor and magnetic field is
(a) 0° (b) 180°
(c) Both (a) and (b) (d) 90°

11 The magnitude of magnetic field (B) produced by a straight current carrying wire at a distance (r) from the wire is given by
(a) $B \propto r$ (b) $B \propto \frac{1}{r}$ (c) $B \propto \sqrt{r}$ (d) $B \propto \frac{1}{r^2}$

12 The direction of magnetic force on a current carrying conductor placed in uniform magnetic field is given by
(a) Maxwell's left hand thumb rule
(b) Maxwell's right hand thumb rule
(c) Fleming's right hand rule
(d) Fleming's left hand rule

13 If number of turns of the circular current carrying wire increases to double, then magnetic field due to circular wire is
(a) increased to double
(b) decreased to half
(c) increased to four time
(d) decreased to one-fourth

14 An electric motor is a device which converts
(a) mechanical energy into electrical energy
(b) electrical energy into mechanical energy
(c) mechanical energy into magnetic energy
(d) magnetic energy into mechanical energy

15 Frequency of alternating current and direct current are respectively
(a) 0 Hz and 50 Hz (b) 50 Hz and 50 Hz
(c) 50 Hz and 100 Hz (d) 50 Hz and 0 Hz

16 An electron is travelling horizontally towards East. A magnetic field in vertically downward direction exerts a force on the electron along
(a) West (b) East
(c) South (d) North

17 A loop of flexible wire of irregular shape carrying current is placed in an external field. Then,
(a) it rotates in a direction perpendicular to its axis
(b) it rotates along an axis perpendicular to its plane
(c) it does not show any change
(d) it assumes a circular shape

18 A large magnet is broken into two pieces, so that their lengths are in the ratio 2 : 1. The pole strengths of the two pieces will have ratio
(a) 2 : 1 (b) 1 : 2
(c) 4 : 1 (d) 1 : 1

19 In which application, the material goes through an AC cycle of magnetisation for a long period?
(a) Transformer cores
(b) Telephone diaphragms
(c) Generator
(d) Both (a) and (b)

20 Electromagnets are made of soft iron because soft iron has
(a) low susceptibility and low retentivity
(b) low susceptibility and high retentivity
(c) high permeability and low retentivity
(d) high permeability and high retentivity

Answers

1 (b)	2 (a)	3 (c)	4 (d)	5 (b)	6 (c)	7 (a)	8 (c)	9 (a)	10 (c)
11 (b)	12 (d)	13 (a)	14 (b)	15 (d)	16 (c)	17 (d)	18 (d)	19 (d)	20 (c)

BIOLOGY

Chapter 01 Basics of Biology

Introduction to Biology

- **Biology** is a natural science concerned with the study of life and living organisms, i.e. plants and animals.
- It is classified into two parts, i.e. Botany and Zoology.
- Study of plants is called Botany and study of animals is called Zoology.
- The term 'Biology' was coined by **Lamarck** and **Treviranus.**
- The scientist who gave his thought for the first time about the life of plants and animals was **Aristotle**. He is also known as the Father of Zoology.
- **Theophrastus** is known as Father of Botany.

The Cell

- The **cell** is the basic structural and functional unit of all known living organisms.
- **Robert Hooke** coined the term cell. However, he only discovered cell wall.
- The first living cell was discovered by **Leeuwenhoek.**
- The branch of biology, which deals with the study of cell is called **cytology**.

Types of Cell

On simplest categorisation, the cells can be

Prokaryotic Cells

(*Pro*-primitive, *karyos*-nucleus) These are primitive cells, lacking a well-defined nucleus and most of other cell organelles.

Eukaryotic Cells

These are advance cells, which have a well-defined nucleus and membrane bound cell organelles.

Structural Organisation of Cell

A typical cell consists of following structures and components

Protoplasm

- It is the living fluid matter of the cell.
- It can be differentiated into the fluid present outside the nuclear membrane, i.e. **cytoplasm** and the fluid present inside the nuclear membrane, i.e. **nucleoplasm.**
- The non-living matter of the cell is called **deutoplasm.**

Cell Wall

- It is the outermost covering of plant cells, bacteria and fungi.
- It is composed of **cellulose** in plants and **chitin** in fungi.
- It is non-living. Its main function is to provide shape and rigidity to the cell.

Plasma Membrane

- It is the outer covering of all cells. However, in plant, bacterial and fungal cells, it is present below cell wall.
- Proteins and phospholipid molecules are main components. It is elastic, living and selectively permeable, i.e. provide passage for various substances.
  A typical cell representing both plant and animal cell organelles are as follows

Mitochondria

- It is a semi-autonomous (can form its own copies) organelle and is also called as **powerhouse of the cell** because in it, stepwise oxidation of fuel, i.e. nutritive substances occurs resulting to release of energy.

- It is bounded by a double membrane. The inner membrane has many folds, called the **cristae**. Fluid (called matrix) is present on interior, which contains many enzymes and coenzymes.
- The energy released by its functioning is stored in the form of ATP.

Plastids

- These are present only in plant cells and are of three types-**chloroplasts** (green), **leucoplasts** (white) and **chromoplasts** (of various colours except green).
- **Chloroplast** is the site of photosynthesis as it contains chlorophyll and is called the **kitchen of the cell.**
- Leucoplasts are storage plastids, while chromoplasts provide various colours like.
- The red colour of tomatoes is due to the presence of **lycopene** pigment, i.e. chromophore.
- The colour of carrot is due to **carotene** pigment.

Endoplasmic Reticulum

- These are hollow membranous system having ribosomes (thus called Rough ER) or no ribosomes (thus called Smooth ER)
- Rough Endoplasmic Reticulum (RER) is the site of **protein synthesis,** while Smooth Endoplasmic Reticulum (SER) is the site of synthesis of **steroids** and **detoxification.**

Golgi Apparatus

- It is made up of sac-like flattened structures and play an important role in secretion, transportation and acrosome formation.
- Their name is attributed to their discoverer, i.e. **Camillo Golgi.**

Ribosomes

- These are minute, non-membranous particles, composed of RNA and protein.
- Their two types, i.e. 70 S type are found in prokaryotes, while 80 S type are found in eukaryotes. These are the site of protein synthesis.

Lysosomes

- These are polymorphic organelles having hydrolytic enzymes.
- These enzymes function at (acidic) pH-5. These are also called as **suicidal bags of the cell.**

Centrosome

- It is composed of two set of centrioles and participate in the formation of mitotic spindle during cell division.

Vacuoles

- These non-living structures mainly belong to plants and are bounded by a membrane called **tonoplast.**
- Pigment anthocyanin is present in the cell vacuole, which provide colour to flowers. It stores toxic metabolic waste and helps in osmoregulation.

Nucleus

- It was discovered by **Robert Brown.** It contains nucleoplasm, nucleolus and chromatin material all covered up by a nuclear membrane.
- Nucleolus is rich in protein and RNA. Chromatin is the main controlling centre of cell as it forms chromosomes.

Chromosome

- It is thread-like structure, found in the nucleus. These are the units of inheritance, i.e. carriers of genetic information from generation to generation, hence also called **genetic vehicles.**
- The number of chromosomes is fixed in each species.

Tissues

- The term **tissue** was coined by **N Grew.**
- It is defined as a group of cells that are structurally similar and constitute together to perform a particular function. e.g., blood, phloem, muscle, etc.
- Tissues are broadly categorised into plant tissues and animal tissues.
- Branch of biology which deals with the study of tissues is known as **histology.**

Plant Tissue

- Most of the tissues present in plants are dead and provide more mechanical strength to them than the living cells because the dead cells of plant do not need so much of maintenance.
- On the basis of the functions they perform, plant tissue can be categorised as

Plant Tissue

- Meristematic tissue
  - Apical meristems
  - Lateral meristems
  - Intercalary meristem
- Permanent Tissue
  - Simple Permanent Tissue (*made up of one type of cells*)
    - Parenchyma
    - Collenchyma
    - Sclerenchyma
  - Complex Permanent Tissue (*made up of many type of cells*)
    - Xylem
    - Phloem

Meristematic Tissue

- It includes group of cells, which remain in continuous state of division or retain their power of division, i.e., they actively divide throughout their life.
- These are living cells which bring an increase in the length and girth (thickness) of the plant. These cells always keep dividing.
- Meristematic tissues are of three types, depending upon the position in the plant body

1. **Apical Meristems** These are found at the apices (growing tips) of main and lateral shoots and roots. It is responsible for height or length of the plants, which is called primary growth.
2. **Lateral Meristems** (Cambium) These are also found on the lateral sides of the stem and roots. These are also responsible for the growth in thickness, i.e., to increase stem or root in diameter called **secondary growth.**
3. **Intercalary Meristems** These are found at the base of the leaves or internodes on twigs (on either side of the node). These meristems help in longitudinal growth of the plant by adding primary tissue. e.g., in stems of various grasses.

Permanent Tissue or Mature Tissue

These are made up of mature cells which have lost their ability of cell division and are already adopted or accommodated to perform some specific work. These tissues are of following two types

1. Simple Permanent Tissue

These are composed of similar type of cells, which have common origin and function. These are further classified under three categories

(i) **Parenchyma** These are the most simple and unspecialised type of permanent tissue, whose cells are usually with intercellular spaces among them, which allows the exchange of gases.

(ii) **Collenchyma** There is no intercellular space as these are elongated in shape due to irregular thickening of cellulose and pectin in the cellular walls. It is basically a mechanical tissue which provides mechanical support and elasticity to the plants.

(iii) **Sclerenchyma** It consists of dead cells and are devoid of protoplasm cells of rigid tissue. Cell walls of such cells are greatly thickened due to lignin or cellulose (or both). It gives mechanical strength, support and rigidity to the plant body.

2. Complex Permanent Tissue

These are another type of permanent tissues, composed of more than one type of cells having common origin. Complex tissues are also of two main types

(i) **Xylem** It is the chief conducting tissue of vascular plants responsible for the conduction of water and inorganic solutes (minerals) from roots to apical parts of the plant. Its main function is to provide mechanical strength and rigidity to the plant.

(ii) **Phloem** It is also the chief conducting tissue of vascular plants responsible for the conduction of organic solutes (food). This conduction may be bi-directional, i.e., from leaves to storage organs or may be from storage organs to growing parts of plants.

Animal Tissue

- Animal tissues have organised layers or masses of structurally similar cells of common embryonic origin and same function.
- All complex animals consist of four basic types of tissues i.e., epithelial, connective, muscular and neural (nervous tissue).

1. Epithelial Tissue or Epithelia

- It is composed of one or more layers of closely packed cells covering the external surface and internal lining of the body organs.
- The epithelium lines all the organs of the body cavity as well as ducts. It also forms a barrier to keep the different body systems separately.

Types of Epithelial Tissues

On the basis of cell layers and shape of cells, epithelial tissues are classified as

(i) **Simple Epithelial Tissue** It is formed from a single layer of cells, resting on the basement membrane. These are mainly found on the secretory and absorptive surfaces.

(ii) **Compound Epithelia** (Multilayered Epithelia) The compound epithelia consists of a few to several layers of cell. Therefore, they are thicker and stronger than the simple epithelia. These have major roles in providing protection to the underlying tissues against chemical, mechanical, thermal or osmotic stresses.

2. Connective Tissue

- These are most abundant and widely distributed in the body of complex animals. These tissues arise from the mesoderm of the embryo.
- They are named so because of their special function of linking and supporting other tissues or organs of the body.
- The basic components of connective tissue are intercellular medium, connective tissue cells and fibres.
- The cells of connective tissue are loosely packed, living, embedded in an intercellular matrix.
- The matrix may be jelly-like fluid, dense or rigid in nature.
- **Functions of connective tissues** Attachment of one tissue to another, supporting cartilage and bone, storage and insulation (by fat storage) transporting materials, etc.

3. Muscular Tissue

- Muscle cells have the feature of contractility.
- Muscles also have the property of electrical excitability, which is due to the energy provided by the electrical potential difference across the plasma membrane.
- Structurally, they consist of long, narrow cells called **muscle fibres** and the cytoplasm which is known as **sarcoplasm**.
- In muscle tissue cells, mitochondria is abundantly present in between the myofibrils and termed as **sarcosomes**.

There are three types of muscular tissue

(i) **Striated (Striped) Muscle** The striated muscle consists of 80% or more of the mass of soft tissues in vertebrates. The cells of this tissue are long, cylindrical, unbranched and multinucleate (having many nuclei).

(ii) **Non-Striated (Smooth) Muscle** The cells of non-striated muscle tissue are thin, long with pin pointed ends (spindle shaped) and uninucleate (i.e., have single nucleus). The conical shaped nucleus is found in the centre of every fibre.

(iii) **Cardiac Muscle** These muscles are mainly confined to the wall of the heart. The muscle cells of the heart are cylindrical, branched and uninucleate.

4. Neural Tissue

- This tissue in an animal receives stimuli and conducts impulses for controlling and coordinating body functions.
- It forms central nervous system (CNS), peripheral nervous system (PNS) and autonomic nervous system (ANS).
- Nervous tissue is mainly composed of nerve cells and glial cells.
- The main function of neural tissue is to accommodate the working of almost all organs according to the specific requirements.

Taxonomic Classification

- A hierarchical system is used for classifying organisms to the species level.
- This system is called taxonomic classification.

The most recent one is that of **RH Whittaker** and is called five kingdom system.

The kingdom were named-Monera, Protista, Fungi, Plantae and Animalia.

Kingdom-Monera (Bacteria)

These are unicellular prokaryotes which may be autotrophic or heterotrophic.

Characteristics of bacteria are as follows

- They have thick cell wall (made up of chitin) and an inner cell membrane (made up of proteins and phospholipids.
- Most bacteria are autotrophic (i.e., can either be photosynthetic or chemosynthetic) and some of them are heterotrophic.
- Bacteria may be saprophytic (derive food from dead plants and animals, e.g., *Pseudomonas*), symbiotic (derive food by living in the body of living beings or hosts, e.g., *Rhizobium*), or parasitic (derive food directly from tissues of living plants or animals). These are responsible for causing various diseases.
- They reproduce asexually by binary fission.
- Sexual reproduction is absent in them but it may occur parasexually by conjugation (two cells fuse and transfer genetic material) and transformation (manipulation of genetic profile by picking up foreign DNA from any external medium).
- Some bacteria that live in liquids have long, thread-like structures called **flagella** for rythmic movement.
- They perform respiratory activities by mesosomes.
- Some bacteria produce methane (from formic acid) and CO_2 and known as methanogenic bacteria, e.g., *Methanococcus.*
- Some bacteria have the ability to live in salt rich media and impart brownish colouration to salt, known as **halophilic**, e.g., *Halococcus.*
- All spore producing bacteria are gram positive and become purple on colouration. The cellular walls of such bacteria are composed of murine.

Kingdom–Protista

The kingdom–Protista was created by **Haeckel** (1886). These were the first eukaryote to evolve about 1000 million years back. This kingdom mostly includes aquatic unicellular eukaryotic cells.

Characteristics of Protista are as follows

- **Cell structure** surrounded by plasmalemma as cell membrane.
- **Cell wall** is composed of cellulose, protein strips (pellicle) and silica.
- **Cell organelles** like mitochondria, Golgi body, endoplasmic reticulum, nucleus, chromosome, etc are present in the fully developed forms.
- **Ribosome** i.e., 80 S are present.
- **Chloroplast** Photosynthetic forms of Protista like dinoflagellates, contain chloroplasts with internal thylakoids.
- **Reproduction** can be both sexual and asexual.
- **Locomotary organs** are cilia and whip-like flagella which occur in a number of forms. They have typical 9 + 2 fibrils.
- **Locomotion** found mostly pseudopodial (e.g., *Amoeba*), flagellar and ciliary.
- **Modes of nutrition** can be autotrophic, heterotrophic or both.

Kingdom–Fungi

These are the most primitive members and show a great diversity in morphology and habitat. Fungi are usually defined as a group of eukaryotic organisms. They may possess a single cell (unicellular) or multiple cells (multicellular). Structurally, they have definite cell wall and true nucleus but lack chlorophyll.

Characteristics of Fungi are as follows

- **Structure** Body is made up of a number of elongated, tubular filaments known as **hyphae.** The body of a fungus having hyphae is known as **mycellium.**
- **Cell Wall** It made up of tough complex sugar, called chitin or **fungal cellulose.**
- **Food Reserve** In the form of glycogen and oil.

Reproduction

- If can be sexual, asexual and vegetative.
  - (a) **Sexual** It includes the formation and union of two gametes or their nuclei.
  - (b) **Asexual** Through the formation of spores. e.g., *Mucor, Rhizopus*, etc.
  - (c) **Vegetative** By fragmentation, budding, fission, etc.
- These are also spore-forming. e.g., yeast, mushrooms, *Aspergillus*, *Penicillium*, *Rhizopus* and *Agaricus.*

Kingdom–Plantae

- Kingdom–Plantae includes green, brown and red algae, liverworts, mosses, ferns and seed plants with or without flowers.
- These are multicellular eukaryotes and generally have chlorophyll in the photosynthetic regions.
- Kingdom–Plantae has been further described under Thallophyta, Bryophyta and Tracheophyta.

Kingdom-Animalia

- There are overall around a million of animals that have been described till now. Therefore, the need of classifying animals becomes very important.
- Animal-kingdom contains animals ranging from sponges to mammals. All members of kingdom Animalia are multicellular, heterotrophic and eukaryotic.
- Animals have four different levels of organisation
  - (a) Protoplasmic grade (e.g., protozoans)
  - (b) Cellular grade (e.g., sponges, mesozoans)
  - (c) Tissue grade (e.g., Platyhelminthes)
  - (d) Organ system (e.g., higher invertebrates and all vertebrates).
- Body symmetry is the similarity of parts in different regions and directions of the body. It may be asymmetrical, radial or bilateral.

Phylum–Protozoa

- These are unicellular animals, i.e., made up of only one cell.
- In these, all the metabolic activity like digestion, respiration, excretion and reproduction takes place in unicellular body, e.g., *Amoeba, Plasmodium, Euglena* etc.

Phylum–Porifera

- These are found in marine water and have porous body. The pores are called **ostia**. These are multicellular animals.
- Their skeleton is made up of minute calcareous or siliceous spicules. e.g., *Sycon*, Sponge, etc.

Phylum–Coelenterata

- These are aquatic animals, have thread-like structures called tentacles around the mouth which help in holding the food.
- They have specialised **cnidoblast** cell to help in catching the food.
- Phenomenon of polymorphism (many forms) and metagenesis (alternation of generation) are associated with coelentrates. e.g., *Hydra*, jellyfish, sea anemone, etc.

Phylum– Platyhelminthes

- Animals of this phylum have alimentary canal with single opening, anus is absent.
- These are hermaphrodite animals (males are not separated from females). e.g., *Planaria*, liverfluke, tapeworm etc.

Phylum–Aschelminthes

- These are long, cylindrical, unsegmented worms.
- Their alimentary canal is complete in which mouth and anus both are present.
- There is no circulatory and respiratory system but nervous system is developed. They are unisexual.
- Most forms are parasitic but some are free-living in soil and water. e.g., *Ascaris*, threadworm, etc.

Phylum-Annelida

- Their body is long, thin, soft and metamerically (truly) segmented.
- Alimentary canal is well-developed.
- These are the first to have proper organ systems.
- Blood (called haemolymph) is red (iron rich haemoglobin).
- Their blood flows in closed vessels.
- They respire through skin.
- Excretion by nephridia.

- They move through setae made up of chitin., e.g. earthworm, *Nereis*, leech etc.

Phylum–Arthropoda

- Arthropoda is the largest phylum (contains maximum number of animals and its existence is recorded for maximum period over the Earth).
- Jointed leg is their main feature.
- Circulatory system is open type.
- Trachea or book lungs, body surface are respiratory organs, e.g., Cockroach, prawn, crab, bug, fly, mosquito, bees, etc.

Phylum–Mollusca

- Their body is soft and divided into head and muscular foot.
- Mantle is always present in it, which secretes a hard calcareous shell.
- Respiration takes place through gills or ctenidia. Blood is colourless.
- Eyes of *Octopus* are similar to chordate eyes e.g. *Pila, Aplysia* (sea rabbit), *Doris* (sea lemon), *Octopus* (Devil fish), *Sepia* (Cuttle fish).

Phylum– Echinodermata

- All the animals in this group are marine. They have water vascular system. Brain is not developed in nervous system.
- They have a special capacity of regeneration.
- These are the only invertebrate animals which contain proper bone like structures (ossicles). e.g., starfish, sea urchin, sea cucumber etc.

Phylum-Chordata

- They have notochord a dorsal hollow tubular nerve cord and paired pharyngeal gill slits at some stage of their lifespan.

Exam Pattern Questions

1 The team 'Biology' was coined by
(a) Aristotle (b) Theophrastus
(c) Lamarck (d) None of these

2 The cell lacking a true nucleus
(a) eukaryotic cells (b) prokaryotic cells
(c) mitotic cells (d) meiotic cells

3 'Protoplasm theory' was proposed by
(a) Schleiden (b) Schwann
(c) Schultze (d) Hooke

4 Which theory explains the structure of protoplasm?
(a) Colloidal theory
(b) Sol-gel theory
(c) Viscosity theory
(d) Surface tension theory

5 Who gave the name cell for the first time?
(a) Robert Hooke (b) Robert Brown
(c) Mendel (d) C Benda

6 Largest organelle of an eukaryotic cell is
(a) nucleus (b) chloroplast
(c) ribosomes (d) mitochondria

7 The role of the mitochondria in a living cell is to
(a) produce energy for the cell
(b) act as the control centre of the cell
(c) store materials in the cell
(d) get rid of the waste materials of the cell

8 Which one of the following has its own DNA?
(a) Mitochondria
(b) Dictyosome
(c) Lysosome
(d) Peroxisome

9 Which is called suicidal bag?
(a) Centrosome (b) Lysosome
(c) Mesosome (d) Chromosome

10 Plant cells are different from animal cells in not having
(a) plastids (b) cell wall
(c) dictyosome (d) lysosome

11 A major site for synthesis of lipid is
(a) RER (b) SER
(c) Symplast
(d) Nucleoplast

12 The Golgi complex plays a major role
(a) in trapping the light and transforming it into chemical energy
(b) in digesting proteins and carbohydrates
(c) as energy transforming organelles
(d) in post transactional modification of protein and glycosidation of lipids

13 Photosynthesis takes place in which cell organelle?
(a) Ribosomes (b) Mitochondria
(c) Chloroplast (d) Golgi body

14 Which of the cell organelle lacks membrane?
(a) Mesosome (b) Mitochondria
(c) Ribosome (d) Liposome

15 RNA plays an important role in
(a) protein synthesis (b) fat synthesis
(c) glucose synthesis (d) Both (a) and (c)

16 Which of the following is known as power house of cell?
(a) Mitochondria (b) Ribosomes
(c) Nucleus (d) RNA

17 Gametes formation takes place through the process of
(a) amitosis (b) mitosis
(c) meiosis (d) fission

18 Which of the following is not a part of epidermal tissue system?
(a) Companion cells (b) Trichomes
(c) Root hairs (d) Guard cells
(e) Subsidiary cells

19 In woody trees, the exchange of gases between the outer atmosphere and the internal tissue of the stem takes place through
(a) aerenchyma (b) stomata
(c) pneumatophores (d) lenticels

20 Cork cambium gives rise to
(a) phellogen and secondary cortex
(b) phellogen, phelloderm and secondary cortex
(c) cork and phellogen
(d) cork and secondary cortex

21 At maturity, the sieve plates become impregnated with
(a) cellulose (b) pectin
(c) suberin (d) lignin

22 Match the following columns.

Column I	Column II
A. Endodermis	1. Companion cells
B. Stomata	2. Lenticels
C. Sieve tube	3. Palisade cells
D. Periderm	4. Passage cells
E. Mesophyll	5. Accessory cells

Codes

	A	B	C	D	E
(a)	4	5	2	1	3
(b)	5	3	1	2	4
(c)	4	5	1	2	3
(d)	4	2	5	3	1

23 The girth of the stem increases due to activity of
(a) apical meristems
(b) intercalary meristems
(c) lateral meristems
(d) parenchyma cells

24 Which of the following plant tissues provides mechanical strength to plants?
(a) Parenchyma
(b) Collenchyma
(c) Sclerenchyma
(d) Aerenchyma

25 The function of a vessel is
(a) conduction of food
(b) conduction of water and minerals
(c) conduction of hormones
(d) All of the above

26 Radial conduction of water takes place by
(a) vessels
(b) vessels and tracheids
(c) phloem
(d) ray parenchymatous cells

27 Which of the following plants shows multiple epidermis?
(a) *Croton* (b) *Allium*
(c) *Nerium* (d) *Cucurbita*

28 The tissue covering the external surface of animal and internal surface of visceral organs is
(a) adipose tissue
(b) connective tissue
(c) cartilaginous tissue
(d) epithelial tissue

29 All the following are examples of connective tissue except
(a) tendons (b) ligaments
(c) muscle (d) adipose tissue

30 Wharton's jelly present in umbilical cord is an example of
(a) adipose tissue
(b) mucus connective tissue
(c) areolar tissue
(d) elastic connective tissue

31 Blood is a kind of
(a) areolar tissue
(b) connective tissue
(c) fluid connective tissue
(d) reticular connective tissue

32 Ligament is mainly made up of
(a) reticulin (b) elastin
(c) myosin (d) collagen

33 The outer covering of cartilage is called
(a) peritoneum (b) periosteum
(c) endosteum (d) perichondrium

34 Cardiac muscle is found in
(a) pericardium (b) endocardium
(c) myocardium (d) peritoneum

35 Smooth muscles are
(a) involuntary, fusiform, non-striated
(b) voluntary, multinucleate, cylindrical
(c) involuntary, cylindrical, striated
(d) voluntary, spindle-shaped, uninucleate

36 Tendons and ligaments are a kind of
(a) muscular tissue (b) connective tissue
(c) epidermal tissue (d) nervous tissue

37 The cavities of alveoli of lungs are lined by
(a) cuboidal epithelium
(b) columnar epithelium
(c) startified cuboidal epithelium
(d) squamous epithelium

38 Fibroblasts, macrophages and mast cells are seen in
(a) epithelial tissue (b) connective tissue
(c) skeletal muscle tissue (d) smooth muscle tissue

39 Choose the wrong statement with reference smooth muscles.
(a) Myofibrils show alternate dark and light bands
(b) They are spindle-shaped uninucleate cells
(c) Their contractions are under the control of autonomous nervous system
(d) They exhibit prolonged contractions

40 Which one is a specialised connective tissue among these?
(a) Adipose tissue (b) Bone
(c) Areolar tissue (d) Fibroblasts

41 Cellular organisation of body is present in
(a) Annelida (b) Platyhelminthes
(c) Porifera (d) Urochordata

42 Collar cells are characteristic of
(a) earthworm (b) roundworms
(c) coelenterates (d) sponges

43 In most simple type of canal system of Porifera, water flows through which one of the following ways?
(a) Ostia → Spongocoel → Osculum → Exterior
(b) Spongocoel → Ostia → Osculum → Exterior
(c) Osculum → Spongocoel → Ostia → Exterior
(d) Osculum → Ostia → Spongocoel → Exterior

44 Radial symmetry is seen in
(a) *Hydra* (b) *Schistoma*
(c) *Taenia* (d) *Fasciola*

45 Animal without anus is
(a) *Unio* (b) *Pheretima*
(c) *Fasciola* (d) *Periplanata*

46 Jellyfish belongs to class
(a) Hydrozoa (b) Scyphozoa
(c) Anthozoa (d) None of these

47 Budding is found in
(a) *Sycon* (b) *Hydra*
(c) *Fasciola* (d) *Obelia*

48 Cavity of coelenterates is called
(a) coelenteron (b) coelom
(c) cavity (d) None of these

49 Medusa is the reproductive organ of
(a) *Hydra* (b) *Aurelia*
(c) *Obelia* (d) Sea anemone

50 Which of the following animal phyla does not possess a coelom?
(a) Platyhelminthes (b) Annelida
(c) Mollusea
(d) Echinodermata

51 Which one of the following kinds of animal are triplobastic?
(a) Flatworms
(b) Sponges
(c) Ctenophores
(d) Corals

52 Earthworms are
(a) ureotelic, when plenty of water is available
(b) uricotelic, when plenty of water is available
(c) uricotelic under conditions of water scarcity
(d) ammonotelie when plenty of water is available

53 Earthworms have no skeleton, but during burrowing the anterior ene becomes turgid and act as a hydraulic skeleton. It is due to
(a) coelomic fluid (b) blood
(c) gut peristalsis (d) setae

54 Which is not correctly matched?
(a) Annelida - Enterocoelomate
(b) Platyhelminthes - Acoelomate
(c) Arthropoda - Schizocoelomate
(d) Nemathelminthes - pseudocoelomate

Answers

1 (c)	2 (b)	3 (c)	4 (a)	5 (a)	6 (a)	7 (a)	8 (a)	9 (b)	10 (a)
11 (b)	12 (d)	13 (c)	14 (c)	15 (a)	16 (a)	17 (c)	18 (a)	19 (d)	20 (d)
21 (d)	22 (d)	23 (c)	24 (c)	25 (b)	26 (d)	27 (c)	28 (d)	29 (c)	30 (b)
31 (c)	32 (b)	33 (b)	34 (c)	35 (a)	36 (b)	37 (d)	38 (b)	39 (a)	40 (b)
41 (c)	42 (d)	43 (a)	44 (a)	45 (c)	46 (b)	47 (b)	48 (a)	49 (c)	50 (a)
51 (a)	52 (d)	53 (a)	54 (a)						

Chapter 02

Ornithology (Science of Birds)

Introduction

- The study related to birds is called **Ornithology**. Dr. Salim Ali is regarded as 'Bird Man of India'.
- The birds belong to phylum Chordata and class Aves. It is related to animal kingdom.

Characteristics of Birds

- The body is boat-shaped (streamlined) and is divisible into head, neck, trunk and tail. On the head a toothless beak or bill is also visible.
- The forelimbs are modified into wings and have powerful flight muscles, which bear three clawless digits.

  Three main categories of flight muscles are
  (i) **Pectoral Muscles** Pectoralis major (most powerful flight muscle) and pectoralis miner.
  (ii) **Accessory Muscles** Coraco-brachialis longus and coraco-brachialis brevis.
  (iii) **Tensor Muscles** Tensor longus, tensor brevis and tensor accessories.
- They have **pneumatic bones**, i.e., contain air cavities to reduce weight. The lower jaw consists of five or six bones and it articulates with the quadrate and have no teeth.
- They are air breathing, **endothermic** or **warm-blooded** (can regulate their body temperature), oviparous, bipedal, feather-covered vertebrates.
- The hindlimbs are adapted for walking, perching and swimming and bear four claws.
- They have **epidermal exoskeleton** in the form of feathers, scales, claws and beaks. Scales (epidermal) are present only on lower legs and feet.
- The skin is dry and skin glands are absent except the cutaneous oil glands or preen glands (uropygial glands) that are located at the root of the tail. These glands are absent in parrot and ostrich.
- The **sternum** is large and it bears a keel for the attachment to flight muscles.
- Two special structures **crop** and **gizzard** are present in alimentary canal. The crop stores and softens the food. The gizzard is muscular to crush the softened food.
- Some birds keep store in the gizzard to effectively crush seeds and grains. Gall bladder is absent.
- Respiration only takes place by lungs. The lungs are provided with **air sacs**. The birds exhibit double-respiration. Air sacs are connected to lungs for supplement respiration.
- A **syrinx** or **sound box** is present at the caudal end of the trachea.
- The heart is **four-chambered** (two auricles and two ventricles) with no sinus venosus, only right systemic arch is present. This keeps the oxygenated and deoxygenated blood separate. RBCs are oval, biconvex and nucleated.
- The females have a **single left ovary** and lay telolecithal (large yolk), cleidoic (with calcareous shell) and amniotic eggs.
- Fertilisation is internal but lack copulatory organs except ratilae, geese and ducks.
- Eyes are powerful and have nictitating membranes, sclerotic ring (bony structure) and pecten (which help in accommodation).

Flight Adaptation in Birds

In birds almost every system is modified to support flight as given under

- The boat-shaped body helps to proper through the air easily.
- The feathers constitute very smooth covering over the body to reduce the friction of the air.
- Wings (remiges) act as main organ of flight with association of feathers. They are responsible for supporting the bird during the flight. Remiges are attached by ligament or directly to the bone.
- Extremely powerful muscles are developed to enable the wings to work during flight. These are **pectoralis major** and **minor**, **coraco-branchialis brevis** and **longus**.
- The bones are light, hollow and provide more space for the muslces attachment.
- Due to pneumatic nature, weight of the body is reduced, which is helpful in flight. The bones are lacking bone marrow. Bones of skull are fused, light and extremely thin. The teeth are absent in beak.
- The first four thoracic vertebrate are fused to form a **fulcrum** for working of the wings. In flightless birds, they are free.
- **Sternum** is well-developed and supports the viscera and provide the surface for the attachment of flight muscles.
- The sternum (breastbone), bears a prominent keel where the flight muscles attach. The last four **caudal vertebrae** are fused to form the pygostyle, which offer a strong attachment to the rectrices.
- The **furcula** (wishbone), serves as a brace during the flight stroke. It is derived from the pectoral girdle in birds.
- The **lungs** are spongy and inelastic. Due to high metabolic rate required for flight, birds have a high oxygen demand. Air sacs of birds reduce the body weight.
- Birds have four-chambered heart, show double circulation and maintain high body temperature.
- Another weight reducing adaptation in birds is the absence of a urinary bladder and a urethra. Water is reabsorbed in urinary tubules and coprodaeum. (chamber of cloaca).
- So, the outcome of the nitrogenous waste is the insoluble uric acid, which is thrown at once with faecal matter.
- Reproductive system has single left **ovary** and **oviduct** to reduce the weight of the body.

Some Common Birds

The common birds found in nearly places of own houses are pigeon and house sparrow.

The general description of these two birds is as follows

Pigeon *(Columba livia)*

- This is an omnivorous bird commonly found in all types of Indian climate. It is 20-25 cm long, grey coloured sometimes white coloured bird.
- It's body is covered with feathers and it has a short tail. It's beak is pointed toothless and is hooked. It's forlimbs are modified into wings for flying purpose.
- It's hindlimbs are clawed having four fingers in each toe. These are unisexual and oviparous animals.

House Sparrow *(Passer domesticus)*

- This is an omnipresent bird and found every where in India. It's body is 10-12 cm long, streamlined.
- It is covered with brownish grey coloured feathers. It is an warm-blooded animal.
- The abnomial region in both male and female animal is covered with white feathers.
- The male's upper body is covered with blackish, greyish coloured feathers, so can be easily distinctively recognised from females.
- Both male and female have strong small beak. The other common birds are crow, parrot, cuckoo, kingfisher, etc.

Exam Pattern Questions

1. The branch of science dealing with the study of birds is
(a) Herpetology (b) Ornithology
(c) Oncology (d) Anthropology

2. Name the 'Bird Man of India'
(a) Karm Narayan Bahl
(b) MI Bhatia
(c) Salim Ali
(d) EM Thillayampalam

3. Birds fly with the help of
(a) patagium (b) wing
(c) feather (d) limbs

4. What is true about birds?
(a) Fertilisation is external
(b) 10 pairs of cranial nerves are present
(c) They excrete mostly urea
(d) They have a beak, but no teeth

5. In birds, the lungs are
(a) spongy
(b) spongy and inelastic
(c) solid
(d) solid and elastic

6. The most important feature of class-Aves is
(a) 4-chambered heart
(b) presence of tail
(c) thermal regulation
(d) exoskeleton of feathers

7. Which one is developed in Aves?
(a) Right systemic arch
(b) Left systemic arch
(c) Both (a) and (b)
(d) A complex of three aorta

8. Flight feathers are
(a) contours
(b) down feathers
(c) coverts
(d) filoplumes

9. Remiges are
(a) flight feathers of wings
(b) flight feathers of tail
(c) small feathers similar to quills
(d) small feathers that cover the body

10. Sternum of birds is prolonged to form boat-shaped structure called
(a) keel (b) retrices
(c) remiges (d) pygostyle

11. Bones of birds are
(a) solid and heavy (b) solid and light
(c) hollow and light (d) spongy and heavy

12. The characters of birds, without oception is
(a) omnivorous
(b) flying wings
(c) beak without teeth
(d) lay eggs with calcarious shell

13. The largest aquatic mammal is
(a) otter (b) sea lion
(c) dolphin (d) blue whale

14. Which of these defines the birds best?
(a) Flying (b) Warm-blooded
(c) Feathered quadrupeds (d) Feathered bipeds

15. Birds do not possess
(a) teeth (b) urinary bladder
(c) gall bladder (d) All of these

16. The avian eyes are peculiar because of the presence of
(a) pecten (b) large number of cones
(c) large pupil (d) sensitive retina

17. Birds possess
(a) right ovary (b) left-systemic arch
(c) urinary bladder (d) None of these

18. Which of the following traits is not characteristic of birds?
(a) air sacs attached to lungs (b) hollow bones
(c) ectothermic (d) amniote egg

19. Air sacs of birds
(a) Keep body warm
(b) Facilitate blood circulation
(c) Maintain body temperature
(d) Reduce body weight

20. What is common among dodo, penguin and rhea?
(a) These are flightless birds
(b) These are running birds
(c) These are migratory birds
(d) These have four toes in their feet

21. Flight muscles of bird are attached to
(a) clavicle (b) coracoid
(c) keel of sternum (d) scapula

22. Bird vertebrate are
(a) heterocoelous
(b) procoelous
(c) acoelous
(d) opisthocoelous

23. Birds differ from bats in the absence of
(a) 4-chambered heart
(b) homoiothermy
(c) diaphragm
(d) tracheae

24. The largest egg belongs to
(a) elephant (b) whale
(c) dinosaur (d) ostrich

25. Both male and female pigeons secrete milk through
(a) mammary glands (b) crop glands
(c) salivary glands (d) gizzard glands

26. Birds have bipedal locomotion as it
(a) reduces body weight
(b) increases rate of locomotion
(c) provides more support to the body
(d) spares forelimbs for flight

27. Bone marrow does not occur in
(a) fishes (b) amphibians
(c) birds (d) reptiles

28. Female have only left functional ovary in
(a) salamander (b) pigeon
(c) rabbit (d) *Uromastix*

29. Two chief features of mammals which distinguish them from other vertebrates are
(a) Hair and viviparity
(b) Viviparity and mammary glands
(c) Viviparity and internal fertilisation
(d) Mammary glands and internal fertilisation

30. If a bird is transferred from 30°C to 10°C. The body temperature true will change to
(a) 10°C (b) 30°C
(c) 15°C (d) remain unchanged

31. Eggs of birds are
(a) alecithal (b) telolecithal
(c) homolecithal (d) isolecithal

32. Which one of the following birds cannot perch?
(a) Sparrow (b) Crow (c) Duck (d) Robin

33. A flying bird lands by
(a) folding the wings back and dropping on the ground or other substratum
(b) folding the wings above and back of the body and coming down
(c) lowering and fanning out the retrices
(d) pronation and forward movements of wings

34. Only cutaneous gland present in bird is
(a) sebaceous gland (b) sweat gland
(c) uropygial gland (d) femoral gland

35. What is the generic name of sparrow?
(a) *Pavo* (b) *Passer*
(c) *Corvus* (d) *Eudynamis*

36. Kiwi is found in
(a) India (b) South America
(c) New Zealand (d) East Indies

37. The smallest bird is
(a) Cuban bee (b) Sun bird
(c) *Passer* (d) None of these

38. The bird that hibernates in winter is
(a) Poorwill *(Caprimulgus)*
(b) Arctic tern *(Sterna)*
(c) Albatross
(d) None of the above

39. Largest living bird is
(a) eagle (b) rhea
(c) humming bird (d) ostrich

Answers

1 *(b)*	2 *(c)*	3 *(b)*	4 *(d)*	5 *(b)*	6 *(d)*	7 *(a)*	8 *(c)*	9 *(a)*	10 *(a)*
11 *(c)*	12 *(c)*	13 *(d)*	14 *(d)*	15 *(d)*	16 *(a)*	17 *(d)*	18 *(c)*	19 *(d)*	20 *(a)*
21 *(c)*	22 *(a)*	23 *(c)*	24 *(d)*	25 *(b)*	26 *(d)*	27 *(c)*	28 *(b)*	29 *(d)*	30 *(d)*
31 *(b)*	32 *(c)*	33 *(b)*	34 *(c)*	35 *(b)*	36 *(c)*	37 *(a)*	38 *(a)*	39 *(d)*	

Chapter 03

Biological Processes

- Life can be defined as a unique aggregation of molecules. These molecules have the tendency to express themselves through various chemical reactions collectively called metabolic reactions.
- The basic purpose of these reactions is to transform (produce) and utilise energy.

The metabolism is of two types

(a) **Anabolism** In this, all those reactions of the body are involved in which complex biomolecules are synthesised, e.g. photosynthesis.

(b) **Catabolism** These are breaking down reactions and form simple molecules form complex ones, e.g. respiration digestion.

Nutrition

- Energy is the basic requirement of all living organisms to perform various vital activities, that are required for their survival.
- Nutrition is a process of intake of nutrients (such as carbohydrates, fats, proteins, minerals, vitamins and water) by an organism as well as the utilisation of these nutrients for the maintenance of different life processes like growth, repair, reproduction, etc.

Types of Nutrition in Plants

There are two main types of nutrition in plants

1. Autotrophic Nutrition

- The word *'auto'* means self and *'trophe'* means nutrition. Thus, autotrophic nutrition is the mode of nutrition in which an organism makes (synthesises) its own food by the utilisation of simple substances like carbon dioxide and water in the presence of sunlight.
- This process is known as **photosynthesis**. It is an enzyme regulated anabolic process of manufacturing organic compounds inside the chlorophyll containing cells, (i.e., chloroplasts) from carbon dioxide and water with the help of sunlight (as a source of energy).
- This process is used by green plants to make their own food.
- In other words, it is defined as the process by which plants can convert light energy to chemical energy and store it in the form of sugars (carbohydrate).
- The oxygen produced is considered as the waste product of photosynthesis.

  The equation of photosynthesis is as follows

$$6CO_2 + 12H_2O \xrightarrow[\text{Radiant energy (686 kcal)}]{\text{Chlorophyll, Enzymes}} C_6H_{12}O_6 + 6O_2 \uparrow + 6H_2O$$

2. Heterotrophic Nutrition

- The word *'heteros'* means *others* and *'trophe'* means *nutrition*. Thus, heterotrophy means 'nutrition obtained from others'.
- Heterotrophic nutrition is that mode of nutrition in which an organism cannot prepare (or synthesise) its own food from simple inorganic materials like carbon dioxide and water and depends on other organisms for it. Such organisms are called **heterotrophs**.

These plants are further categorised into two types

(i) **Parasitic Plants** These plants derive some or all of its nutritional need from other living plants.

e.g., *Cuscuta, Orobanche, Viscum, Loranthus, Santalum, Hyobanche, Sanguinea,* dodder, *Rafflesia,* Western Australian Christmas tree, etc.

(ii) **Saprophytic Plants** These are the plants that grow and live on dead and decaying matter of animals and plants and take their nutrition by secreting digestive juices on these matter and converting them into a solution.
The plants that follow saprophitic mode of nutrition are known as **saprotrophs**. e.g., fungi, bacteria, etc.

Digestion

- Food is the basic requirement of all living beings. It provides energy and organic materials for growth and repair of tissues. The major components of the food are carbohydrates, proteins and fats.
- Vitamins and minerals are also required in small quantities. The water we take in also plays an important role in body's metabolic processess.
- There are two types of digestion
  (i) **Digestion in Unicellular Organisms**
  It occurs in the cell itself in the food vacuoles. So it is called as **intra cellular digestion**. The examples of unicellular organism carrying snin type of digestion are *Amoeba, Paramecium, Euglena* etc.
  (ii) **Digestion in Multicellular Organisms**
  It occurs in a tubular digestive system and is associated digestive glands. The food get digested is different part of this tubular system in the help of digestive secretions. It is found in higher vertebrates e.g. monkey, man, etc.

Respiration

- All living beings obtain energy *via* oxidation of nutrients taken. The process of nutrient oxidation is called **respiration.**
- The obtained energy is stored in an individuals body as ATP (Adenosine Triphosphate). It is a compound known to occur in all living cells and referred to as universal energy currency.
- This usually takes place in the presence of oxygen and energy is released in the process as ATP. During the process of breakdown of food molecules, carbon dioxide gas (which is toxic to the body cells) is also released.

Types of Respiration

Based on the mode of oxidation of nutrients respiration is of following two types

(i) **Aerobic Respiration** It occurs when the cells utilise molecular oxygen for oxidising nutrient. It occurs in the mitochondria of the cells. It produces a lot of ATP per glucose molecule. It is done under normal circumstances by an animal, when heart rate and breathing rates are normal.

(ii) **Anaerobic Respiration** It occurs, when nutrients are oxidised without using molecular oxygen. It is also called **fermentation.**
It occurs in the cytoplasm of the cells. It produces less ATP per glucose molecule. It is done during oxygen deficient situations, i.e. like the first 1-2 minutes of exercise.

Respiration in Plants

- It occurs by all body cells of plant present in root, stem, leave etc.

Respiration in Animals

- The lower animals breath through their body surfaces i.e. skin, while higher animals have respiratory system for exchange of gases (CO_2 and O_2).

Circulatory System

- All living cells require nutrients, oxygen and other essential materials for their growth and survival.
- These substances take part in various metabolic processes of the cell.
- It is therefore, essential to have an efficient mechanism for the movement of these substances to and from the cells.

The animals have two types of circulatory system

(i) **Open Circulatory System** In this type the tissue remain suspended and bathing in the blood which is present in the body cavity. It occurs in insects and cephalopod animals.

(ii) **Closed Circulatory System** It occurs in higher vertebrates like rabbit, earthworm and man. In this the blood flows in tubular system called **blood vessels** (Arteries, Veins and Capillaries).

Transport in Plants

- The plants transport and circulate mineral salt/water through special tissue called **conductive tissue** (Xylem for Water and Mineral, phloem for food).

Excretion

- Certain waste products are formed as a result of metabolic reactions in the body of organisms. The biological process which eliminates such materials from the body is called **excretion.**
- The nitrogenous waste products like ammonia (NH_3), urea and uric acid etc., get dissoluted in water and thrown out from body of an individuals.

Excretion in Plants

The excretion in plants occurs in the following ways

- Through gaseous wastes
- Through water soluble wastes
- Through solid wastes
- Some useful excretory products of plants are Tannin, Essential oil, Gum, Resin, Rubber and many other medicinally useful products.

Excretion in Animals

There are three types of exception, based on the type of nitrogenous waste

- **Ammonotelic** (bony fishes, Amphibians)
- **Ureotelic** (mammals and other vertebrates)
- **Uric acid** or **Uricotelic** (Birds, Reptiles, insects).

Movement and Locomotion

- Movement is a change in posture or position of any body part of a living organism. It is an essential and significant feature of living organisms.
- When movement results in change of place or location it is termed as locomotion. Animals show both movement and locomotion, while plants show movement only. Locomotion is rare in them.

Types of Movements

Living beings show following two basic types of movements

1. Non-muscular movements

These movements do not involve any kind of muscular tissue in them. They are further of following types

(i) **Amoeboid or Pseudopodial Movement** It occurs with the help of pseudopodia, which are formed by cytoplasm. It is found in protozoans, leucocytes and macrophages for capturing food and change their place.

(ii) **Ciliary Movement** This type of movement occurs in protozoans and in the internal tubular organs of higher animals, which are lined by ciliated epithelium, e.g. ciliated movement in trachea helps us in removing waste substances inhaled.

(iii) **Flagellar Movement** This type of movement occurs in protozoans like *Trypanosoma, Euglena*, etc. along with sponges. In sponges, flagella of choanocyte cells maintain a regular current of water through the canal system.

2. Muscular Movement

- It is the basic type of movement used in majority of vertebrates including humans. It takes place through muscle fibres of muscular tissue.

Movement in Plants

The movement in plants occurs through growth. It is of the types

- Movements of locomotion which includes rotation and circulation.
- Movements of curvature occurs due to light, gravity, water stimulation.

Control and Coordination

- Multicellular animals have structurally complex body organisation. Due to this, there arises a need to have a system for coordinating various metabolic and homeostatic activities of different parts, organs, organ systems in the body.

- This is achieved by nervous and endocrine systems present in the body. Both these systems jointly coordinate and integrated all such activities.

Reproduction

The process of producing the new individuals of their own kind by living organisms is called reproduction. It is of two types :

(i) **Asexual Reproduction** In thus, the new individuals are produced without any act of fertilisation.
It occurs by the following methods
(a) Binary fission e.g. Bacteria, *Euglena*
(b) Fragmentation e.g. *Spirogyra, Rhizopus*
(c) Budding e.g. Yeast, *Hydra*
(d) Regeneratin e.g. *Hydra, Planaria.*
(e) Sporulation e.g. *Mucor, Rhizopus*
(f) Vegetative reproduction Rose, Grapes.

(ii) **Sexual Reproduction** In this kind of reproduction, two parents are involved and formation and fusion of gametes takes place. The offsprings produced by this method are different from their parents. This process is main source of evolution in organisms.

Reproduction in Plants

- The higher plants (angiosperms) have special structures specially meant for the reproduction.
- These structures are found in the flower of plants. It is a modified shoot which has outer and inner whorls having four essential organs named calyx, corolla, androecium and gynoecium.

The following steps are involved in sexual reproduction in plants

(i) **Gametogenesis** The male and female gametes are formed as result of meiotic cell division. These are haploid structures. Pollens are male gametes and egg cell is female gamete.
(ii) **Pollination** Transfer of pollen from anther to stigma of ovary is called pollination. It is brought about by various agencies like wind, insects etc.
(iii) **Fertilisation** It is an act of union of male and female gametes. After fertilisation the zygote formed develops into an embryo, ovary into **seeds** and **fruits.**

Reproduction in Animals

The reproduction in higher animals is mainly by sexual methods. It involves the following steps

(i) **Gametogenesis** The process of formation of gamete is called gametogenesis. The haploid male and female gametes are formed in male and female organs of an animal. The formation of sprem is called spermatogenesis and formation of egg is called **oogenesis.**
(ii) **Fertilisation** There are two types of fertilisation in animals
(a) **External fertilisation** e.g. fishes, frogs etc.
(b) **Internal fertilisation** e.g., Reptiles, birds, mammals.
(iii) **Development of Embryo** The formed zygote by the act of fertilisation divide by mitotic cell division. Which later develops into an fully grown individuals either outside or inside female body of organism.

Exam Pattern Questions

1 Which of the following combines with O_2 in our body to provide energy?
(a) Amino acids (b) Glucose
(c) Fatty acids (d) Glycogen

2 Which of the following is not required for photosynthesis?
(a) Oxygen (b) Carbon dioxide
(c) Sunlight (d) Water

3 The breathing organ in the plants is
(a) lungs (b) stomata
(c) gills (d) seeds

4 Green plants make their food in the presence of
(a) sunlight, water, carbon dioxide
(b) oxygen and water

(c) water and carbon dioxide
(d) None of the above

5 Photophosphorylation takes place in which cell organelle?
(a) Ribosomes (b) Mitochondria
(c) Chloroplast (d) Golgi body

6 The tubes which carry water and minerals to the leaf are called
(a) stomata (b) veins
(c) petiole (d) cells

7 The food factories of plant are
(a) leaves (b) flowers
(c) seeds (d) fruits

8 Which part of a plant respires?
(a) Root (b) Leaf
(c) Seed (d) All of these

9 Digestive system
(a) gives message to the body
(b) helps to burn food
(c) makes the food into simple form
(d) None of the above

10 Protein which catalyse or helps in biochemical reactions are called
(a) hormones (b) structural protein
(c) protective protein (d) enzymes

11 Saliva helps in the digestion of
(a) fats (b) proteins (c) fibres (d) starch

12 What should be given to an athlete for instant energy?
(a) Protein (b) Vitamin
(c) Carbohydrate (d) None of these

13 Which of the following is the component of balance diet?
(a) Carbohydrate (b) Minerals
(c) Water (d) All of these

14 Stomach in vertebrates, is the chief site for digestion of
(a) fats (b) proteins
(c) carbohydrates (d) All of these

15 In mammals, the digestion of starch starts from
(a) mouth (b) stomach
(c) oesophagus (d) duodenum

16 Glycogen is stored in
(a) liver and muscles (b) liver
(c) epidermis (d) muscles

17 Emulsification is the function of
(a) bile (b) lipases
(c) esterases (d) proteases

18 Respiration can be defined as
(a) a catabolic process by which animal cells utilise carbon dioxide, produce oxygen and convert the released energy to ATP
(b) a catabolic process by which animal cells utilise oxygen, produce carbon dioxide and convert the released energy to ATP
(c) an anabolic process by which animal cells utilise oxygen and carbon dioxide to form ATP
(d) an anabolic process by which animal cells utilise oxygen, produce carbon dioxide and convert the released energy to ATP

19 Exchange of gases in lungs is by
(a) simple diffusion (b) active transport
(c) passive transport (d) osmosis

20 Haemoglobin most strongly combines with
(a) carbon monoxide (b) oxygen
(c) carbon dioxide (d) ozone

21 The affinity of carbon monoxide for Hb is .... more than oxygen.
(a) 2 times (b) 20 times
(c) 200 times (d) 1000 times

22 The mammal with nucleated RBC's is
(a) rabbit (b) camel
(c) monkey (d) rat

23 Blood pressure in measured by
(a) Sphygmomanometer (b) Stethoscope
(c) Electrocardiogram (d) Phonocardiogram

24 Which is the protein, present in human blood?
(a) Myosin (b) Insulin
(c) Haemoglobin (d) Trypsin

25 Blood plasma has a pH of
(a) 7.4 (b) 7.8
(c) 6.9 (d) 6.3

26 Smallest blood vessel in the body is
(a) capillary (b) artery
(c) vein (d) vena cava

27 The normal blood pressure of human beings is in one of the following ranges

(a) 140/80 mm (b) 110/70 mm
(c) 120/80 mm (d) 110/75 mm

28 The body organ which is not present in pair is
(a) kidney (b) testes
(c) ovary (d) heart

29 Blood is formed in the human adult by the
(a) heart (b) spleen
(c) red bone marrow (d) yellow bone marrow

30 Circulatory system
(a) gives oxygen to the body
(b) helps to burn food
(c) makes the food into simple form
(d) None of the above

31 Veins carry blood
(a) away from the heart (b) towards the heart
(c) towards the brain (d) None of these

32 Which of the following is made up of muscular walls?
(a) Blood (b) Bone (c) Heart (d) Skin

33 Kidney is a part of
(a) digestive system (b) skeleton system
(c) nervous system (d) excretory system

34 Which of the following is the most toxic waste matter?
(a) Urea (b) Uric acid
(c) Ammonia (d) Hippuric acid

35 Animal, which excretes urea produced during metabolism of amino acid is
(a) ureotelism (b) uricotelism
(c) ammonotelism (d) aminotelism

36 The main function of kidney is
(a) ultrafiltration (b) passive absorption
(c) selective reabsorption (d) Both (a) and (c)

37 Accessory excretory human organ is
(a) skin (b) skin and liver
(c) skin and lungs (d) All of these

38 In which of the following part largest muscle is found in human body?
(a) In hand (b) In nitambh
(c) In neck (d) In legs

39 Tendons are made up of
(a) collagen (b) elastin
(c) keratin (d) All of these

40 Total number of bones in the body of man is
(a) 28 (b) 206 (c) 108 (d) 218

41 In old age, stiffness of joints is due to the
(a) hardening of bones
(b) inefficiency of muscles
(c) decreases in synovial fluid
(d) enlargement of bones

42 Nervous system
(a) helps to produce babies
(b) helps us to breathe
(c) controls our actions
(d) None of the above

43 The brain
(a) pumps blood to all parts of the body
(b) is the main control centre of the body
(c) helps to breath in air
(d) None of the above

44 Memory is the responsibility of
(a) grey matter (b) white matter
(c) cerebrum (d) cerebellum

45 The master control centre of the human body in
(a) brain (b) heart
(c) stomach (d) liver

46 Which muscle type is moved voluntarily?
(a) Cardiac (b) Skeletal
(c) Smooth (d) All of these

47 Which harmone is produced by the testes of male?
(a) Testosterone
(b) Progesterone
(c) Melatonin
(d) Thyroxine

48 The hormone which is not directly associated with reproduction is
(a) testosterone (b) oestrogen
(c) progesterone (d) parathormone

49 Goitre or abnormal enlargement of the thyroid gland is caused by the deficiency of
(a) iodine (b) iron
(c) calcium
(d) potassium

50 Which gland secretes the most kinds of hormones?
(a) Adrenal (b) Pineal
(c) Pituitary (d) Thyroid

51 The number of floating ribs in the human body is

(a) 6 pairs (b) 5 pairs
(c) 3 pairs (d) 2 pairs

52 During which of the following types of reproduction do the fully matured tiny individuals detach from the parent body and become new independent individuals?
(a) Multiple fission
(b) Fission
(c) Budding
(d) Regeneration

53 New individual develops from buds :
(a) *Amoeba* (b) *Paramecium*
(c) Bacteria (d) *Hydra*

54 The number of chromosomes in a human female germ cells is
(a) 46 (b) 48
(c) 23 (d) 24

55 Male germ cells are produced an ....
(a) testes (b) epididymis
(c) ovary (d) prostrate

56 Gametes formation takes place through the process of
(a) amitosis (b) mitosis
(c) meiosis (d) fission

57 The pitch of the voice in females is in general
(a) much lower than that of men
(b) marginally lower than that of men
(c) higher than that of men
(d) the same as that of men

58 Wind pollination is common in
(a) lilies (b) grasses
(c) orchids (d) legumes

59 If you want to develop hybrid seeds within a bisexual flower, the following part needs to be removed from the same flower
(a) stigma (b) ovary (c) anther (d) oviduct

60 Plants with ovaries having only one or a few ovules, are generally pollinated by
(a) bees (b) butterflies
(c) birds (d) wind

61 Male gametes in angiosperms are formed by the division of
(a) microspore (b) generative cell
(c) vegetative cell
(d) microspore mother cell

62 Cross pollination through insect agent is called
(a) anthropophily (b) malacophily
(c) entomphily (d) ornithophily

63 Zygote is resulted by the process
(a) Isogamy (b) Anisogamy
(c) Monogamy (d) Syngamy

64 Testa of a seed is produced from
(a) ovary wall (b) hilum
(c) outer integument of ovule
(d) funicle

Answers

1 *(b)*	2 *(a)*	3 *(b)*	4 *(a)*	5 *(c)*	6 *(b)*	7 *(a)*	8 *(d)*	9 *(c)*	10 *(d)*
11 *(d)*	12 *(c)*	13 *(d)*	14 *(b)*	15 *(a)*	16 *(a)*	17 *(a)*	18 *(b)*	19 *(a)*	20 *(a)*
21 *(c)*	22 *(b)*	23 *(a)*	24 *(c)*	25 *(a)*	26 *(a)*	27 *(c)*	28 *(d)*	29 *(c)*	30 *(a)*
31 *(b)*	32 *(c)*	33 *(d)*	34 *(c)*	35 *(b)*	36 *(d)*	37 *(d)*	38 *(b)*	39 *(a)*	40 *(b)*
41 *(a)*	42 *(c)*	43 *(b)*	44 *(c)*	45 *(a)*	46 *(b)*	47 *(a)*	48 *(d)*	49 *(a)*	50 *(c)*
51 *(d)*	52 *(c)*	53 *(d)*	54 *(c)*	55 *(a)*	56 *(c)*	57 *(c)*	58 *(b)*	59 *(c)*	60 *(d)*
61 *(b)*	62 *(c)*	63 *(d)*	64 *(a)*						

Chapter 04 Human Body and System

- Various organs in the body specialised to perform specific functions, work together in coordination to maintain the body.
- These systems include digestive system, respiratory system, circulatory system, excretory system, skeletal system, nervous system, endocrine and reproductive system.

Digestive System

The human digestive system consists of **alimentary canal** and **digestive glands**. The alimentary canal consists of mouth (having teeth and tongue), oesophagus, stomach, small intestine and large intestine.

Dentition

- The oral or buccal cavity of vertebrates contains masticatory organs called **teeth**. Mammal contains two sets of teeth.
- The first set is called **milk teeth** and second set is called **permanent teeth**.
- These are of following four types
  (i) **Incisors** (for cutting) four in each jaw.
  (ii) **Canines** (for tearing) two in each jaw.
  (iii) **Premolars** (for grinding) four in each jaw.
  (iv) **Molars** (for grinding) six in each jaw.
- The number of teeth are different in different animals.

  Dental Formula In adults

  $$I\frac{2}{2}, C\frac{1}{1}, Pm\frac{2}{2}, M\frac{3}{3} = \frac{8}{8} \times 2 = 32$$

- Tooth has three regions, i.e. crown, neck and root. Enamel covering the outer part of teeth is the hardest substance in the body.
  In elephants, tusks are the incisors of the upper jaw.

Digestive Glands

Various glands are associated with alimentary canal, serving the process of digestion of food. These are given below

- **Salivary Glands** These glands secrete saliva containing an enzyme called **salivary amylase** (ptyalin). Three pairs of salivary glands that secrete saliva are parotid (present below the pinna) submaxillary (present on inner side of lower jaw) and sublingual (present below the tongue).
- **Gastric Glands** These are found in the wall of the stomach. The gastric glands release digestive juice containing HCl, pepsin, mucous, etc.
- **Liver** It is known as the largest gland of the body, which secretes bile juices. They act on large fat molecules to form smaller globules thus, increasing the efficiency of enzyme action. Gall bladder stores bile juice for the further use.
- **Intestinal Glands** Walls of small intestine contain numerous glands that secrete intestinal juice containing **amylolytic, proteolytic** and **lipolytic** enzymes.
- **Pancreas** It secretes **pancreatic juice**, which contains enzymes like **amylase, trypsin** and **lipase.** It is connected to the small intestine through its main duct called **pancreatic duct.**

Mechanism of Digestion

In human beings, the digestion of food starts in the buccal cavity and continues till the anus present at the end of large intestine.

The mechanism of digestion continues in the following steps

- **Digestion in Buccal or Oral Cavity** Digestion starts in oral cavity by the chemical hydrolytic action of the carbohydrates splitting enzyme, salivary amylase (ptyalin).

- **Digestion in Stomach** The food mixes thoroughly with the acidic gastric juice secreted in the stomach by the **churning movements** of its muscles and becomes semi-digested, acidic, pulpy mass called **chyme**. The enzymes of stomach and their actions are given below
  - **Pepsin** converts proteins into proteases and peptones (peptides).
  - **Rennin** Its secretion helps in the digestion of milk proteins.
  - **Gastric Lipases** It acts on emulsified fats and also helps in digesting around 25% of milk fat (in infants).
- **Digestion in Small Intestine** The contractions of muscles in the small intestine allow the further churning and kneading of the chyme and finally pushing it into the large intestine.
- **Digestion in Large Intestine** The last stage of digestion of food occurs in large intestine. This is carried out by bacterial action.
- Glands of this region tend to secrete mucus, i.e. enzymes are not secreted into this part of the digestive system.

Respiratory System

It is an oxidising and energy liberating process, during which nutrient molecules in tissues are broken down to form CO_2 and H_2O and release energy (ATP).

It is brought about by respiratory organs. Respiratory organs are different in different animals

(i) **Lungs** In man, frog, birds, lizards, camel and cattles, etc.
(ii) **Skin** In frog, earthworm.
(iii) **Gills** In fishes, prawn.
(iv) **Trachea** In insects.
(v) **General Body Surface** In *Amoeba, Euglena, Spirogyra* and *Chlamydomonas*.

Types of Respiration

Respiration is of two types based on the presence or absence of O_2.

- **Anaerobic Respiration** It is the process in which the respiratory substrates are incompletely oxidised into CO_2 and alcohol.

  It occurs in the absence of oxygen. It is also called as **fermentation**.

  $$C_6H_{12}O_6 \xrightarrow{\text{Yeast}} 2CO_2 + 2C_2H_5OH + 56 \text{ kcal}$$

  It occurs in lower organisms such as bacteria and fungi and in higher organisms under the condition when O_2 is limiting.
- **Aerobic Respiration** It is the process in which respiratory substrates are oxidised into CO_2, water and energy, in the presence of oxygen.
- This is common in higher organisms.

  $$C_6H_{12}O_6 + 6O_2 \rightarrow 6CO_2 + 6H_2O + 2870 \text{ kJ}$$

  The aerobic respiration involves the following two steps
  - **External Respiration** It involves exchange of oxygen from the atmosphere with CO_2 produced in the cells. This process is also called **breathing.** It gets accomplished in the following steps
    - **Inhalation** The process of taking in oxygen from the atmosphere.
    - **Exchange of Oxygen and Carbon Dioxide in Alveoli** The walls of alveoli contain an extensive network of blood vessels. The squence of exchange of oxygen and carbon dioxide, which occurs between blood vessels and alveoli.
    - **Exhalation** The process of giving out carbon dioxide from lungs to the atmosphere.
  - **Internal or Cellular Respiration** It is a basic biological process of stepwise burning of food substrate.

Human Respiratory System

It consists of two parts, i.e. **conducting** and **exchanging** portion. The conducting portion consists of nostrils, pharynx, larynx, trachea and bronchi, while exchanging portion consists of lungs in which numerous alveoli are present.

These are primary sites of exchange of gases.

- In human beings, air is taken in through nostrils through the throat reaches the lungs. Rings of cartilage are present in the trachea in the throat to prevent it from collapsing.

- Within the lungs, the respiratory tract finally terminates into balloon-like structures called **alveoli** which provides large surface area for gaseous exchange.
- When we breath in (**inhalation**), the ribs get raised and diaphragm flattens to increase the chest cavity and air is drawn in.
- When we breath out (**exhalation**), the ribs and diaphragm return to normal position reducing the thoracic cavity and the air is thrown out.
- The lungs always contain certain volume of air, i.e. residual volume.
- Respiratory pigment haemoglobin present in the blood takes up oxygen from air in the lungs and carries it to the tissues.
- Carbon dioxide from the tissues is mostly transported in dissolved form in our blood.

Circulatory System

- It is a transport system that supplies the useful material and removes the waste from the body cells.
- Blood circulation was discovered by **William Harvey.**

Blood

- Blood is a fluid connective tissue and composed of blood corpuscles and plasma.
- It is slightly alkaline in nature (pH 7.2).
- Its volume in an adult is 5.8 L.
- Plasma consists of albumin, globulin, fibrinogen and prothrombin proteins.

Blood corpuscles are as follows

- **Erythrocytes** (RBCs) It contain the respiratory pigment called **haemoglobin**, which distributes oxygen.
- At the foetal stage, RBC is formed in the liver and after birth it is formed in the bone marrow.
- The average lifespan of RBC is 120 days.
- **Leucocytes** (WBCs) These are part of the body's immune system, attack infectious agents and foreign substances.
- **Thrombocytes** (Platelets) It is responsible for blood clotting (coagulation). It changes fibrinogen into fibrin.
- During blood clotting, fibrinogen changes into fibrin by thrombin which is obtained from thromboplastin in the presence of Ca^{2+}.

Blood Groups

- Father of blood groups : **Karl Landsteiner.**
- He discovered A, B and O blood groups.
- **Decastello** and **Sturle** discovered AB blood group.
- Blood transfusion technique was developed by **James Blundell.**
- People of 'O' Blood group called universal donor and 'AB' universal **recipient**.

Blood Group	Can donate to	Can receive from
A	A, AB	A, O
B	B, AB	B, O
AB	AB	A, B, AB, O
O	A, B, AB, O	O

Heart

- This is a thick, muscular, contractile, automatic pumping organ of blood vascular system.
- Human heart is four-chambered. The chambers which receive the blood from body tissues are called **auricles** and the chambers of heart which pump blood to body tissues are called **ventricles.**
- There is a thin two-layered sac around the heart known as **pericardium,** filled with a watery fluid called **pericardial fluid,** which allows frictionless movements of heart and protects it from mechanical shocks.
- To pump out blood, the heart chamber undergoes alternate contraction called **systole** and relaxation called **diastole.**
- The regular sequence of these systole and diastole causes the heart sound **lubb and dupp.**
- Human heartbeat is **myogenic** in nature, i.e. initiated by a patch of modified heart muscles itself without requiring an external stimulation. This patch is called **SA node** (Sino-Auricular node) or **pacemaker.**
- The normal rate of heartbeat at rest is about 70-72 times per minute. In a newly born baby heartbeat rate is about 140 per minute.

Blood Vessels

These are of three types

- **Arteries** These are thick-walled blood vessels, which carry the blood away from the heart to various body parts.
- **Veins** These are thin-walled blood vessels and carry blood away from various body parts towards the heart.
- **Capillaries** These are the thinnest blood vessels and connect arteries to the veins.

Lymph

- It is another types of tissue fluid that is formed by plasma and blood cells that escape into intercellular spaces.
- Lymph carries digested food from the intestine.

Excretory System

- It is composed of organs that are involved in the removal of nitrogenous wastes generated by the metabolic activities.
- In human beings, the nitrogenous waste is in the form of urea, hence they are **ureotelic**.
- The animals that excrete the wastes in the form of ammonia are called **ammonotelic**, e.g. fish, etc., and those which excrete the nitrogenous wastes in the form of uric acid are called **uricotelic** animals.

Human Excretory System

It consists of the following parts

- A pair of **kidney** is present on either side of vertebral column. Every kidney contains numerous tubular functional units called **nephrons** or uriniferous tubule which form urine by removing waste materials from the blood.
  A nephron consists of
  - A cup-like Bowman's capsule, enclosing a bunch of capillaries, formed by afferent arteriole called **glomerulus.**
  - A Proximal Convoluted Tubule (PCT).
  - U-shaped loop of Henle.
  - A Distal Convoluted Tubule (DCT).
  - A collecting tubule.

  Collecting tubules of many nephrons open into a large collecting duct. Several adjacent collecting tubules converge to open into a short and thick structure called duct of Bellini.
- A pair of **ureter** arising from each kidney and takes urine to urinary bladder.
- **Urinary bladder** is a muscular bag where urine is stored temporarily.
- **Urethra** is the opening by which urine is thrown out.
- In case of kidney failure, artificial kidney is used to remove nitrogenous waste products. This process is called **dialysis.**

Skeletal System

Skeletal system is of two types

- **Exoskeleton** It is found on the surface of the body, e.g. nails, hair, etc.
- **Endoskeleton** It is found inside the body and provides structural framework of the body.
- It is made up of bones and cartilages.
  - Human body consists of 206 bones.
    In childhood, the number of bones is 213.
  - The skull consists of 29 bones (cranium 8, facial 14, 3 pairs of auditory bone and 1 hyoid bone) of ear ossicles.
  - The number of bones in the vertebral column of an adult is 26 and the ribs contain 24 bones.
  - **Tendons** join the muscles and bones.
  - The muscles which join bone to bone are called **ligaments.**

Muscular System

- Human body has about 639 types of muscles.
- Muscles specialised to contraction are of three types, i.e. striated, unstriated and cardiac.
  - **Striated Muscles** These are also called skeletal muscles or voluntary muscles. They are present in limbs, tongue, pharynx, etc.
  - **Unstriated Muscles** These are involuntary muscles and present in urinary bladder, in the walls of large blood vessels and alimentary canal.
  - **Cardiac Muscles** These are involuntary, striated and non-fatigued fibres which are found in the wall of heart.

Nervous System

The nervous system provides the fastest means of communication within the body, so that suitable response to stimuli can be made at once.

Nervous system is found only in animals and absent in plants. Nervous system controls the body by using a series of tissues throughout the body formed by a network of electrically conducting cells called **neurons or nerve cells.**

Neuron

It is the structural and functional unit of nervous system. Neurons are of three types

- **Motor** conducts messages from central nervous system to effector organs.
- **Sensory** conducts information from sensory organ to central nervous system.
- **Mixed** works both as sensory and motor neurons.

Human Neural System

It is derived from embryonic ectoderm.

It is composed of

Central Nervous System (CNS)

It includes

(a) Brain (b) Spinal cord

Brain

- Brain lies in the cranium of skull.
- **Cerebrum** governs consciousness, storage of memory having information. It is a site of intelligence speech sight, smell and taste.
- **Thalamus** deals with touch, visual system, sleep wakefulness, temperature, water balance in body, behavioural patterns of sex, sleep, stress, emotions, etc.
- **Midbrain** deals with visual and auditory, analysis.
- **Cerebellum** controls coordination of accurate movements and balancing.
- **Medulla oblongata** is long connecting part of brain to spinal cord. It deals with control of heartbeats, blood vessels, breathing, salivary secretion and mostly reflex and involuntary (uncontrolled) movements like blood pressure, salivation and vomitting.

Spinal Cord

- An elongated cylindrical structure forming the posterior part of CNS.
- It is made up of two types of nervous tissue, i.e. grey matter and white matter.
- It conducts impulses to and fro from the brain. It controls most of the reflex activities of the brain.
- It also acts as a means of communication between the spinal nerves and the brain.

Reflex Action and Reflex Arc

- It is the involuntary functioning or movement of any organ or part of the body to a stimulus.
- The nervous pathway taken by nerve impulses in a reflex action is called **reflex arc.**

Peripheral Nervous System (PNS)

The peripheral nervous system is one of two components that make up the nervous system of bilateral animals with the other part being the central nervous system. It consists of

1. **Somatic Nervous System** (SNS) It transmits impulse from CNS to skeletal muscle *via* the cranial (12 pairs) and spinal nerves (31 pairs).
2. **Autonomic Nervous System** (ANS) It transmits impulse from CNS to skeletal muscle or organs under involuntary control.

Endocrine System

It is formed by ductless glands which secrete hormones to regulate the activities of the body. Various endocrine glands in human body are as follows

- **Pituitary Gland** It is also called **master gland** as it control the secretion of various other endocrine glands.
- Growth hormone is secreted by the pituitary which is involved in the body growth. Its deficiency causes **dwarfism** and if released in excess it causes **gigantism.**
- **Thyroid Gland** It releases hormone thyroxine. Due to the deficiency of this hormone, the person suffers from **goitre.**

- **Parathyroid Gland** It influences calcium and phosphorus metabolism.
- **Pancreas** It has both exocrine and endocrine glands. Endocrine part contains **islets of Langerhans**, which produce hormones insulin (beta cells) and glucagon (alpha cells).
- Insulin controls the amount of sugar in the blood.
- Deficiency of insulin causes **diabetes mellitus** in the person.
- **Adrenal Glands** It contains two parts cortex and medulla.
  - **Adrenal medulla** secretes the hormones adrenalin and nor-adrenalin which are the hormones of emergency.
  - **Adrenal cortex** secretes mineralocorticoids and glucocorticoids.
- **Testis and Ovaries** It produces gametes, sperms in males and ova in females. Testis produces male sex hormone **testosterone** and females produce hormones **oestrogen** and **progesterone**.

Reproductive System

The various organs which constitute the male and female reproductive system and their functions are tabulated below

Male Reproductive Organs

Reproductive Organ	Number	Function
Testes	2	Produce sperm and testosterone
Sperm duct	2	Conduct the sperm from the testes to urethra
Seminal vesicles	2	Secrete seminal plasma
Prostate gland	2	Secrete an alkaline fluid to neutralise the acidity of urethra and make the spermactive
Penis (urethra) (have rich blood supply	2	Pass urine and deposite sperm in female genital tract.

Female Reproductive Organs

Reproductive Organ	Number	Function
Ovaries	2	To produce ova and hormones (Estrogen and progesterone).
Oviducts	2	To move the ovum towards uterus.
Uterus	1	To provide space for developing child.
Vagina	1	To receive the sperms

Human Body (At a Glance)

Total number of muscles in the body	639
Total number of bones in the human body	206
Longest bone	Femur (thigh bone)
Smallest bone	Ear ossicle–stapes
Largest organ of human body	Skin
Number of cells in body	75 trillion
Weight of brain	1424 g
Blood volume	6.8 L (in 70 kg body)
Normal BP	120/80 mm Hg
Hb content in body	500-700 gm
Blood platelets	200000-400000 per cubic mm
Universal blood donor	O Blood Group
Universal blood recipient	AB Blood Group
Blood clotting time	2-5 minutes
Normal body temperature	98.4° F or 37°C
Breathing rate	16-20/minute
Dental formula	Adult : 2123/2123 = 32 Child : 2120/2120 = 20 milk teeth
Largest endocrine gland	Thyroid
Largest muscle in the body	Gluteus maximus (Buttock muscle)
Largest Cell	Nervw Cell (Neuron)
Greatest regeneration power	In liver
Minimum regeneration power	In brain cells
Minimum distance for proper vision	25 cm
Pulse rate	72/minute

Exam Pattern Questions

1 Digestive system
(a) gives message to the body
(b) helps to burn food
(c) makes the food into simple form
(d) None of the above

2 Saliva helps in the digestion of
(a) fats (b) proteins (c) fibres (d) starch

3 Which of the following is called the complete food?
(a) Cereal (b) Milk
(c) Vegetables (d) Chapati

4 Which one of the following organs does not secrete digestive juices?
(a) Oesophagus (b) Small intestine
(c) Liver (d) Stomach

5 Gastric juice contains
(a) hydrochloric acid and pepsin
(b) bicarbonates
(c) sucrose
(d) lipids and sucrose

6 Ram wants to bite into an apple. Which type of teeth will he use?
(a) Incisors (b) Canines
(c) Premolars (d) Molars

7 Hardest part in human body is
(a) dentine (b) enamel (c) keratin (d) chitin

8 Maximum absorption of food takes place in
(a) stomach (b) small intestine
(c) large intestine (d) oesophagus

9 All of the following molecules are carbohydrates except
(a) lactose (b) haemoglobin
(c) cellulose (d) glycogen

10 For immediate energy production in cells, which should be supplied?
(a) Fatty acid (b) Ammonia acid
(c) Vitamin-C (d) Glucose

11 While cooking food, the compounds lost to the maximum are
(a) vitamins (b) carbohydrates
(c) proteins (d) fats

12 What should be given to an athlete for instant energy?
(a) Protein (b) Vitamin
(c) Carbohydrate (d) None of these

13 Milk teeth are
(a) teeth which are permanent
(b) teeth which do not grow at all
(c) teeth which grow twice in life
(d) the teeth which are temporary

14 Which of the following does not contain carbohydrates?
(a) Wax (b) Cellulose
(c) Wheat flour (d) Starch

15 Oxygen (O_2) is utilised by an organism to
(a) directly breakdown the nutrient molecules
(b) indirectly breakdown the nutrient molecules
(c) obtain nourishment from the food
(d) burn the organic compounds indirectly

16 Larynx is present in between
(a) epiglottis and glottis
(b) trachea and bronchiole
(c) epiglottis and trachea
(d) bronchus and epiglottis

17 Which portion of the human respiratory system is called sound box?
(a) Larynx (b) Trachea
(c) Nasopharynx (d) Glottis

18 Friction on the lungs surface is reduced by
(a) double layered pleura
(b) single layered pleura
(c) epiglottis upto trachea
(d) mucous membrane surrounding the lungs

19 Inspiration is initiated by the
(a) extension of diaphragm
(b) contraction of diaphragm
(c) extension of lungs
(d) contraction of lungs

20 During expiration, the diaphragm becomes
(a) normal (b) flattened
(c) dome-shaped (d) oblique

21 Which one of the following types of blood cells is responsible for clotting of blood?
(a) Erythrocytes (b) Lymphocytes
(c) Monocytes (d) Thrombocytes

22 Haemoglobin is dissolved in the plasma of
(a) man (b) fish
(c) frog (d) earthworm

23 Which of the following proteins, is present in human blood?
(a) Myosin (b) Insulin
(c) Haemoglobin (d) Trypsin

24 Blood plasma has a pH of
(a)7.2 (b) 7.8 (c) 6.9
(d) 6.3

25 Mast cells secrete
(a) hippurin (b) myoglobin
(c) histamine (d) haemoglobin

26 Which of the following organs is called graveyard of RBC?
(a) Kidney (b) Spleen
(c) Liver (d) Pancreas

27 Smallest blood vessel in the body is
(a) capillary (b) artery
(c) vein (d) vena cava

28 The normal blood pressure of human beings is in one of the following ranges
(a) 140/80 mm (b) 110/70 mm
(c) 120/80 mm (d) 110/75 mm

29 The body organ which is not present in pair is
(a) kidney (b) testis
(c) ovary (d) heart

30 Blood is formed in the human adult by the
(a) heart (b) spleen
(c) red bone marrow (d) yellow bone marrow

31 What is Rh in blood?
(a) Hormone in body (b) Antibody
(c) Antigen (d) Gene

32 Circulatory system
(a) gives oxygen to the body
(b) helps to burn food
(c) makes the food into simple form
(d) None of the above

33 Veins carry blood
(a) away from the heart (b) towards the heart
(c) towards the brain (d) None of these

34 Which of the following is made up of muscular walls?
(a) Blood (b) Bone
(c) Heart (d) Skin

35 In one minute, heartbeats
(a) 60 times (b) 62 times
(c) 72 times (d) 82 times

36 Pacemaker of heart is
(a) auricles (b) SA node
(c) ventricles (d) AV node

37 The process of excretion involves the
(a) removal of useful substances from the body
(b) removal of metabolic wastes from the body
(c) removal of the substances which have never been used by the body
(d) byproducts removal formed during useful activities in the body

38 In ureotelic animals, ammonia produced by metabolism is converted into urea in
(a) kidney (b) liver (c) spleen (d) lungs

39 Excretion of nitrogenous products in the semisolid form is performed by
(a) ammonotelic organisms
(b) ureotelic organisms
(c) uricotelic organisms
(d) All of the above

40 Structural and functional unit of the kidney is
(a) medulla (b) nephridia
(c) nephron (d) hilum

41 Kidney is a part of
(a) digestive system (b) skeleton system
(c) nervous system (d) excretory system

42 In which of the following parts largest muscle is found in human body?
(a) In hand (b) In nitambh
(c) In neck (d) In legs

43 Which of the following is not an element of the bone?
(a) Carbon (b) Phosphorus
(c) Calcium (d) Oxygen

44 Tendons are made up of
(a) collagen (b) elastin
(c) keratin (d) All of these

45 Muscular tissue is differentiated into
(a) striped and cardiac
(b) unstriped, striated and cardiac
(c) cardiac and unstriped
(d) striped and unstriped

46 Bifocal lenses are used by people suffering from
(a) myopia and hypermetropia
(b) hypermetropia but not myopia
(c) myopia but not hypermetropia
(d) myopia or hypermetropia

47 Which of the following is not correct for cerebellum?
(a) It controls movements, speech, sight, smell, taste, hearing and intelligence
(b) It maintains equilibrium of the body
(c) It lies in the posterior region of the brain
(d) It is a part of hindbrain

48 .... fills the space inside the organs and supports the internal organs and helps in repair of tissue.
(a) Adipose (b) Tendons
(c) Areolar (d) Ligament

49 Our body has many organs. Which of the following organs is the largest?
(a) The brain (b) The stomach
(c) The kidneys (d) The skin

50 Involuntary actions including blood pressure, salivation and vomiting are controlled by the .... .
(a) spinal cord (b) pons
(c) cerebellum (d) medulla

51 The brain
(a) pumps blood to all parts of the body
(b) is the main control centre of the body
(c) helps to breath in air
(d) None of the above

52 The unit of nervous system is
(a) nephron (b) neuron
(c) neuroglia (d) axon

53 Nervous system
(a) helps to produce babies
(b) helps us to breathe
(c) controls our actions
(d) None of these

54 Which of the following is the correct group of sense organs?
(a) Eyes, nose, lips, ear, tongue
(b) Nose, ear, teeth, hair, eyes
(c) Nose, ear, eyes, skin, tongue
(d) Ear, eyes, nose, lips, teeth

55 Memory is the responsibility of
(a) grey matter (b) white matter
(c) cerebrum (d) cerebellum

56 The master control centre of the human body in
(a) brain (b) heart
(c) stomach (d) liver

57 The working of the human eye is like that of a
(a) camera (b) telescope
(c) microscope (d) periscope

58 What is the outermost layer of the skin called?
(a) Epidermis (b) Mucus
(c) Fibre (d) None of these

59 The skin is
(a) excretory organ (b) sense organ
(c) breathing organ (d) None of these

60 Which of the following is not the part of nervous system?
(a) Brain (b) Nerves
(c) Blood (d) Spinal cord

61 Of the following human organs, which one is least susceptible to harmful radiations?
(a) Brain (b) Heart
(c) Eyes (d) Lungs

62 The colour of the human skin is due to
(a) keratin (b) melanin
(c) myelin (d) myoglobin

63 The sensory organ that has reached its highest level of evolution in birds is the
(a) ear (b) skin
(c) nose (d) eye

64 Which of the following hormones brings about changes in appearance seen in boys at the time of puberty?
(a) Testosterone (b) Thyroxin
(c) Insulin (d) Animal hormone

65 Endocrine gland is also called ....
(a) liver gland (b) ductless gland
(c) pituitary gland (d) thyroid gland

66 Which of the following hormones is secreted by the pituitary to start the ovulation process?
(a) Luteinizing hormone (b) Thyroid
(c) Progesterone (d) Oestrogen

67 Human insulin is being commercially produced from a transgenic species of
(a) *Mycobacterium* (b) *Rhizobium*
(c) *Saccharomyces* (d) *Escherichia*

68 Which hormone is produced by the testes of male?
(a) Testosterone (b) Progesterone
(c) Melatonin (d) Thyroxine

69 The hormone which is not directly associated with reproduction is
(a) testosterone (b) oestrogen
(c) progesterone (d) parathormone

70 Goitre or abnormal enlargement of the thyroid gland is caused by the deficiency of
(a) iodine (b) iron
(c) calcium (d) potassium

71 Which gland secretes the most kinds of hormones?
(a) Adrenal (b) Pineal
(c) Pituitary (d) Thyroid

72 The process of dialysis is used when there is malfunctioning of
(a) heart (b) kidney
(c) stomach (d) lungs

73 The number of bones present in human body is
(a) 206 (b) 200 (c) 205 (d) 220

74 The basic frame work of human body is formed by
(a) bones (b) cartilages
(c) Both (a) and (b) (d) None of these

75 The number of bones in the vertebral column is
(a) 24 (b) 28 (c) 31 (d) 33

76 Cardiac muscles are present in
(a) digestive tract (b) limbs
(c) heart (d) respiratory tract

77 The master gland is
(a) pancreas (b) parathyroid gland
(c) pituitary gland (d) ovaries

78 Dwarfism is caused to the deficiency of
(a) growth hormone (b) thyroxine
(c) insulin (d) adrenalin

79 Male reproductive system does not have
(a) testes (b) vas deferens
(c) penis (d) Fallopian tube

80 Female reproductive system comprises of a pair of
(a) ovaries (b) uterus (c) vagina (d) testes

81 Male germ cell are produced a/an
(a) testes (b) epididymis
(c) ovary (d) prostrate

82 In human, the development of fertilised egg takes place in the
(a) ovary (b) testis (c) oviduct (d) uterus

83 After fertilisation, the resulting cell which gives rise to a new individual is the
(a) embryo (b) ovum (c) foetus (d) zygote

84 The multicellular organism which reproduces by budding is
(a) *Amoeba* (b) Yeast
(c) *Paramecium* (d) *Hydra*

85 The production of an exact copy of an animal by asexual reproduction is known as
(a) budding (b) mating
(c) cloning (d) hatching

86 The male gamete in plants is
(a) anther (b) stamen
(c) pollen grain (d) pollen sac

87 Conidia are asexual structures found in
(a) Algae (b) Fungi
(c) Lichen (d) Protozoa

88 Budding is found in
(a) *Hydra* (b) yeast
(c) Both (a) and (b) (d) *Paramecium*

Answers

1 (c)	2 (d)	3 (b)	4 (a)	5 (a)	6 (a)	7 (b)	8 (b)	9 (b)	10 (d)
11 (a)	12 (c)	13 (d)	14 (a)	15 (b)	16 (c)	17 (a)	18 (a)	19 (b)	20 (c)
21 (d)	22 (d)	23 (c)	24 (a)	25 (c)	26 (b)	27 (a)	28 (c)	29 (d)	30 (c)
31 (c)	32 (a)	33 (b)	34 (c)	35 (c)	36 (b)	37 (b)	38 (b)	39 (c)	40 (c)
41 (d)	42 (d)	43 (a)	44 (a)	45 (b)	46 (a)	47 (a)	48 (c)	49 (d)	50 (d)
51 (b)	52 (b)	53 (c)	54 (c)	55 (c)	56 (a)	57 (a)	58 (a)	59 (b)	60 (c)
61 (a)	62 (b)	63 (d)	64 (a)	65 (b)	66 (a)	67 (d)	68 (a)	69 (d)	70 (a)
71 (c)	72 (b)	73 (a)	74 (c)	75 (d)	76 (c)	77 (c)	78 (a)	79 (d)	80 (a)
81 (a)	82 (d)	83 (d)	84 (d)	85 (c)	86 (c)	87 (b)	88 (c)		

Chapter 05

Nutrition, Health and Diseases

Nutrition

The substances that provide nourishment essential for the maintenance of life and for growth are called nutrients. The process by which body obtains and uses these nutrients is called **nutrition**.

Balanced Diet

- It is a combination of all the essential constituents of food in proper proportion, which is necessary for the growth and maintenance of the body.
- The various components of food are carbohydrates, fats, proteins, minerals, vitamins, water and roughage.
  These are described below

Carbohydrates

- One gram of carbohydrate gives 17 kJ of energy. They are better source of energy than proteins and fats.
- They are made up of carbon (C), oxygen (O) and hydrogen (H).
- They are of three types–monosaccharides, disaccharides and polysaccharides.
  - **Monosaccharides** are simplest sugars such as glucose, fructose and galactose.
  - **Disaccharide** consists of two units of monosaccharides, e.g. sucrose, lactose and maltose.
  - **Polysaccharides** consist of more than three units of monosaccharides, e.g. glycogen, starch, cellulose, etc.

Proteins

- These are made up of carbon, hydrogen, oxygen, nitrogen and sulphur.
- It is important for growth, development and repair of the body.
- Proteins are made of basic units called **amino acids.**
- Out of 20 amino acids, some are synthesised in our body are called **non-essential amino acids**, e.g. alanine, etc.
- Rest are not synthesised in our body and have to be supplemented by food.
- These are **essential amino acids**, e.g. isoleucine, methionine, valine, etc.
- Proteins liberate energy in the absence of fats and carbohydrates.
- Due to the deficiency of protein in children, diseases such as **kwashiorkor** and **marasmus** occur.
- Some important food sources of proteins are milk, egg, meat, pulses, soybean, etc.

Fats

- These are also called lipids, they are made up of carbon, hydrogen and oxygen.
- These provide much more energy (about twice) than carbohydrates.
- These are saturated fatty acids, which are solid at room temperature and unsaturated fatty acids, that are liquid at room temperature.
- Excess of saturated fatty acids is bad for health and can cause heart attack.
- The chief sources of fats are butter, ghee, cooking oil, etc.
- The process by which unsaturated fatty acids are converted into saturated fatty acid by the addition of hydrogen is called **hydrogenation**.

Vitamins

- Vitamin term was coined by **Funk**. They are not the sources of energy but are required to regulate various metabolic activities.
- Vitamins are **fat-soluble** like vitamin–A D, E and K or **water-soluble** like vitamin–B and C.
- Some of the sources of various vitamins and the diseases caused due to their deficiency is given below

Vitamins, their sources and deficiency symptoms

Vitamins	Sources	Effect of Deficiency
(i) **Fat-Soluble Vitamins**		
A (Retinol)	Milk, butter, egg yolk, liver	Xerophthalmia, Night blindness
D (Cholecalciferol)	Synthesised in skin cells	Rickets, osteomalacia
E (Tocopherol)	Green vegetables	Causes sterility, muscular dystrophy
K (Phylloquinone)	Carrots, lettuce	Haemorrhages, delayed blood clotting
(ii) **Water-Soluble Vitamins**		
B_1 (Thiamine)	Rice bran, whole wheat flour	Beri-beri
B_2 (Riboflavin)	Cheese, eggs, yeast	Cheilosis keratitis of cornea
B_3 (Nicotinic acid)	Fresh meat, liver, fish	Pellagra, muscle atrophy
B_6 (Pyridoxine)	Milk, cereals, fish, meat, liver	Dermatitis, convulsions, nausea, mental disorders
B_5 (Pantothenic acid)	Yeast, liver, kidneys, eggs, meat	Dermatitis, anaemia, fatigue, nausea
B_7 (Biotin)	Yeast, vegetables, fruits, eggs	Skin lesions, loss of appetite, hair fall
B_{12} (Cyanocobalamin)	Meat, fish, liver, Eggs	Pernicious anaemia
C (Ascorbic acid)	Lemon, orange	Scurvy (bleeding of gums)

Minerals

- These are inorganic substances required for many metabolic functions in our body.
- Most of them are required in minute quantities.
- Minerals are of two types : Macro-nutrient Elements e.g. (Ca, P, K, S, Na, Cl and Mg) and Micronutrient elements (e.g. I, Fe, Co, F, Mo and Fe)
- Some of the important minerals, their sources, functions and deficiency diseases are given below

Minerals	Sources	Functions	Deficiency
Macroelements			
Calcium	Milk, cheese, green vegetables, eggs, fish, etc.	Formation of teeth and bones, muscle contraction	Weak teeth and bones
Sodium	Table salt, milk, eggs, meat, seafood, etc.	Maintains body fluid balance, transmission of nerve impulses	Low blood pressure, loss of appetite
Potassium	Most vegetables, fruits, meat, etc.	Body fluid balance, muscle contraction transmission of nerve impulses	Weak muscles, risk of paralysis
Phosphorus	Milk, meat, etc.	Component of bones and teeth, nucleic acids, etc.	Weak teeth, bones, retarded growth
Iron	Spinach, liver, banana, jaggery, etc.	Important component of haemoglobin	Anaemia, weakness, etc.
Iodine	Seafood, green leafy vegetables, iodised salt, etc.	Essential for synthesis of thyroxine hormone	Goitre, cretinism
Sulphur	Proteins of food	Component of amino acids	Disturbed protein metabolism
Chlorine	Table salt	Acid-base balance	Loss of appetite, muscle cramps
Microelements			
Fluorine	Drinking water, pea, seafood	Maintenance of bones and teeth	Weak teeth
Manganese	Dry fruits, cereals	Cofactor of some enzymes	Irregular growth of bones, cartilages

Water

- It is the main component of the body. Human body contains about 65% water and about 70% of this water is protoplasm.
- Water do not yield energy, yet it is so vital for the body that a person dies if he is deprived of water.
- Functions of water are as follows
  (i) To control the body temperature.
  (ii) To act as an important medium in the excretional activities.
  (iii) To regulate almost all biochemical reactions, which actually occur in aquatic environment (atmosphere).

Roughage

- Indigestable fibrous material present in the food is called roughage.
- It provides bulk to the diet for satisfying appetite.
- Bulk amount of roughage helps in expanding gut and also stimulates peristalsis to eliminate the faecal matter.

e.g. cellulose present in the cell walls of plant material such as vegetables, fruits and bran all contain roughage.

Health

- According to World Health Organisation or WHO (1948) health is a state of complete mental, physical and social well-being and not merely absence of disease.
- There are some basic factors which contribute to our good health. Balance diet is one of them.

Diseases

- Any change in the normal functioning of body causing discomfort or disability is called **disease**.
- It is a condition of the body or some organs of the body in which their normal functions are disturbed or dearranged.
- The disease may be congenital, i.e. present in organism since birth or it could be acquired, i.e. present in organism after birth.
- The acquired diseases can be of two types
  (i) **Non-Communicable or Non-Infectious diseases** These diseases cannot be transferred from an affected person to a normal healthy person. e.g. Rellagra, Souevy, Goietre etc.
  (ii) **Communicable Diseases or Infectious Diseases** These are transmitted from infected person to a healthy person. They are caused by some infectious agents like virus, bacteria, fungi, protozoan, worm, etc. These are called **pathogens**. e.g. Hepatitis, TB, Cholers phenmonia etc.

List of Various Diseases, their Symptoms and Prevention

Viral Diseases

Diseases (caused by)	Symptoms	Prevention and Control	Body Part Affected
AIDS (HIV) (Epidemic disease)	• Weight loss and loss of breathe • Cough, headache • Shaking chills • Soaking night sweats	• Use of condom • Safe sex • AIDS vaccine	Damage immune system
Hepatitis (Hepatitis virus)	• Jaundice • Anorexia acute malaise • Body and headache • Chills and fatigue	• Avoid infection transmission from infected to healthy persons. • Vaccines are available for hepatitis 'A', 'B' and 'C'.	—
Influenza or **Flu** (Influenza viruses A and B)	Fever, chill, muscular aches, uneasiness, etc.	• Vaccination with live attenuated virus vaccines. • Antibiotics such as terramycine, etc.	—
Smallpox (Variola virus) (Epidemic disease)	High fever, headache, backache, skin rashes on the third day passing through bright red spots, pustules, papules and vesicles scabs which fall off from skin leaving pitted pock marks.	• Vaccination • Diseased person should remain isolated from healthy person.	—

Diseases (caused by)	Symptoms	Prevention and Control	Body Part Affected
Swine flu (H1N1, fluvirus) (Epidemic disease)	Headache, tiredness sore throat, vomiting, breathing problems.	• Frequently washing hands with soap fearly flu, vaccination	Whole body (muscles)
Rabies (Rabies virus)	• Severe headache, high fever with alternating stages of excitement and depression. • Difficulty in swallowing, paralysis, convulsions, etc.	• Use of antirabies vaccine invented by Louis Pasteur. • Series of antibiotics are followed. • Cleaning of wound with pure carbolic acid or nitric acid.	—
Dengue or Break bone fever	• High fever, rashes on face and head. • Severe pain in eyes, muscle and joint pain.	• Use of mosquito repellents, bed rest. • Hygiene to control mosquitoes.	—
Mumps (Paramyxovirus)	• Fever, swelling in glands particularly salivary gland, parotid gland or organs. • Severe pain when mouth is opened.	• Vaccination with live attenuated virus like MMR vaccine. • Mouth wash with a soft warm water relaxes the suffering in people up to a great extent.	—
Measles (Rubella virus)	Fever, inflammation of respiratory mucous membranes, sensitive to light, loss of appetite, vomiting, rashes on the skin.	• Inoculation of gamma globulin. • Light intake of food. • Drinking boiled, filtered water.	—

Bacterial Diseases

Diseases (caused by)	Symptoms	Prevention and Control	Body Part Affected
Tuberculosis (*Mycobacterium tuberculosis*)	• Low grade fever • Coughing • Lethargy/weakness • Weight loss	• BCG vaccination. • Personal and domestic hygiene. • Keeping patient in isolation.	Lungs
Typhoid (*Salmonella typhii*)	• High fever • Weakness • Stomach pain, etc.	• Maintaining personal/domestic food hygiene habits.	Intestines/Whole body
Tetanus/ Lockjaw (*Clostridium tetani*)	• Muscular tetany. • Body arched because of muscle malfunction.	• Can be easily prevented through vaccination.	Heart failure
Cholera (*Vibrio cholerae*)	• Vomiting, acute diarrhoea, muscular cramps, etc. • Slow down of blood circulation.	• Drink pure water or boiled water, eat light food and careful disposal of wastes. • Vaccine is available for immunisation.	Mainly intestine
Diphtheria (*Corynebacterium diphtheriae*)	Mild fever, sore throat, patches on false membrane in the throat.	• Immunisation vaccine or to take the injection of antitoxin diphtheria within 12-24 hours of its appearance in the system.	Throat
Plague (*Yersinia* or *Bacillus pestis*) (Epidemic disease)	Acute body pain, reddish eyes, increase in body temperature, inflammation of glands in the neck, armpit and thigh.	• Exit of infected rats from the diseased zone. • Proper vaccination. • Usage of sulphur drugs and streptomycin.	Swelling of lymph node.

Diseases (caused by)	Symptoms	Prevention and Control	Body Part Affected
Pneumonia (*Streptococcus pneumoniae*)	Chills, chest pain, production of sputum, breathing problems, abdominal pain, etc.	• Protection from excessive cold must be taken. • Antibiotic drugs must be used.	Rapid shallow breathing.

Protozoan Diseases

Diseases (Caused by)	Symptoms	Prevention and Control	Body Part Affected
Kala-azar (*Leishmania donovini*)	• Enlargement of organs like spleen, liver. • Fever, jaundice and skin pigmentation.	Control of sandfly by using pesticides.	Weight loss, darkeing of skin, infection.
Sleeping sickness (*Trypanosoma brucei*)	• Fever, headache. • Enlargement of glands at the back of the neck, rashes on the back and chest, pain in the joints, swelling in ankles and hands, mental disturbance, lethargy, etc.	No specified drug recommended.	Loss of appetite, anaemia.
Amoebic dysentery or **Amoebiasis** (*Entamoeba histolytica*)	• Mild diarrhoea, in severe cases, mucosa and blood appears in the stools.	• Drink filtered water. • No immunisation is available.	Small intestine
Pyorrhoea (*Entamoeba gingivalis*)	• Pus in teeth emerges through the gums of the teeth. • Sometimes wounds also occur in the roots of the teeth.	Regular dental checkup, regular cleaning of teeth gums, flossing and brushing, use of antiseptic mouthwashes.	Gum, teeth, Buccal cavity

Organ Related Diseases

Organs	Diseases
Teeth and gums	Scurvy, Pyorrhea.
Liver	Jaundice
Stomach	Gastritis, Bloating
Intestine	Constipation, Colitis
Nasal chambers	Rhinites
Larynx	Laryngitis
Bronchioles	Bronchitis, Asthma
Lungs	Emphysema, Tuberculosis
Blood	Anaemia, Leukemia.
Heart	Coronary artery disease, Myocardial Infarction (MI)
Kidney	Kidney failure, Renal-Calculi (Kidney stone), Uremia.

Organs	Diseases
Bone	Arthritis, Rickets, Paget's disease, Tuberculosis.
Muscle	Muscular dystrophy, Myasthenia gravis, Tetany
Nerves	Paralysis, Polio
Brain	Meningitis, Encephalitis
Skin	Ringworm, Dermatitis, Eczema
Eyes	Hypermetropia, Myopia, Presbyopia, Astigmatism, Glaucoma, Xeropthalmia, Night blindness.
Ears	Tinnitus, Meniere's disease.

Exam Pattern Questions

1 Daily food intake with adequate quantity of all nutrient substances is called
(a) nutrition (b) health food
(c) junk food (d) balanced diet

2 What are the best source of fuel in our body ?
(a) Fats (b) Carbohydrates
(c) Proteins (d) Minerals

3 Which of the following is the best source of carbohydrates ?
(a) Carrot (b) Apple
(c) Strawberry (d) Rice

4 Which of the following pairs are both monosaccharides ?
(a) Glucose, sucrose (b) Maltose, lactose
(c) Fructose, galactose (d) Glucose, lactose

5 The sugar found in the milk is
(a) glucose (b) fructose
(c) lactose (d) maltose

6 Which of the following should be in the highest quantity in your plate ?
(a) Pulses (b) Eggs (c) Fish (d) Rice

7 Sweetest sugar is
(a) D-fructose (b) glucose
(c) D-maltose (d) D-sucrose

8 In which form is the sugar stored for future use of energy in animals ?
(a) Starch (b) Glycogen
(c) Glucose (d) Glucagon

9 Typical honey mostly consists of
(a) galactose (b) maltose (c) fructose (d) sucrose

10 Which form of sugar is present in germinating seeds ?
(a) Glucose (b) Maltose
(c) Sucrose (d) Fructose

11 Carbohydrate found in the cell wall of plants is
(a) starch (b) cellulose
(c) glycogen (d) None of these

12 The monomer of proteins is
(a) amino acid (b) monosaccharides
(c) glycerol (d) disaccharides

13 Which substances are present in proteins besides carbon(C), hydrogen (H) and oxygen(O) ?
(a) Ca and Mb (b) Na and K
(c) N and S (d) Ca and P

14 Essential amino acids are
(a) synthesised in our body
(b) not synthesised in our body
(c) only required in children
(d) the ones that form proteins

15 A body builder requires to eat lots of
(a) proteins (b) fats (c) vitamins (d) minerals

16 A child suffering from kwashiorkor disease should eat lots of
(a) rice (b) green vegetables
(c) pulses (d) apples

17 Richest source of protein is
(a) pulse (b) peas (c) mushroom (d) soybean

18 Highest amount of energy is released by
(a) carbohydrates (b) fats
(c) proteins (d) minerals

19 Form of food which is dangerous for health is
(a) saturated fatty acids (b) unsaturated fatty acids
(c) mineral salt (d) mannose sugar

20 Unsaturated fatty acids are
(a) solid at room temperature
(b) liquid at room temperature
(c) sometimes solid
(d) can be either solid or liquid

21 Term vitamin was first given by
(a) Funk (b) Leeuwenhoek
(c) C Benda (d) Altmann

22 Which of the following is not a fat soluble vitamins ?
(a) A (b) B (c) E (d) K

23 Xerophthalmia is caused due to the deficiency of
(a) Vitamin-B (b) Vitamin-C
(c) Biotin (d) Vitamin-A

24 The deficiency of vitamin-B_1 causes
(a) cheilosis (b) beri-beri
(c) pellagra (d) anaemia

25 Which of the following pair of diseases and cause of deficiency is wrong ?
(a) Night blindness– Vitamin-A
(b) Beri-beri– Vitamin-B
(c) Scurvy– Vitamin-C
(d) Sterility– Vitamin-B_5

26 It is important to eat iodised salt because it
(a) improves sight (b) improves digestion
(c) controls thyroid gland (d) increases fertility

27 Which of the following are important components of bone ?
(a) Calcium and sodium
(b) Calcium and potassium
(c) Iron and phosphorus
(d) Calcium and phosphorus

28 Disease causing biological agents are called
(a) agents (b) pathogens
(c) source (d) vectors

29 Which amongst the following pair represents the disease caused by bacteria ?
(a) Tuberculosis and cholera
(b) Cholera and smallpox
(c) Smallpox and dengue
(d) Smallpox and kala-azar

30 Diphtheria is caused by
(a) poisons released by living bacterial cells into the host tissues
(b) poisons released from dead bacterial cells into the host tissues
(c) poisons released by virus into the host tissues
(d) excessive immune response by the host's body

31 *Salmonella* is related with
(a) typhoid (b) polio (c) TB (d) tetanus

32 BCG vaccine is used against
(a) TB (b) leprosy
(c) food poisoning (d) None of these

33 Letter 'B' in BCG vaccine represents
(a) bacteria (b) brown (c) bacillus (d) big

34 Dengue spread by mosquito bite is caused by
(a) virus (b) bacteria
(c) fungi (d) helminth

35 The vector for malaria is
(a) male *Anopheles* (b) female *Culex*
(c) female *Aedes* (d) female *Anopheles*

36 Which of the following is a bacterial disease transmitted by sexual contact ?
(a) Mumps (b) Syphilis
(c) Myelitis (d) Rabies

37 Who discovered the malarial parasite?
(a) Salk and Sabin (b) Ronald Ross
(c) Robert Hooke (d) Funk

38 Which one of the following is a protozoan disease ?
(a) Polio (b) AIDS
(c) Taeniasis (d) Malaria

39 African sleeping sickness in caused by
(a) *Trypanosoma* (b) *Leishmania*
(c) *Latimeria* (d) *Plasmodium*

40 Polio vaccine was invented by
(a) Dr. Salk (b) Jenner
(c) Fleming (d) Bohr

Answers

1 (d)	2 (b)	3 (d)	4 (c)	5 (c)	6 (d)	7 (a)	8 (b)	9 (c)	10 (b)
11 (b)	12 (a)	13 (c)	14 (b)	15 (a)	16 (c)	17 (d)	18 (b)	19 (a)	20 (b)
21 (a)	22 (b)	23 (d)	24 (b)	25 (d)	26 (c)	27 (d)	28 (b)	29 (a)	30 (a)
31 (a)	32 (a)	33 (c)	34 (a)	35 (d)	36 (b)	37 (b)	38 (d)	39 (a)	40 (a)

Chapter 06 Animal Habitat and Adaptations

The living organisms are found at places where there is plenty of food and environmental conditions are favourable.

The organisms live on earth's water bodies, land and branches of trees etc.

Habitat

- The place where an organism lives, is called a habitat.
- It is a part of the total environment of the region.
- It provides the living organism with food, shelter and favourable climate conditions to survive, breed and flourish.
- Several kinds of plants and animals may share the same habitat.

The three types of habitats known are

(i) **Terrestrial habitats** The plants and animals that live on land are said to live in terrestrial habitats, e.g. forests, grasslands, deserts, coastal and mountain regions.

(ii) **Aquatic habitats** The habitats of plants and animals that live in water are called aquatic habitats, e.g. ponds, swamps, lakes, rivers and oceans.

There are large variations in forests, grasslands, deserts, coastal and mountain regions located in different parts of the world. This is true for all aquatic habitats as well.

(iii) **Arboreal Habitats** The animals which live on branches of trees make the arboreal habitat. Some epiphytes (plants), monkey, lemur, birds makes arboreal habitats.

Ecological Adaptations

- It is the quality of an organism of having certain specialised features that enhances its capacity to withstand a particular ecological condition.
- Adaptations may be morphological, physiological, behavioural or combination of all.
- These develop through the natural selection of suitable variations appearing in living beings through mutations and recombinations.

Ecological Adaptations in Plants

Depending upon the climate conditions.

These are as follows

Hydrophytes

The plants growing in abundance of water or wet place are called hydrophytes. These plants may be partially or wholly submerged in water.

The aquatic habit provides the following to the plant to grow

- Availability of nutrients in the water
- Plant growth matrix
- Approximate constant temperature (with least variation)
- Availability of light
- Movement of water (waves strong or weak).

Based on the relation of plants to water and air, the hydrophytes are grouped into the following categories

Ecological Adaptations in Hydrophytes

- Adaptation in hydrophytes can be discussed under three headings, i.e. morphological, anatomical and physiological.
- Roots may be entirely absent e.g. *Wolffia, Salvinia* or poorly developed, e.g. *Hydrilla* but the roots in *Ceratophyllum, Lamna*. There are unbranched with root hairs.
- The stems are long slender spongy which do not break with water currents.
- The leaves are dissected in *Vallisneria* and are ribbon shaped.

Mesophytes

These are plants which grow in moist, habitats and need well-aerated soils.

Ecological Adaptation in Mesophytes

These show the following characteristics

- Root system is well-developed. They are branched, with root caps and root hairs.
- Stems are aerial and freely branched.
- Leaves are large, broad and thin.
- Cuticle in all aerial parts is moderately developed.
- The stomata are dorsiventral in dicotyledons and isobilateral position in monocot leaves.
- The photosynthetic are in leaf, i.e. mesophyll tissue in differentiated into palisade, parenchyma and spongy parenchyma.
- Water and food conductive tissue (vascular tissue) and mechanical tissue (collenchyma and sclerenchyma are well-developed).

Xerophytes

These are the plants which are adapted to drier regions and have high rate of transpiration than absorption of water.

Ecological Adaptations in Xerophytes

- The roots of the plant are very well developed, reach deeper in soil in reach of water.
- Stem of these plants is thick, woody succulent which conserves water.
- The leaves and stems are covered with thick hairs and spines to reduce water loss by transpiration.
- In *Opuntia* stem become flat thickened green, succulent and is called phylloclade. The leaves get modified into spines to reduce transpiration.
- In some plants, leaves have multi-layered epidermis which prevents loss of water.

Halophytes

These plants grow in soil having high content of NaCl, $MgCl_2$ and $MgSO_4$ salts. These soils are called **saline soils.**

Ecological Adaptations in Halophytes

- These plants have two types of roots-underground and aerial.
- Some plants develop from special subterranean roots which become negatively geotropic and respire. These are called pneumatophores e.g. *Rhizophora, Sonneratia, Aricinia.*
- These plants have succulent leaves with thick cuticle.
- The mangrove plants show vivipary in which seed germinate while still attached in parent plants.

Ecological Adaptations in Animals

The animals are adapted to different types of climates and whether conditions. This makes their survival. These adaptations are morphological, physiological and behavioural.

(i) **Structural adaptations** Adaptation of special body parts of an organism that helps it to survive in its natural habitat, e.g. skin colour, shape, body covering.

(ii) **Behavioural adaptations** Adaptation of special ways in a particular organism that helps it to survive in its natural habitat.
It usually occurs in response to some external stimuli, e.g. frogs and bear undergoes hibernation or winter sleep during hard winter season.

(iii) **Physiological adaptations** Adaptation of body systems presents in an organism that allows it to perform certain biochemical reaction, e.g. warm-blooded animals are able to keep a constant body temperature.

Adaptation in Aquatic Animals

- The body of these animals is covered with scales and is streamlined which help in swimming, e.g. fishes.
- The appendages take shape of fins which help in swimming.
- These animals use dissolved O_2 in water for respiration and respire through clomes.
- The animals possess air bladder to maintain buoyancy and bear pressure in deeper region of water bodies.
- These are mostly cold-blooded animals.

Adaptation in Animals for Cold Climate

Polar bear is a large and white bear that lives in North polar region of the Earth.

The polar bear mainly feeds on fishes and seal and can survive in extremely cold climate of polar regions due to the following adaptations

- Their body is covered by a thick coat of white fur. It helps them to blend with their surrounding snow white background and cannot be noticed by their predators.
- Polar bear is a good swimmer which has wide and large paws that help it to swim. These paws also help bear to walk on the snow easily.
- They have a strong sense of smell so that they can locate their prey easily. They also possess small ears to keep the body surface area to the minimum and reduce the heat loss from the body.
- The thick layer of fat beneath the skin also stores food in winter when food is scarce. This stored food (fat) also helps the mother polar bear to survive in the winter when they undergo hibernation beneath the snow with their newborn cubs.

Ecological Adaptations in Xeric Animals

- These animals show adaptation in two ways
  (i) By reducing use of water
  (ii) By bearing heat condition
- These animals use water present in fatty tissues.
- The xeri animals need less water because they can make use of metabolic water.
- The Kangaroo rat hardly drink any water in his life time as it uses metabolic water and excrete very less water in urine.
- Camel an desert animal can store 50 L of water, excrete concentrated urine.
- Many other animals show summer sleep to avoid heat eg. crocodile, frog etc.

Exam Pattern Questions

1 Which of the following cannot be called a habitat?
(a) A desert with camels
(b) A pond with fishes
(c) A jungle with wild animals
(d) Cultivated land with grazing cattle

2 Which of the following constitute the biotic components of the habitat?
(a) Plants and animals
(b) Soil and minerals
(c) Air and water
(d) Sunlight and temperature

3 Choose the set that represents only the biotic components of a habitat
(a) tiger, deer, grass, soil
(b) rocks, soil, plants, air
(c) sand, turtle, crab, rocks
(d) aquatic plant, fish, frog, insect

4 Animals and plants have certain features which make them capable to survive in a particular habitat. This is called
(a) adaptation (b) speciation
(c) specialisation (d) evolution

5 Select those who are all the types of aquatic habitats?
(a) Freshwater, coastal and rainforest
(b) Marine, tundra and desert
(c) Mountain, grassland and coastal
(d) Marine, freshwater and estuaries

6 Among the following, which is not a type of terrestrial habitat?
(a) Desert (b) Grassland
(c) Freshwater (d) Tundra

7 Carbon dioxide in air is used by plants to
(a) breathe
(b) make food
(c) remove waste
(d) trap energy of the sun for photosynthesis

8 Upper part of sea/aquatic ecosystem contains
(a) plankton (b) nekton
(c) Both (a) and (b) (d) benthos

9 In an aqueous environment, microscopic animals and plants are collectively known as
(a) plankton (b) herbivore
(c) commensals (d) flora and fauna

10 Which one lacks both roots and stomata?
(a) Hydrophytes (b) Mesophytes
(c) Hygrophytes (d) Halophytes

11 Amongst hydrophytes finely dissected leaves occur in
(a) rooted floating leaved plants
(b) submerged plants
(c) emerged plants
(d) free-floating plants

12 *Eichhornia crassipes* is a
(a) xerophyte (b) hydrophyte
(c) mesophyte (d) parasite

13 Submerged hydrophytes exchange gases through
(a) stomata (b) hydathodes
(c) lenticels (d) aerenchyma

14 Stem of submerged hydrophytes is soft and weak because of the
(a) absence of phloem
(b) absence of stomata
(c) absence of xylem
(d) feebly developed supporting tissue and xylem

15 Submerged hydrophytes have a well-developed
(a) vascular system (b) aerenchyma
(c) root system (d) stomatal system

16 Aquatic plants generally have a
(a) well-developed vascular system
(b) reduced vascular system
(c) well-developed root system
(d) well-developed stomatal system

17 The floating leaves of an aquatic plant has
(a) stomata on the upper surface
(b) stomata on the lower surface
(c) stomata on both the surface
(d) no stomata

18 A plant devoid of roots is
(a) *Wolffia*/*Ceratophyllum*
(b) *Vallisneria*
(c) *Hydrilla*
(d) *Azolla*

19 *Typha* is a
(a) submerged hydrophyte
(b) floating hydrophyte
(c) emergent hydrophyte
(d) attached hydrophyte with floating leaves

20 Which character is not present in the hydrophytes?
(a) Poor roots
(b) Plentiful xylem and sclerenchyma
(c) Leaves with stomata on the upper surface or absent
(d) Abundant aerenchyma

21 Mechanical tissue in undeveloped in
(a) xerophytes (b) hydrophytes
(c) halophytes (d) mesophytes

22 Sun loving plants are
(a) halophytes (b) sciophytes
(c) heliophytes (d) autotrophs

23 Formation of tropical forests needs mean annual temperature and mean annual precipitation
(a) 18-25°C and 150-400 cm
(b) 5-15°C and 50-100 cm
(c) 30-50°C and 100-150 cm
(d) 5-15°C and 100-200 cm

24 Xeric environment is characterised by
(a) precipitation
(b) low atmospheric humidity
(c) extremes of temperature
(d) high rate of vapourisation

25 What is wrong about xerophytes?
(a) Sunken stomata
(b) Small spiny leaves
(c) Thick cuticle
(d) Larger number of stomata

26 Water storage tissue has
(a) large-sized, thin-walled cells
(b) mucilage
(c) large-sized vacuoles
(d) All of the above

27 The type of plants having adaptations to check transpiration is
(a) xerophytes (b) lithophytes
(c) halophytes (d) epiphytes

28 Ephemerals are a type of xerophytes, which are
(a) drought-escaping (b) drought-resisting
(c) drought-enduring (d) None of these

29 Succulents occur in
(a) deserts (b) tundra
(c) temperate deciduous forests
(d) tropical rainforests

30 Stomata are sunken types in
(a) mesophytes (b) xerophytes
(c) hygrophytes (d) hydrophytes

31 Which character is not present in the xerophytes?
(a) Thick cuticle
(b) Well-developed mechanical tissue
(c) Well-developed conducting tissue
(d) Spongy parenchyma

32 Respiration in aquatic animals occurs by
(a) lungs (b) gills (c) nostrils (d) legs

33 An aquatic adaptation is depicted by which one of the following?
(a) Streamline body
(b) Light and hollow bones
(c) Hair on body
(d) Gills

34 A student comes across in a laboratory with an animal having a streamlined and slippery body. What is the habitat of the animal?
(a) Water (b) Desert
(c) Grassland (d) Mountain

35 Match the Column I with Column II.

Column I	Column II
A. *Hydrilla*	1. Aquatic plant
B. Cat	2. Flight adaptation
C. Bird	3. Living thing
D. Bacteria	4. Non-living thing
E. Aeroplane	5. Terrestrial

Code

	A	B	C	D	E
(a)	5	3	2	4	1
(b)	2	1	3	4	5
(c)	1	5	2	3	4
(d)	1	5	2	3	4

36 Most of the tree dwellers are found in which of the forests?
(a) Northern conifer forest
(b) Deciduous forest
(c) Mediterranean scrub forest
(d) Tropical rainforest

37 If you happen to go to a desert, what changes do you expect to observe in the urine you excrete? You would
1. excrete small amount of urine
2. excrete large amount of urine
3. excrete concentrated urine
4. excrete very diluted urine
Which of the above would hold true?
(a) 1 and 3 (b) 2 and 4
(c) 1 and 4 (d) 1 and 2

38 A terrestrial mammal who seldom drink water is
(a) hippopotamus (b) rhinoceros
(c) kangaroo rat (d) camel

39 Which of the following is the most important cause for animals and plants being driven to extinction?
(a) Drought and floods
(b) Economic exploitation
(c) Alien species invasion
(d) Habitat loss and fragmentation

40 Ram, a student of biology went to a wildlife sanctuary, where she saw dense vegetation of trees, shrubs, herbs and also a variety of animals like monkeys, birds, elephants, snakes, frogs, etc. The most likely location of this sanctuary is in the
(a) temperate region (b) tropical region
(c) polar region (d) coastal region

41 The arboreal animal among the following is
(a) elephant (b) lion
(c) butterfly (d) lion-tailed macaque

42 Match the Column I with Column II.

Column I	Column II
A. Cockroach	1. Aquatic animal
B. Camel	2. Nocturnal
C. Snow bear	3. Desert plant
D. Cactus	4. Desert adaptation
E. Whale	5. Found on mountain

Codes

	A	B	C	D	E
(a)	2	4	5	3	1
(b)	1	2	3	4	5
(c)	5	4	3	2	1
(d)	1	3	5	4	2

43 Which of the following statements is incorrect for penguins?
(a) They huddle together
(b) They cannot swim
(c) They have webbed feet
(d) They have streamlined body

44 The climate at higher altitude like at Himalaya is
(a) hotter (b) temperate
(c) cooler (d) moderately hot

45 Polar bear lives in
(a) north polar region of the earth
(b) south polar region of the earth
(c) east polar region of the earth
(d) west polar region of the earth

46 When the water droplets come in the form of crystals of ice, it is called
(a) fog (b) snowfall
(c) rainfall (d) smog

47 The coldest region of the earth is the
(a) polar region (b) tropical region
(c) temperate region (d) coastal region

48 Choose the odd one from the following options
(a) Thick layer of fat under the skin
(b) White fur
(c) Long grasping tail
(d) Wide and large feet with sharp claws

Answers

1 (d)	2 (a)	3 (d)	4 (a)	5 (d)	6 (c)	7 (b)	8 (a)	9 (a)	10 (a)
11 (b)	12 (b)	13 (d)	14 (d)	15 (b)	16 (b)	17 (a)	18 (a)	19 (c)	20 (b)
21 (b)	22 (c)	23 (a)	24 (b)	25 (d)	26 (d)	27 (a)	28 (a)	29 (a)	30 (b)
31 (d)	32 (b)	33 (a)	34 (a)	35 (d)	36 (d)	37 (a)	38 (c)	39 (d)	40 (b)
41 (d)	42 (a)	43 (b)	44 (c)	45 (a)	46 (b)	47 (a)	48 (c)		

Chapter 07

Ecological Balance and Cycling of Nutrients

Environment

- Environment means the surrounding and everything around us and it can also be defined as the composition of the physical and biological conditions in which we live.
- It includes physical conditions like air (atmosphere), water (hydrosphere) and land (lithosphere) and the biological conditions like plants, animals, human beings, microorganisms (like bacteria, fungi, etc.,) and their inter-relationships.
- Human beings are highly responsible in disturbing the environmental balance for fulfilling their need of food, clothing, housing, industry, transport, etc.

Ecological Balance

- The all communities remains in a equilibrium is any ecosystem with its environmental components.
- Any disturbance is any of the component be it abiotic or biotic leads to collapse of functioning of any ecosystem.
- The sun is the only source of energy which enters into ecosystem by green plants (producers).
- Thus are eaten up by herbivores and then by consumers. This way energy flows in one direction and homeostasis is maintained.
- The anthropogenic (man-made) activities create a kind of imbalance in the cycling of matter, food chain etc by deforesting the lands. Many important animals and plant species are getting lost because of their loss of habitat.

Causes of Imbalance in Ecosystem

- There are certain main causes of imbalance like natural, diasters, introduction of invasive species in a ecosystem, human activities.
- Because of there reasons, there is a constant pressure on natural resources, few of them are on verge of elimination (fossil fuels).

Ecosystem

- The term **Ecosystem** was first used by **AG Tansley** in 1935.
- An ecosystem is a functional unit consisting of all the living beings of an area and the non-living components of their environment, interacting to form a stable system.

Types of Ecosystem

These ecosystem are broadly divided into following two categories

(i) **Natural Ecosystem** The natural ecosystems are forests, deserts, grassland (terrestrial) and ponds, lakes, wetland (aquatic), etc.

(ii) **Artificial** (Man-made) **Ecosystem** The man-made ecosystem are gardens, aquariums, crop fields, etc.

Components of Ecosystem

An ecosystem consists of two components as described below

1. Abiotic Components

Abiotic components mean non-living factors and some of these are mentioned below

(i) **Temperature** The temperature directly affects the physiology of the organisms and their activities like reproduction, etc. For the biotic activity to occur, the average required temperature is 10–45°C.

The temperature dependent activities in the plants are called **thermoperiodism**. It is observed that on increasing the temperature, the rate of evaporation increases and *vice-versa*.

(ii) **Light** The organisms directly depend on the plants for the food. The plants prepare their food by the process of photosynthesis in the presence of light. Some other activities are also affected by the light like locomotional activities in plants, seed sprouting, respiration, evaporation, etc.

(iii) **Wind** The wind directly shows its effect in soil erosion, binding of plants, in pollination and in scattering of the seeds, etc.

(iv) **Humidity** It is directly related to the evaporation. If the humidity is low, then evaporation is high and *vice-versa.*

(v) **Topographic** Topographical factors such as expansion of land, mountains altitude, latitude, etc also affect the organisms.

(vi) **Edaphic** It is a nature related to soil. All vegetations directly interact with soil structure, soil wind, soil water, etc.

(vii) **Availability of Food-Stuffs** It was observed that organisms reside at the places where food-stuffs are easily available, while they exist in fewer number where these availabilities are not easy.

2. Biotic Components

Biotic components include all the living organisms present in ecosystem.

These components are broadly divided into following three categories

(i) **Producers** (Autotrophs) These are organisms which can prepare their own food (from simple inorganic substances like carbon dioxide and water) by using sunlight in the presence of chlorophyll.

The organic materials produced by plants is called **biomass** and the rate at which producers form biomass is called **primary productivity.**

e.g., green plants and certain blue-green algae.

(ii) **Consumers** (Heterotrophs) These are organisms which feed on other organisms or their parts. These are categorised into two broad groups, i.e., herbivores and carnivores. e.g., rabbit, mouse, squirrel, goat, cattle, etc, (herbivores), birds, jackal, snakes, fox, etc (carnivores).

Consumers are categorised into three main types i.e., primary, secondary and tertiary.

- **Primary Consumers** Those organisms that consume mainly producers are called as primary consumers or herbivores.
- **Secondry Consumers** Those organisms that consume mainly primary consumers are called secondary consumers or carnivores.
- **Tertiary Consumers** Those organisms that consume secondary consumers are called tertiary consumers or carnivores.

(iii) **Omnivores** Those organisms that consume both producers and other consumers.

(iv) **Detritivores** Those organisms that consume detritus (the tissues of dead organisms, either producers or consumers and organic wastes.)

(v) **Decomposers** (Reducers) These are organisms which feed on dead bodies of organisms and organic wastes of living organisms.
e.g., termites, beetles, becteria, saprophytic bacteria, fungi (mushrooms), etc.

Functions of Ecosystem

The main functions of an ecosystem are

- Material or nutrient cycle.
- Biological or ecological regulation including both regulation of organisms by environment and regulation of environment by the organisms.

Energy Flow in Ecosystem

- The flow of energy is unidirectional, *i.e.,* it flows from the sun to the producers and then to the consumers, thus maintaining the first law of thermodynamics.
- The energy flow in an ecosystem occurs in the form of food which is converted into energy during metabolic process and is stored as biomass.

Food Chain

- A food chain is the sequence of who eats whom in a biological community to obtain nutrient. It basically starts with the primary energy source (sun) **primary producers** and then to consumers.

- Each food chain ends with a top predator and animal with no natural enemies. Hence, the flow of energy is always unidirectional i.e., it can only flow from producer to carnivores but not *vice-versa.* i.e., as the energy moves forward through various levels, it is unavailable for the previous trophic levels.

  e.g., a simple food chain follows the given manner.

  Grass > Insect > Frog > Snake > Hawk

Food Web

- A network of food chains or feeding relationships by which energy and nutrients are passed on from one species of living organism to another, is called food web.
- It is represented by a graphical description of feeding relationships among species in an ecological community.
- It is also a mean of showing how energy and materials (e.g., carbon) flow through a community of species as a result of these feeding relationships.

Nutrient Flow in Ecosystem

- The term nutrient cycle or biogeochemical cycle is used for the exchange/circulation of biogenetic nutrients between the living and non-living components of the biosphere.
- Biogenetic nutrients or biogeochemicals are essential elements required by the organism for their body building and metabolism.
- The biogeochemical cycles are classified into two gaseous cycle (carbon, nitrogen, oxygen) and sedimentary cycle (sulpher, phosphorus) main types

Nitrogen Cycle

This transformation can be carried out through both biological and physical processors. Important processors in the nitrogen cycle include fixation, mineralisation, nitrification and denitrification.

Carbon Cycle

The carbon cycle is the biogeochemical cycle by which carbon is exchanged among the biosphere, pedosphere, geosphere and atmosphere of the earth. The carbon cycle was initially discovered by **Joseph Priestley** and **Antoine Lavoisier.**

Oxygen Cycle

It is the biogeochemical cycle that describes the movement of oxygen within its three main reservoirs, the atmosphere, the total content of biological matter within the biosphere and the lithosphere.

Phosphorus Cycle

It is the biogeochemical cycle that describes the movement of phosphorus through the lithosphere, hydropshere and biosphere. Unlike other biogeochemical cycles, atmosphere does not play a significant role in the movement of phosphorus.

Sulphur Cycle

Sulphur is considered as a secondary element along with calcium and magnesium. The process of sulphur availability is same as the process of nitrogen avalibility. Most of the sulphur present in soil is in the form of organic matter. Sulphur is an essential element being a constituent of many proteins and co-factors.

The sulphur cycle is the collection of processors by which sulphur moves to and from minerals and living systems. Steps of sulphur cycle include mineralisation of organic sulphur into organic forms such as hydrogen sulphide, oxidation of hydrogen sulphide to sulphate reduction of sulphate to sulphide and lastly incorporation of sulphide into organic compounds.

Water Cycle (Hydrological Cycle)

The water cycle is also known as the hydrological cycle or H_2O cycle. The water constantly circulates through evaporation, condensation and precipitation and the nutrients dissolved in water also circulates within it. It describes the continuous movement of water on, above and below the surface of the earth.

The water cycle influences climate which leads to temperature changes. Human activites that alter the water cycle includes agriculture, industry, dams, urbanisation, use of ground water, etc.

Exam Pattern Questions

1 The word 'ecosystem' was first used by
(a) Elton (b) Tansley (c) Odum (d) Billing

2 Green Plants → Grasshopper → Frog
Frog is a
(a) primary producer (b) herbivore
(c) primary carnivore (d) top consumer

3 Largest ecosystem in the world is contributed by
(a) forests (b) rivers
(c) oceans (d) grasslands

4 An ecosystem resists change because it is in a state of
(a) imbalance (b) homeostasis
(c) shortage of components
(d) deficiency of light

5 How many of the solar energy that falls on the leaves of a plant is converted to the chemical energy?
(a) 1% (b) 10% (c) 30% (d) 50%

6 Creating force of any ecosystem is
(a) organic fuels, carbohydrates
(b) biomass
(c) solar energy (d) producers

7 In an ecosystem, the population of
(a) primary producer is larger than primary consumers
(b) secondary consumer is largest
(c) primary consumers are more than primary producers
(d) primary consumers are least dependent upon primary producers

8 In an ecosystem, which one shows one way passage
(a) free energy (b) carbon
(c) nitrogen (d) potassium

9 A sequence of species through, which the organic molecule in a community pass is called
(a) pyramid of energy (b) food chain
(c) food web (d) nutrient cycle

10 In parasitic food chain, the pyramid of number is
(a) linear (b) upright
(c) inverted (d) inverted upright

11 A food chain consists of
(a) producers (b) consumers
(c) decomposers (d) All of these

12 A food chain always starts with
(a) photosynthesis (b) respiration
(c) nitrogen fixation (d) decay

13 Most food chains are composed of
(a) 1 or 2 species (b) 3 to 4 species
(c) 90 or 10 species (d) more than 16 species

14 Best arrangement of an energy system consists of hawks, snakes, mice and grasses is
(a) grasses → mice → snakes → hawks
(b) grasses → snakes → mice → hawks
(c) grass → mice → hawks → snakes
(d) hawks → snakes → mice → grasses

15 Detritus food chain in comparison to grazing food chain is generally
(a) longer (b) equal
(c) shorter (d) None of these

16 In the food chain, the saprophytic organisms are
(a) producers (b) consumers
(c) predators (d) decomposers

17 At each trophic level of a food chain (pyramid), the energy not used or passed along is given off as a
(a) matter (b) free energy
(c) heat (d) water

18 Energy transfer from organism to organism in a natural community develops
(a) biological control (b) food chain
(c) natural barriers (d) food web

19 The first trophic level in any kind of food chain is always a green plant because
(a) of wide distribution
(b) they alone have the capacity to fix atmospheric N_2
(c) their richness is chlorophyll
(d) their capacity to convert light energy to chemical energy

20 Transducer organisms in the food chain are called
(a) herbivores (b) carnivores
(c) decomposers (d) producers

21 Decomposition takes place in which layer of soil at maximum rate
(a) upper layer of soil (b) middle layer of soil
(c) lower layer of soil (d) None of these

22 Detritus includes
(a) dead plant parts (b) remains of animals
(c) animal excretions (d) All of the above

23 Ecological factor important for determining various ecosystem is/are
(a) light (b) soil
(c) temperature and precipitation
(d) All of the above

24 Amount of light is used in the production process by plants?
(a) 1-5% (b) 5-10%
(c) 20-40% (d) More than 70%

25 Last organisms of the food chain are generally
(a) photosynthetic plant (b) herbivores
(c) carnivores (d) decomposers

26 Suppose all bacteria and fungi are destroyed. What will happen?
(a) There will no disease and death
(b) No antibiotics will become available
(c) Dead bodies and excretions will pile up
(d) Soil will become depleted of all nutrients

27 Decomposers are also called
(a) microconsumers (b) osmotrophes
(c) Both (a) and (b) (d) macroconsumers

28 Biotic components include
(a) producers (b) consumers
(c) producers and consumers
(d) producers, consumers and decomposers

29 Energy flow in an ecosystem is
(a) unidirectional (b) bidirectional
(c) multidirectional (d) None of these

30 Concentration of nitrogen remains constant by
(a) nitrogen cycle (b) thundering
(c) lightening (d) enzymes

31 What is the source of energy that flows through the living world?
(a) Photosynthesis (b) Chemical bond
(c) Green plant (d) The Sun

32 Energy and nutrients enter a community by the way of
(a) producer (b) consumer
(c) scavenger (d) detritivores

33 Sedimentary cycle having a small gaseous component is found in
(a) phosphorus (b) nitrogen
(c) carbon (d) sulphur

34 Which one is sedimentary cycle?
(a) Oxygen cycle (b) Nitrogen cycle
(c) Hydrogen cycle (d) None of these

35 Purefying (O_2 Produced) organisms are
(a) producer organisms
(b) reducer organisms
(c) consumer organisms
(d) parasitic organisms

36 The phosphorus cycle is unusual in that it is entirely
(a) within aquatic systems
(b) within terrestrial ecosystem
(c) sedimentary
(d) gaseous

37 A group of interconnected food chain in called a
(a) pyramid of energy (b) complex food chain
(c) food web (d) food cycle

38 The main nitrogen reservoir in the biosphere is the
(a) atmosphere (b) ocean
(c) organism (d) rocks

39 The phosphorus cycle lacks .... component.
(a) an atmospheric (b) an organic
(c) a mineral (d) an aquatic

40 Which of the following atoms typically cycles within the most localised area?
(a) Carbon (b) Water
(c) Nitrogen (d) Phosphorus

41 Which of the following atoms most often limits the primary productivity of an ecosystem?
(a) Carbon (b) Nitrogen
(c) Sulphur (d) Phosphorus

Answers

1 (b)	2 (c)	3 (c)	4 (b)	5 (a)	6 (c)	7 (a)	8 (a)	9 (b)	10 (c)
11 (d)	12 (a)	13 (b)	14 (a)	15 (c)	16 (d)	17 (c)	18 (b)	19 (b)	20 (d)
21 (a)	22 (d)	23 (d)	24 (a)	25 (d)	26 (c)	27 (c)	28 (d)	29 (a)	30 (a)
31 (d)	32 (a)	33 (d)	34 (d)	35 (a)	36 (c)	37 (c)	38 (a)	39 (a)	40 (d)
41 (a)									

Chapter 08

Natural and Non Natural Resources

Resources

The things/materials which are of some important usage for mankind and which are used for making useful items for humans are called resources.

- Those resources which are derive/get from nature are called **natural resources** like air, water, soil, mineral salts, animals and plants etc. These resources are renewed naturally.
- Artificial or **non-natural resources** are man-made and can not be recycled naturally e.g. plastic paper, hard board, rubber etc.
- The fresh water (Drinkable/Pot table water) comes from glaciers.

Biotic Resources

These are as follows

Forests

In ancient times, we used to live in forests. It met all our requirements for leading a normal life at that time. Now-a-days, we live in cities and towns far off from forests, so we really do not know the important of forests in our life.

Some other benefits we get from forests are as follows

- Plants in the forest release oxygen during photosynthesis. This provides all animals including us with oxygen to breathe and helps to maintain the ratio of oxygen to carbon dioxide in the atmosphere. That is why, forests are called green lungs.
- If amount of carbon dioxide increases in the atmosphere, it would result in increase in earth's temperature.
- Forests give us a large number of useful products. Some of the important products which we get from the forests are wood, honey, gum, sealing wax (or lac), catechu (kattha), fruits, oils, spices, natural rubber, cork, dyes, medicinal plants and fodder for cattle.
- These provide raw materials for paper, hard board, tarpin oil, sports apparatus etc.
- Medicines are obtained from many important medicinal plants.
- Provide resources for small scale cottage industries like silk, honey, wax, birds, rope, basket etc. It helps people to increases their income.
- It provides sites for ecotourism and attracts people from all over the world.
- It helps in preventing flood, soil erosion, climatic changes. So, its conservation is the need of hour.
- The classic exemplary attempt war made by Amrita Devi in 1726 in Jodhpur Village to protect trees and forest. She sacrificed her life for this.
- Chipko Andolan was headed by Sundarlal Bahuguna in 1973 to protect trees in Uttarakhand.
- 21 March is celebrated as World Forest Day every year.
- Van Mahotsav in celebrated all over India in first week of July in which mass tree plantation is done.

Wild Life

- The different types of vegetation present in a forest provide food and shelter to animals, birds and insects which live in the forest.
- It is a natural renewable resource a habitat (home) to many forms of wildlife like bear, bison, jackal, deer, porcupine, elephant, etc.

- Many trees like sal, teak, semal, sheesham, neem, palash, khair amla, bamboo, kachnar and many others are also found in the forests.
- The forest also contains insects, butterflies, honeybees and birds which help in pollination in the flowering plants of the forest in pollination.

Coal

- It was formed from the remains of vegetation. Due to natural processes like flooding, dense forests got buried under the soil.
- Over millions of years, absence of air, high temperature and high pressure transformed the dead vegetation into coal (carbonisation).
- Coal contains about 60-90% carbon or its compounds, while compounds of nitrogen, sulphur, etc., present in small quantities.

Types of Coal

It generally occurs in following four varities

- **Peat coal** (50-60% C) is obtained in the first phase of extraction.
- **Lignite coal** (60-70% C) is also called brown coal.
- **Bituminous coal** (78-86% C) is most common very soft and is used for domestic purpose.
- **Anthracite coal** (94-98% C) [best coal, produce high heat with no smoke] is obtained in last phase of coal extraction.

Petroleum

- It is a dark oily liquid also called **black gold or crude oil or rock oil**. It has an unpleasant odour. It is infact, a mixture of several hydrocarbons and sulphur, calorific value of which is very high.
- It was formed from living organisms in the sea.
- As these organisms died, their bodies settled at the bottom of the sea and got covered with layers of sand and clay.
- Over millions of years, absence of air, high temperature and high pressure transformed the dead organisms into petroleum and natural gas.

Natural Gas

- It is a mixture of 83% methane and 16% ethane. It is generally present at the exporation sites of the petroleum substance.
- Because of the inflammable nature of its constituents, natural gas is considered as a best fuel. It is used in the production of artificial chemical fertilizers.

Abiotic Resources

- The resource we get from non-living things are called abiotic resources. These are also called in **exhaustible resources**. Some examples are water, soil, air, sunlight etc.
- The every ecosystem on planet of earth depends on solar radiation for energy. Only 1% of the solar energy is used by plants through the process of photosynthesis 70% of the area of earth surface is covered by sea water.
- It is not a source of any resource but is integral part of hydrogeocycle.

Exam Pattern Questions

1 Which of the following is not an in exhaustible resource?
(a) Air (b) Soil
(c) Water (d) Coal

2 The artificial/natural resource is
(a) metal (b) plaster
(c) oil (d) coal

3 The exhaustibal natural resource is
(a) coal
(b) solar energy
(c) wind energy
(d) hydrothermal energy

4 Which of the following inexhaustible components of air is present in the largest amount in the atmosphere?
(a) Nitrogen (b) Oxygen
(c) Water vapour (d) Carbon dioxide

5 Which one of the following changes may occur due to decertification?
(a) Decrease in atmospheric temperature
(b) Increase in water holding capacity of soil
(c) Increased chances of floods
(d) Conversion of fertile land into a desert

6 Planting new trees which regenerate exhaustible forest resource is called
(a) species (b) deforestation
(c) desertification (d) reforestation

7 The place of living of an organism in environment is called
(a) home (b) resort
(c) habitat (d) reservoir

8 In our country, large patches of forests are being cleared for cultivation of crops. The environmental impact of such a practice will lead to finish which natural resources to
(a) soil (b) soil pollution
(c) wildlife (d) water

9 5th June is celebrated as
(a) World Forest Day
(b) World Environment Day
(c) World Red Cross Day
(d) World Food Day

10 Which of the following is a renewable natural resource
(a) fossil fuel (b) natural gas
(c) natural vegetation (d) petroleum

11 The natural resources can be renewed by
(a) natural cycles (b) physical cycles
(c) artificial cycles (d) None of the above

12 The raw materials are usually obtained from forests. Which of the following is not a raw material?
(a) Turpentine oil (b) Rubber
(c) Plastic (d) Wood

13 Petroleum is
(a) a natural resources which can not be renewed
(b) a natural resource which can be renewed
(c) synthetic product
(d) water resource

14 About one fifth of ordinary air is
(a) nitrogen (b) carbon dioxide
(c) water vapour (d) oxygen

15 Nitrogen is needed by the plants to make
(a) fats (b) carbohydrates
(c) proteins (d) minerals

16 Deforestation increases the level of which of the natural resource of the atmosphere?
(a) Ozone (b) Carbon dioxide
(c) Oxygen (d) Water vapour

17 Amrita Devi Vishnoi is known as
(a) forest conservation activist
(b) aquatic life conservation activist
(c) social activist
(d) None of the above

18 Kanha National Park is located in ……… and is famous for ……… .
(a) Madhya Pradesh, elephant
(b) Madhya Pradesh, tiger
(c) Odisha, tiger
(d) Asom, elephant

19 What do black duck, elephant, python and golden cat together represent in a forest?
(a) Fauna (b) Ecosystem
(c) Flora (d) Species

20 Identity the odd combination of the habitat and the particular animal concerned.
(a) Dachigam National Park - Snow Leopard
(b) Sundarbans - Bengal Tiger
(c) Periyar - Elephant
(d) Rann of Kutch - Wild Ass

21 Wildlife conservation means the protection and preservation of
(a) ferocious wild animals only
(b) wild plants only
(c) non-cultivated plants and non-domesticated animals
(d) All the above living in natural habitat

22 Kaziranga National Park is located in the state of
(a) Asom (b) Paschim Bangal
(c) Kerala (d) Karnataka

23 World Wildlife Week is observed during
(a) first week of October
(b) last week of October
(c) third week of October
(d) first week of September
(e) first week of September

24 World Water day is celebrated
(a) 22 March (b) 4 October
(c) 21 March (d) 20 March

25 What is the main cause for the extinction of some species in tropical forest?
(a) Deforestation (b) Afforestation
(c) Pollution (d) Soil erosion

26 Which of the following soil is best for cultivation?
(a) Clay
(b) Silt
(c) Loam mixture with silt clay
(d) Loamy soil

27 Most of the tree dwellers (wildlife animals) are found, in which of the forests?
(a) Northern conifer forest
(b) Deciduous forest
(c) Mediterranean scrub forest
(d) Tropical rainforest

28 The 70% freshwater resource come from
(a) polar ice (b) glaciers
(c) Antarctica (d) Green lands

29 The main source of energy for planet earth is
(a) Petrol (b) Diesel
(c) Sun (d) Biogas

30 Which one is not the renewable energy of natural resources?
(a) Tidal energy (b) Wind energy
(c) Fossil fuel (d) Solar energy

31 Land mass occupied by forest is
(a) 40% (b) 22%
(c) 30% (d) 17%

32 Which of the following is an inexhaustible resource?
(a) Fossil fuel (b) Solar energy
(c) Coal (d) Petroleum

33 Which one of the following is non-renewable exhaustible natural resource?
(a) Water (b) Wildlife
(c) Soil fertility (d) Minerals

34 The percentage of forest cover recommended by The National Forest Policy (1988) is
(a) 33% for plains and 67% for hills
(b) 37% for plains and 63% for hills
(c) 20% for plains and 70% for hills
(d) 23% for plains and 77% for hills

Answers

1 (d)	2 (b)	3 (a)	4 (a)	5 (d)	6 (d)	7 (c)	8 (c)	9 (b)	10 (c)
11 (a)	12 (c)	13 (b)	14 (d)	15 (c)	16 (b)	17 (a)	18 (b)	19 (a)	20 (b)
21 (d)	22 (b)	23 (a)	24 (a)	25 (c)	26 (d)	27 (d)	28 (b)	29 (c)	30 (c)
31 (c)	32 (b)	33 (d)	34 (a)						

Chapter

09 Food Production

- Living organisms require food for their growth and survival. Plants are known to prepare their own food while animals obtain their food from plants.
- In order to provide food for a large population, regular production, proper management and distribution of food is necessary.

Crop Production

- When plants of same type are grown and cultivated in a field at large scale, it is called a crop (fasal in Hindi). e.g. wheat crop, paddy crop, etc.
- Accordingly, there is a rich variety of crops grown in different parts of the country.
- Despite this diversity, two broad cropping patterns can be identified on the basis of particular season in which they grow.

Classification of Crops on the Basis of Seasons

On the basis of growing seasons, the crops are classified as follows

Kharif Crops

- The crops that are sown in rainy season are called kharif crops or summer crops.
- These are sown in June-July and harvested at the end of monsoon season, i.e. during September, e.g. paddy (rice), maize, soybean, cotton, groundnut, millets, etc.

Rabi Crops

- The crops that are grown in winter season are called rabi crops or winter crops.
- These are sown during October-November are harvested by March, e.g. wheat, gram, pea, mustard and linseed.

Zaid Crops

- These crops are grown in the month of March and harvested in June.
- These can bear high temperature and bright sunlight e.g. All cucumber crops.

Classification of Crops on the Basis of Food Category

On the basis of category of food obtained from plants crops are categorised as follows

Cereal Crops

- The word 'cereal' is derived from cerealia munera (the Roman Goddess of Agriculture). Cereals are most important source of food.
- These are rich in carbohydrates, but also contain considerable amount of proteins, fats, vitamins and minerals. e.g. rice, wheat, barley, maize, etc.

Pulse Crops

- Legumes or pulses belong to family Leguminosae (Fabaceae) sub-family Papilionaceae. These provide proteins to the vegetarian population.
- The higher protein content is due to presence of nodules on the roots, which contain nitrogen-fixing bacteria (*Rhizobium*).
- Pulses also contain up to 60% carbohydrates. Other crops are Arhar, Rajma, Chane, Moong, Urd, etc.

Oil Yielding Crops

Oil is obtained from the following plants

(a) **Groundnut or Peanut** Oil obtained from cotyledons of *Arachis hypogaea* (Family-Leguminosae).

(b) **Mustard** (*Brassica* sp. Family-Cruciferae) It is most important vegetable oils of India used as cooking oil.

Pungent smell and taste of mustard due to presence of sulphur.

(c) **Soyabean** (*Glycine max* family Leguminosae) It is most important oilseeds crop of the world.

(d) **Coconut** Oil obtained from seeds of *Cocos nucifera* (Family-Palmae). It is also called Kalpvriksha.

Vegetable Crops

- Vegetables are parts of plants that are consumed by humans on other animals as food.
- These crops provide minerals vitamins and some proteins etc. e.g., cabbage, carrot, cowpea etc.

Fruit Crops

Fruit crop any one of a group of wild and cultivated trees, shrubs, sub-shrubs and undershrubs that yield fleshy or hard edible fruits.

Various season fruits provide plenty of vitamins and minerals, e.g. mango, apple, pineapple etc.

Fibre Crops

Fibre crops are filled crops grown for their fibres, which are traditionally used to make paper, cloth, etc. These are as follows

(a) **Cotton** It (Family-Malvaceae) is most important commercial crop of the world.

The fibre is almost pure cellulose. Cotton fibre is thin walled and without lignin.

(b) **Jute** It (Family-Tiliaceae) is second most important fibre and most affordable natural fibres. Jute fibres are composed primarily of the plant materials cellulose and lignin.

Food from Animals

Besides plants, some animals also provide us food. The food obtained by animals are rich in protein (that are not present in plants), good amount of fats but less amount of carbohydrates. There are many types of food and animals are as follows

(a) **Cattle Farming** The animals are reared for various products like milk, also for draught labour at field like ploughing, tilling and carting etc. e.g. cow, buffalo, sheep etc.

(b) **Poultry Farming** Certain birds are reared for egg, broilers for meat etc. These are chicken goose, fowls etc.

(c) **Apiculture** This word is derived from the honey bee's zoological name *Apis*. For apiculture, large place called apiaries or been farms are arranged.

(d) **Pisciculture** It deals with the cultivation of fishes. Fishes are regarded as a valuable and easily available source of protein rich food. Pisciculture involves the exploitation of aquatic animals for various purposes of human welfare.

Food/Agricultural Wastes Management

The waste materials are left over in the field after to harvest of crop as well as domestication of animals. These are bio degradable waste and can be decomposed by fungi and bacteria.

Method of Food/Agricultural Wastes Management

- Agriculture operations just like any other process, produces wastes as well. The agricultural wastes are mainly organic wastes.
- If these wastes are not properly handled. These can pollute earth surface, ground water and surrounding air.
- The proper management of these wastes can contribute in a significant way to farm operations. The methods of food/agricultural waste materials are as follows

Biogas

- **Biogas** is a complex mixture of gases, like CH_4, CO_2 and H_2, but its major content is methane gas. It is produced by the microbial activity during anaerobic digestion of biomass mainly agricultural wastes. Biogas is used as fuel.
- **Methanogenesis** Certain bacteria, which grow anaerobically on cellulosic material, produce large amount of methane gas along with CO_2 and H_2 by the process called methanogenesis.

- **Gobar Gas** The excreta of cattle, commonly called **gobar**, is rich in methanogenic bacteria. Thus, cattle dung can be used for the generation of biogas, commonly called gobar gas.
- **Cattle Dung** As cattle dung is available in large quantities in rural areas this method of biogas production is mostly functional in those areas.

Manure Production

The organic waste of agriculture produce are turned into the manure by the following methods

Vermicomposting

- It is a method of using worms to transform organic waste into a nutrients-rich fertiliser.
- It is a healthy and clean way to eliminate wastes going into our landfills, which improves the environment.
- Vermicomposting is inexpensive and only takes two to three months to produce results. Vermicomposting is easy, requires very few supplies and can be done by anyone.

Green Manure

- It is a type of cover crop grown primarily to add nutrients and organic matter to the soil.
- Green manure crops may include legumes such as cowpeas, soyabeans, annual sweet clover, vetch, sunn hemp. *Sesbania* and velvet beans, as well as non-leguminous crops such as sudangrass, millet, sorghum and buckwheat.

Exam Pattern Questions

1 Which of the following statements is correct?
(a) Pulses contains 80% carbohydrates
(b) Rice contains 90% carbohydrates and 8-10% proteins
(c) Rice contains 60% carbohydrates and 35-40% proteins
(d) Rice contains 70% carbohydrates and 25-30% proteins

2 The aroma and flavour of tea is due to
(a) caffeine and thiol
(b) the eternal oil and thiol
(c) vegetable oil and thiol
(d) essential oil and thiol

3 Match the List I (spice name) and List II (constituents) and choose the correct option from the codes given below

List I	List II
A. Pepper	1. Zingiberene, cineol
B. Turmeric	2. Non-volatile oleoresin
C. Ginger	3. Eugenol
D. Clove	4. Volatile oil

Codes

	A	B	C	D		A	B	C	D
(a)	4	1	2	3	(b)	2	1	3	4
(c)	1	4	2	3	(d)	3	1	4	2

4 Saffron is obtained from which part of the plant?
(a) Leaf
(b) Stem
(c) Anther and whole flower
(d) Stigma and style

5 Which one of the following is responsible for the stimulating effect of tea?
(a) Tannin (b) Steroid
(c) Alkaloid (d) Flavonoid

6 Soft drinks such as cola contain significant quantities of
(a) caffeine (b) nicotine
(c) tannin (d) renin

7 Which one of the following plants is used for green manuring in India?
(a) Wheat (b) Sunnhemp
(c) Cotton (d) Rice

8 Which one of the following plants preferred for mixed cropping in order to enhance the bioavailability of nitrogen?
(a) Wheat (b) Gram
(c) Maize (d) Barley

9 Consider the following crops of India.
I. Groundnut II. Sesamum
III. Pearl mullet

Which of the above is/are predominantly rain fed crop/crops?
(a) I and II (b) II and III
(c) Only III (d) I, II and III

10 Consider the following crops
I. Cotton II. Groundnut
III. Rice IV. Wheat
Which of these are Kharif crops?
(a) I and IV (b) II and III
(c) I, II and III (d) II, III and IV

11 ....is second most important fibre and most affordable natural fibres.
(a) cotton (b) jute
(c) 'a' and 'b' (d) None of these

12 The term 'livestock' means
(a) domestic animals
(b) poultry animals
(c) bee culture
(d) Both (b) and (c)

13 Which one is of most recent domestication?
(a) Buffalo (b) Sheep
(c) Turkey (d) Silkworm

14 Sheep are reared mainly for
(a) meat (b) mutton
(c) wool (d) milk

15 The cross breed of cattle is
(a) Ongole (b) Sunandini
(c) Tharparkar (d) Kangayam

16 High milk yielding varieties of cows are obtained by
(a) superovulation
(b) artificial insemination
(c) use of surrogate mothers
(d) All of the above

17 Cows and buffaloes remain in heat for
(a) 24-36 h (b) 24-36 days
(c) 7-10 days (d) 15-20 days

18 The birds, which are reared for eggs are called
(a) broilers (b) layers
(c) cocks (d) hen

19 The birds, which are reared for meat purpose are called
(a) layers (b) broilers
(c) cocks (d) hen

20 A nutritional disease, which is found in poultry birds is
(a) Rickets (b) Ranikhet
(c) Fowl cholera (d) Aspergillosis

21 Which of the following species of honeybee is reared in artificial hives?
(a) *Apis indica* (b) *Apis dorsata*
(c) *Apis florea* (d) None of these

22 Honey is
(a) acidic (b) neutral
(c) alkaline (d) basic after some days

23 In honeybees, the drones develop from
(a) fertilised egg (b) unfertilised egg
(c) schizogony (d) asexual reproduction

24 In bees, dance in meant for
(a) only reproduction (b) communication
(c) recreation (d) Both (b) and (c)

25 The drones in honeybee are
(a) fertile males (b) fertile females
(c) sterile males (d) sterile females

26 The wax glands in honeybee are present on the
(a) ventral side of the last segment
(b) ventral side of second to fifth abdominal segments
(c) dorsolateral of first two abdominal segments
(d) lateral side of last two abdominal segments

27 Which one of the following is a marine fish?
(a) Rohu (b) Hilsa
(c) *Catla* (d) Common carp

Answers

1 (b)	2 (a)	3 (a)	4 (d)	5 (c)	6 (a)	7 (b)	8 (b)	9 (b)	10 (c)
11 (b)	12 (a)	13 (c)	14 (c)	15 (b)	16 (d)	17 (a)	18 (b)	19 (b)	20 (a)
21 (a)	22 (a)	23 (b)	24 (b)	25 (c)	26 (b)	27 (b)			

CHEMISTRY

Chapter 01

Matter and its States

Matter

- Anything that has mass, occupy volume, show physical resistance and can be realised by the sense organs is called matter.
- It includes stones, water, wood, food, air, large celestial objects etc.

States of Matter

- There are **five states** in which matter exists, namely solid, liquid, gas, plasma and Bose-Einstein Condensate (BEC).
- Out of these, first three are most prominent.
- In **solid state**, shape and volume of matter is fixed. e.g. Ice, wood block, etc.
- In **liquid state**, volume of matter is fixed, but have no definite shape. e.g. Water, oil, etc.
- In **gaseous state**, neither shape nor volume of matter is fixed. e.g. Water vapour, air, etc.
- At absolute zero temperature ($T = 0\,K$), the gas molecules stop their movement.
- **Plasma** is the fourth and **BEC** is the fifth latest discovered state.
- Plasma state and BEC are achieved only under certain conditions.
- **BEC** is a state of matter of a dilute gas of low densities called boson cooled to nearly absolute zero temperature.
- The sun and other stars exist in plasma state because of very high temperature.

Interconversion of States of Matter

- The states of matter are interconvertible. They can be interchanged by changing temperature or pressure as

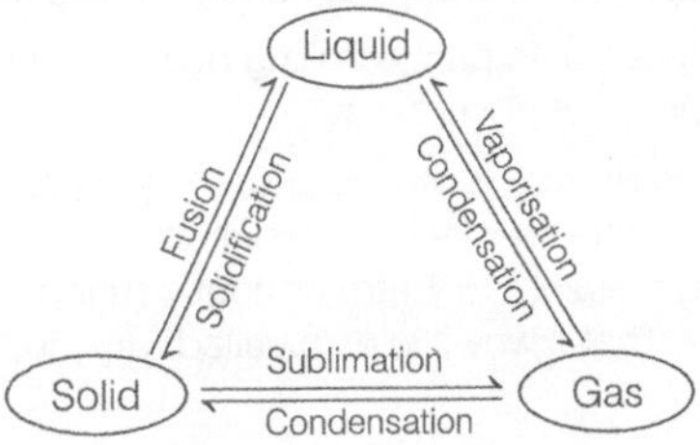

Various terms related to interconversion of states of matter are

- **Fusion** The process of melting, i.e., change of solid state into liquid state is also known as fusion.
- **Melting Point** The temperature at which a solid starts to melt to become a liquid at the atmospheric pressure is called its melting point. Higher the melting point of solid, higher will be the force of attraction between the particles of solid. Melting point of ice is 0°C.
- **Sublimation** It is the process used for those solids which convert directly into vapours on heating without converting into liquid phase and the vapours upon cooling give back the solid. Such solids are called **sublimates.**
- **Vaporisation** The process in which a liquid substance changes into a gas rapidly on heating is called vaporisation. The same phenomenon is called evaporation when heating is categorised to be done below the boiling point of the liquid.
- **Boiling Point** The temperature at which a liquid starts boiling at the atmospheric pressure is known as its boiling point. Boiling is a bulk phenomenon and varies from place to place. Boiling point of water at normal pressure is 100°C.

- **Condensation** It is the process in which gas changes into the liquid state or liquid changes to solid state i.e., **solidification.**

Important Observation Related to Interconversion of States

- At high altitudes, atmospheric pressure is low, therefore, the vapour pressure of a liquid becomes equal to atmospheric pressure at low temperature, i.e., water boils at a temperature less than 100°C and hence, food requires more time to cook.
- Inside the pressure cooker, pressure is high and hence, water boils at a temperature higher than 100°C. Thus, less time is required to cook the food.
- In the presence of impurity, boiling point increases and freezing point decreases.
- Solid carbon dioxide is stored under high pressure. It gets converted directly to gaseous state on decreasing pressure to 1 atm without coming into liquid state. That's why it is also called 'dry ice' or 'dry kold'.

Classification of Matter

On the basis of chemical composition, matter can be classified as :

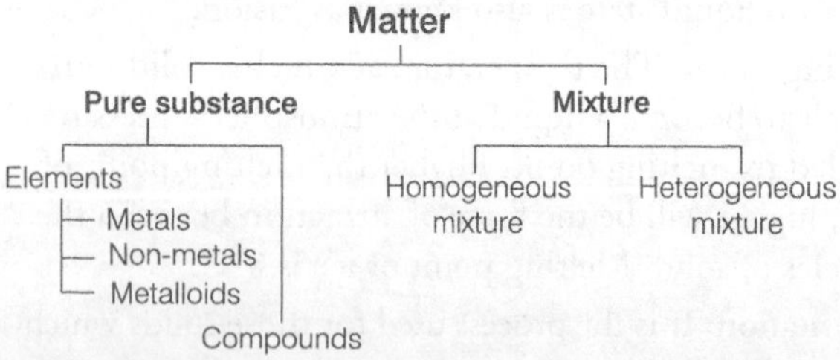

Pure Substances

These are substances, which are made up of only one kind of constituent particles, which cannot be broken down by simple physical means.

- **Element** is made up of only one kind of atoms. e.g. Sodium (Na), carbon (C), oxygen (O), etc.
- On the basis of variation in properties, elements can be broadly classified as metals, non-metals and metalloids.
- **Compound** is made up of two or more elements, chemically combined with one another in fixed proportion. e.g. Water (H_2O), carbon dioxide (CO_2).

Mixtures

Mixtures are constituted by more than one kind of pure form, known as a substance.

- Most of the matter around us exist as mixtures of two or more pure components. e.g. Sea water, minerals, soil, etc., are all mixtures.
- Depending upon the nature of the components that form a mixture, we have two different types of mixture, which are as follows
  - **Homogeneous mixture** is the one that has uniform composition through out the mixture. e.g. Salt in water solution, clean air (gas in gas), etc.
  - **Heterogeneous mixture** does not have uniform composition through out the mixture. e.g. Mud water, polluted air (dust in air), mixture of two powders, colloidal solution (like milk), etc.

Separation of Mixture

The various techniques for the separation of components of a mixture are as follows

(i) **Evaporation** This method can be used to separate a volatile component (solvent) from a non-volatile component (solute) of a mixture.

(ii) **Centrifugation** Two components having difference in densities can be separated by this method.

(iii) **By the use of separating funnel** This method is used to separate a mixture of two immiscible liquids.

(iv) **Sublimation** By this process, the mixture of those two solids is separated in which one solid is sublimate. Examples of solids that sublime are camphor, ammonium chloride, naphthalene, anthacene, etc.

(v) **Distillation** It is based on the difference in the boiling points of the liquids in the given mixture. It can be further divided into two types

- **Fractional Distillation** This method is used to separate a mixture of two or more miscible liquids for which the difference in boiling points is less than 25K. e.g. Separation of different gases from air.

- **Steam Distillation** This technique is applied to separate substances which are steam volatile and are immiscible with water.

(vi) **Crystallisation** It is a process that separates a pure solid in the form of its crystals from a solution.

(vii) **Chromatography** This technique is used for the separation of those solutes that dissolve in the same solvent.

Particles of Matter

- **Atom** The smallest unit of an element that takes part in a chemical reaction is called atom. It is the smallest particle that consists all the chemical properties of its element.
- **Molecule** The smallest particle of a substance, which is capable of independent existence and which has all the properties shown by the substance is called molecule. e.g. H_2, N_2, Ne, H_2O etc.

Mass Terms Related to Matter

The various mass terms related to matter are as follows :

Mass and Weight

- **Mass** (m) is the amount of matter present in a substance. It remains constant for a substance at all the places. Its unit (SI unit) is kilogram (kg), but in laboratories usually gram (1 kg = 1000 g) is used.
  - Analytical balance or electrical balance is used to measure the mass of a substance.
- **Weight** (w) is the force exerted by gravity on an object. It varies from place to place due to change in gravity. Its unit is Newton (N).

Atomic Mass (Weight)

Atomic mass is defined as a number that expresses as to how many times an atom of the element is heavier than 1/12th of the mass of carbon atom (^{12}C). Therefore,

$$\text{Atomic mass} = \frac{\text{mass of an atom}}{(1/12)\times \text{mass of a carbon atom } (^{12}C)}$$

Molecular Mass (Weight)

- Molecular mass is the sum of atomic masses of the elements present in a molecule.
- Thus, it is obtained by multiplying the atomic mass of each element by the number of its atoms and then adding them together. e.g.
  Molecular mass of methane can be calculated as
- $CH_4 = 1 \times \text{atomic mass of C} + 4 \times \text{atomic mass of H}$
  $= (12.011\text{ u}) + 4(1.008\text{ u}) = 16.043\text{ u}$

Equivalent Mass (Weight)

It is the mass of an element or a compound, which would combine with or displace (by weight) 1.008 part of hydrogen or 8 parts of oxygen or 35.5 parts of chlorine.

$$\text{Equivalent mass} = \frac{\text{Molecular mass}}{n}$$

Physical Change

- In a physical change, a substance undergoes a change in its physical properties such as shape, size, colour and state.
- It is generally reversible, i.e. the original substance is further obtained by reversing the reaction conditions.
- Conversion of matter from one state to another, like evaporation of water, melting of ice, freezing of water, boiling of water, formation of clouds, stretching of spring, rubber, etc., are the examples of physical change.

Chemical Change

- A change in which one or more new substances are formed is called chemical change.
- In a chemical change, the internal molecular composition of original substance is deformed.
- Most of the chemical changes are irreversible.
- Burning of magnesium ribbon, coal, wood or leaves, ripening of fruits, rusting of iron, curdling of milk, etc., are the examples of chemical change.
- During burning of a candle, both physical and chemical changes take place.

Exam Pattern Questions

1 Which of the following is the latest discovered state of matter?
(a) Solid (b) Gas
(c) Plasma (d) BEC

2 Which of the following is/are in the plasma state?
(a) Mars (b) Jupiter
(c) Sun (d) All of these

3 Which of the following consists of ionised gas?
(a) Plasma (b) BEC
(c) Carbon monoxide (d) Oxygen

4 If a gas having density equal to one hundred thousandth the density of normal air, is cooled to a very low temperature, what kind of state will it achieve?
(a) Solid state (b) Liquid state
(c) Plasma state (d) BEC

5 On the basis of conversion of state, pick the odd one out
(a) naphthalene (b) ice
(c) dry ice (d) iodine

6 The water kept in a pitcher becomes cool. This is due to
(a) melting (b) evaporation
(c) sublimation (d) None of these

7 Carbon when burns, produces carbon dioxide gas which is a/an
(a) element
(b) compound
(c) homogeneous mixture
(d) heterogeneous mixture

8 Clean air is the example of
(a) element
(b) compound
(c) homogeneous mixture
(d) heterogeneous mixture

9 In which of the following case, a homogeneous mixture is not formed?
(a) When sugar is dissolved in water
(b) When two gases are kept in the same container
(c) When alcohol is mixed into water
(d) When kerosene is mixed into water

10 Brass, a alloys of copper and zinc is a
(a) compound
(b) homogeneous mixture
(c) heterogeneous mixture
(d) a kind of colloidal solution

11 When ice melts, its
(a) volume increases (b) volume decreases
(c) mass increases (d) mass decreases

12 Smallest unit of a substance is
(a) molecule (b) atom
(c) elements (d) All of these

13 What will be the mass of one atom of C-12 in gram?
(a) 1.99×10^{-23} g (b) 0.199×10^{-23} g
(c) 19.92×10^{-23} g (d) 1.99×10^{-20} g

14 Calculate molecular mass of glucose ($C_6H_{12}O_6$) molecule
(a) 18.16 u (b) 180 u
(c) 180.162 u (d) 182.162 u

15 Which changes take place during burning of a candle?
(a) Physical change (b) Chemical change
(c) Both (a) and (b) (d) None of these

16 Which of the following is an example of physical change?
(a) Curdling of milk (b) Freezing of water
(c) Rusting of iron (d) Ripening of fruits

Answers

1 (d)	2 (c)	3 (a)	4 (d)	5 (b)	6 (b)	7 (b)	8 (c)	9 (d)	10 (b)
11 (a)	12 (b)	13 (a)	14 (c)	15 (c)	16 (b)				

Chapter 02 Structure of Atom

Atomic Theory

- Dalton proposed that every substance is made up of indivisible particle called **atom.**
- The theory failed with the discovery of smaller particles called **sub-atomic particles.**

Structure of Atom

- More than 30 sub-atomic particles are known, among which three, namely electron, proton and neutron, are considered as fundamental particles.

Sub-atomic particles	Charge	Mass (in u and kg)	Position	Discovery
Electron	Negative	$1/1836 \simeq 0\ (9.1 \times 10^{-31}\text{kg})$	in the orbits around the nucleus	By J.J. Thomson as the constituent of cathode rays
Proton	Positive	$\simeq 1\ \text{u}\ (1.672 \times 10^{-27}\text{kg})$	in the nucleus	By E. Goldstein as the constituent of anode or canal rays
Neutron	Neutral	$\simeq 1 (1.674 \times 10^{-27}\ \text{kg})$	in the nucleus	By J. Chadwick

Atomic Models

To explain the distributions of various sub-atomic particles (i.e. electrons, protons and neutrons) in an atom, several models have been proposed. These were called atomic models.

Thomson Model

- J.J. Thomson proposed an atomic model called **plum pudding model** or **the watermelon model.**
- In this model, he suggested that electrons (negative particles) are embedded in positive sphere like seeds are embedded in watermelon.
- This model could explained the electrical neutrality of atom, but it could not explain the results of gold foil scattering experiment by Rutherford.

Rutherford's Model of an Atom

- With discovery of proton, Rutherford through his 'gold-foil experiment' suggested that protons are present in the nucleus and electron revolves around it.
- The positive charge and most of the mass of the atom was densely concentrated in extremely small region, called the **nucleus** by Rutherford.
- The nucleus is surrounded by electrons that move around the nucleus with a very high speed in circular paths, called **orbits.**
- Electrons and the nucleus are held together by electrostatic forces of attraction.

- This model does not tell about the distribution of electrons around the nucleus.

Composition of Nucleus

After the formulation of various theories, it is now accepted that protons and neutrons are found in nucleus. While electrons are present outside nucleus.

Bohr Atomic Model

In order to overcome the drawback of Rutherford's model of an atom and to explain the line spectrum of hydrogen, **Neils Bohr** proposed a new model of atom based upon Planck's quantum theory. This model is called **Bohr's atomic model.**

- The electron in the hydrogen atom can move around the nucleus in a circular path of fixed radius and energy (i.e. energy of an electron is quantised).
- These paths are called **orbits, stationary states** or **allowed energy states.**
- These orbits are arranged concentrically around the nucleus. The stationary states for electron are numbered $n = 1, 2, 3$ or $K, L, M \ldots$ The integral numbers are known as **principal quantum number.**
- The energy of an electron is certain in the orbit, i.e. it does not change with time.
- However, the energy is absorbed or emitted when electron jumps from lower to higher or higher to lower stationary states.
- The energy change does not take place in a continuous manner.

Characteristics of an Atom

An atoms is characterised by an atomic and mass number

Atomic Number

It is defined as the number of protons in the nucleus of an atom. All the atoms of the same element have the same number of protons in their nuclei and hence, they have the some atomic number.

Atomic number (z) = number of protons = number of electrons

Mass Number

It is defined as the sum of number of protons and neutrons present in the nucleus of an atom. Protons and neutrons together are called as **nucleons.**

Mass number (A) = Number of protons + number of neutrons.

Different Atomic Species

(i) **Isotopes** are species of same element having same atomic number but different mass number. e.g. ${}_1H^1$, ${}_1H^2$, ${}_1H^3$

(ii) **Isobars** are species of different elements having different atomic number but same mass number. e.g. ${}_{32}Ce^{76}$, ${}_{34}Se^{76}$

(iii) **Isotones** are the atoms of chemically different elements having same number of neutrons but different mass number as well as atomic number. e.g. ${}^{36}S$, ${}^{37}Cl$, ${}^{38}Ar$, ${}^{39}K$.

Structural Features of An Atom

In the present perspective, the structural features of an atom are as follows

Shell and Subshell

- The orbits or paths of different and definite energies in which the electrons revolve, are called **shells.**
- Each orbit or shell consists of one or more **subshells.**
- Each subshell is associated with one or more **orbitals.**
- Each orbital is associated with 2 electrons.

Shapes of Orbitals

- The *s*-orbitals are spherical in shape
- The *p*-orbitals are three in number and dumb-bell shaped with two lobes of same size on each side of nucleus.
- The *d*-orbitals are five in number. Four of these have a double dumb-bell shape whereas fifth is dumb-bell in shape with collar of high electron density.
- The *f* orbitals are 7 in number and have diffused *s*.
- The location of an electron in an atom can be traced through quantum numbers.

Exam Pattern Questions

1 Atomic theory of matter was given by
(a) Avogadro (b) Dalton
(c) Newton (d) Pascal

2 What particles move around the nucleus of an atom and are negatively charged?
(a) Electrons (b) Protons
(c) Positrons (d) Neutrons

3 The three basic components of an atom are
(a) protons, neutrons and ions
(b) protons, neutrons and electrons
(c) protium, deuterium and tritium
(d) protons, electrons and ions

4 The ratio of charge and mass would be greater for
(a) proton (b) electron (c) neutron (d) α-particle

5 The charge on the proton
(a) is equal to the charge of electron
(b) is opposite to the charge of electron
(c) Both (a) and (b)
(d) None of the above

6 Existence of nucleus first of all shown by
(a) Dalton (b) Rutherford
(c) J.J. Thomson (d) Pascal

7 Rutherford's α-particle scattering experiment eventually concluded that
(a) mass and energy are related
(b) neutrons are burried deep in the nucleus
(c) electrons occupy space around the nucleus
(d) the point of impact with matter can be precisely determined

8 Which of the following is not present in the nucleus of an element?
(a) Proton (b) Electron
(c) Neutron (d) All of these

9 The maximum energy is possessed by an electron, when it is present
(a) in nucleus
(b) in ground energy state
(c) in first excited state
(d) at infinite distance from the nucleus

10 The integral number are known as
(a) principle quantum number
(b) orbits
(c) energy states
(d) stationary states

11 The number of proton in the nucleus of an atom is
(a) mass number (b) atomic number
(c) atomic mass (d) All of these

12 The sum of numbers of protons and neutrons can be known as
(a) atomic number (b) isotopes
(c) isobars (d) mass-number

13 The mass number of a nucleus is
(a) always less than its atomic number
(b) always more than its atomic number
(c) always equal to its atomic number
(d) sometimes more and sometimes equal to its atomic number

14 An atom has 10 protons in its nucleus. The number of electrons in said atom are
(a) 5 (b) 20 (c) 10 (d) 15

15 Two atoms are said to be isotopes, if they have
(a) same atomic number, but different mass numbers
(b) same number of neutrons, but different mass numbers
(c) the sum of the number of protons and neutrons same
(d) same number of neutrons, but different modes of radioactive decay

16 Isotopes have similar
(a) chemical properties (b) physical properties
(c) number of neutron (d) mass number

17 Isobars are the elements have
(a) same atomic number but different mass number
(b) different atomic number but same mass number
(c) different atomic and mass number
(d) same atomic and mass number

18 An element has atomic masses 35 and 37 respectively. These are
(a) isotopes (b) isotones
(c) isobars (d) All of these

19 ${}_{32}Ce^{76}$, ${}_{34}Se^{76}$ are the example of
(a) isotopes (b) isotones
(c) isobar (d) All of these

20 Elements having different atomic number different mass number but same number of neutrons is known as
(a) isotopes (b) isobars
(c) isotones (d) None of these

21 How many subshels are their in 4th shell

(a) 1 (b) 2
(c) 3 (d) 4

22 The maximum number of electrons in an orbital is/are

(a) 1 (b) 2
(c) 3 (d) 4

Answers

1 (b)	2 (a)	3 (b)	4 (b)	5 (c)	6 (c)	7 (d)	8 (b)	9 (d)	10 (a)
11 (b)	12 (d)	13 (d)	14 (c)	15 (a)	16 (a)	17 (b)	18 (a)	19 (c)	20 (c)
21 (d)	22 (b)								

Chapter 03 Classification of Elements

- At present, 118 elements are known to us, out of which 98 are naturally occurring while remaining are synthesised artificially by man.
- Main objective of classification of elements is to make the study of 118 elements more convenient, systematic and organised.

Periodic Classification

- The arrangement of elements in which elements reappear at a regular interval, is called **periodic classification** or **periodic arrangement** of elements.
- **Dobereiner** grouped the elements into **triads** and said that the atomic weight and properties of the middle element is the average of atomic weights or properties of other two elements.
- **Newland** gave the law of octaves and told that when elements are arranged in increasing order of their atomic weights, every eighth element resembles in properties with the first one just like musical notes.

But all these were unable to arrange all the known elements. The first impressive attempt in this direction was made by **Mendeleev**.

Mendeleev's Periodic Table

- Mendeleev's studied the formula and properties of hydrides and oxides of different elements.
- On the basis of their comparative study, he gave a law called the **Mendeleev's periodic law.**
- It states that the properties of elements are the periodic function of their atomic masses or atomic weights.
- Mendeleev's periodic table is the tabular representation of elements.
- It contains vertical columns called **groups** and horizontal rows called **periods.**
- In this table, there were 8 groups and 7 periods.
- Mendeleev placed elements with similar nature in the same group with respect to atomic weight.

Modern Periodic Table

- It is based on modern periodic law, according to which, "the physical and chemical properties of the elements are the periodic function of their atomic numbers".

Numerous forms of periodic table have been devised from time to time.

A modern version, so called **long form of the periodic table** of elements, which is based on the electronic configuration of elements, is the most convenient and widely used.

Characteristics of Long Form of Periodic Table

- The horizontal rows are called **periods** and the vertical columns are called **groups**.
- The groups are numbered from 1 to 18 and there are altogether 7 periods.
- Elements having similar outer electronic configurations in their atoms are arranged in the vertical columns, i.e. groups or families. That's why elements of a group possess similar chemical properties.
- The first period contains 2 elements and the subsequent periods consist of 8, 8, 18, 18 and 32 elements respectively and seventh period is incomplete.
- In this form of the periodic table, 14 elements of both sixth and seventh periods (lanthanoids and actinoids respectively) are placed in separate panels at the bottom.

Characteristics of Periods

- The number of valence electrons in elements increases from 1 to 8 on moving from left to right in a period.
- The elements in a period have consecutive atomic numbers.
- The atoms of different elements with same number of shells are placed in the same period.
- As the number of valence shell electrons change, the chemical properties of the elements also change.

Characteristics of Groups

- All the elements of a group of the periodic table have the same number of valence electrons and hence, have almost similar chemical properties.
- The number of shells increases as use go down the group.
- The physical properties of the elements such as melting point, boiling point and density vary gradually.

Prediction of Number of Group and Period of an Element

- Number of shells in an atom determines period number of an element.
- Number of valence electrons determines group number of an element.
- If more than 2 valence electrons are present, then group number is equal to number of valence electrons plus 10.

Periodic Properties

The properties which are repeated at regular intervals are known as **periodic properties.** These properties show a regular order along a group and period.

- **Valency** The combining power of an element is called its **valency**.
  - It generally increases from 1 to 7 in a period with respect to hydrogen but with respect to oxygen, it first increases from 1 to 4 and then decreases to 0.
  - For alkali metals (i.e. Na, K etc) it is 1, for alkaline earth metals (i.e. magnesium, calcium, etc) it is 2, for aluminium it is 3 and for nitrogen it varies from – 3 to + 5.
- **Atomic Size** It refers to the radius of an atom.
  - It generally increases on moving down the group because new shells are being added as we go down the group.
  - It decreases along a period from left to right.
- **Ionisation Energy** It is the energy required to remove an electron from an isolated gaseous atom in its ground state.
  - It generally increases along a period from left to right due to increase in effective nuclear charge but ionisation energy of group-2 elements (Be, Mg, Ca, Sr) is larger than the ionisation energy of group-3 (B, Al, Ga, In) elements.

- It generally decreases along a group on moving downwards due to increase in atomic size.

- **Electron Gain Enthalpy** ($\Delta_{eg} H$) It is defined as the enthalpy change accompanying the process when an extra electron is added to neutral gaseous atom to convert it into an anion.
  - The energy released during the process is called **electron affinity** (EA).
  - EA increases across a period from left to right but EA of group-2, group-15 and group-0 is zero or positive.
  - It decreases on moving down the group. It is highest for chlorine.
- **Electronegativity** It is the tendency of an atom in a molecule to attract the shared pair of electrons towards itself.
  - It increases regularly along a period from left to right and decreases on moving down a group. It is highest for **fluorine**.
- **Metallic Character** It is the tendency of an element to form cation by the loss of electrons.
  - It decreases along a period from left to right and increases in a group on moving downwards.
  - Thus, metallic elements occupy the left hand columns of the periodic table.
- **Non-Metallic Character** It is the tendency of an element to form anion by the gain of electrons.
  - It increases along a period from left to right and decreases in a group on moving downwards.
- **Density** It is defined as mass per unit volume.
  - It increases on moving down a group as well as along a period from left to right but density of gold is higher than that of mercury.
  - The order of density of steel, mercury and gold is steel < mercury < gold.

Some Elements with Highest and Lowest Properties in the Periodic Table

Highest/Lowest Properties	Elements	Highest/Lowest Properties	Elements
Lightest element (non-metal)	Hydrogen	Element having least ionisation potential	Caesium
Heaviest element	Osmium	Metal having highest melting point	Tungsten
Lightest metal	Lithium	Element having highest electron affinity	Chlorine
Liquid metal	Mercury	(i.e. electron accepting tendency)	
Liquid non-metal	Bromine	Most electronegative element	Fluorine
Best conductor (metal)	Silver	Strongest oxidant	Fluorine
Second best conductor	Copper	Strongest reductant	Lithium
Best non-metallic conductor	Graphite (an allotrope of carbon)	Monoatomic gases	Inert or noble gases
Most ductile and malleable metal	Gold	Group of gaseous elements	zero group
Most reactive metal	Caesium	Element stored in kerosene oil	Sodium
Most reactive non-metal	Fluorine	Element present in bones and teeth	Calcium
Element having highest ionisation potential	Helium	Most poisonous metal	Plutonium

Exam Pattern Questions

1 How many elements are found naturally?
(a) 18 (b) 98 (c) 108 (d) 118

2 The heaviest naturally occurring element is
(a) osmium (b) uranium
(c) mercury (d) polonium

3 Who classified elements into triads on the basis of their atomic weights?
(a) Mendeleev (b) Newlands
(c) Mosley (d) Dobereiner

4 Whose classification system resembled to musical notes?
(a) Mendeleev (b) Newlands
(c) Dobereiner (d) Mosley

5 In Mendeleev's periodic table, the space left for an unknown element called eka-aluminium was later filled by
(a) silicon (b) scandium
(c) gallium (d) germanium

6 How many elements were discovered at the time of Mendeleev?
(a) 43 (b) 54 (c) 63 (d) 76

7 In modern periodic table, which of the following properties is considered as fundamental property?
(a) Atomic size (b) Density
(c) Atomic weight (d) Atomic number

8 Lanthanoids and actinoids, respectively belong to
(a) 5th and 6th periods
(b) 6th and 7th periods
(c) 6th and 7th periods
(d) 7th and 6th periods

9 Which of the following elements from 3rd period will have the highest number of valence electrons?
(a) Sodium (b) Aluminium
(c) Sulphur (d) Chlorine

10 Which of the following pair of elements have same number of valence electrons?
(a) Sodium and magnesium
(b) Carbon and sulphur
(c) Fluorine and chlorine
(d) Oxygen and silicon

11 All of these radicals have a valency of 2, except
(a) SO_4 (b) CO_3
(c) NH_4 (d) $MgCO_3$

12 In CuO, valency of copper is
(a) 1 (b) 2
(c) 3 (d) 4

13 Which of the following metals will be most reactive?
(a) Lithium (b) Sodium
(c) Potassium (d) Caesium

14 Which of the following has largest atomic size?
(a) Sodium (b) Magnesium
(c) Sulphur (d) Chlorine

15 The energy required to remove an electron from an isolated gaseous atom in its ground state is called
(a) ionisation energy
(b) electron gain enthalpy
(c) electron affinity
(d) electronegativity

16 Which of the following element has highest electron affinity in the periodic table?
(a) Oxygen (b) Fluorine
(c) Chlorine (d) Caesium

17 The most electronegative element among the following is
(a) sodium (b) chlorine
(c) oxygen (d) fluorine

18 Arrange the following elements in the increasing order of their metallic property : Li, Na, K,
(a) Na, Li, K, (b) K, Na, Li
(c) Li, Na, K (d) None of these

19 The hightest metal among the following is
(a) H (b) Li
(c) Cs (d) Na

20 Liquid metal at room temperature is
(a) gold (b) silver
(c) lithium (d) mercury

Answers

1 (b)	2 (a)	3 (d)	4 (b)	5 (c)	6 (c)	7 (d)	8 (b)	9 (d)	10 (c)
11 (c)	12 (b)	13 (d)	14 (a)	15 (a)	16 (c)	17 (d)	18 (c)	19 (b)	20 (d)

Chapter 04 Symbols of Elements, Chemical Formula, Chemical Reactions and Their Equations

- Dalton introduced symbols for representing elements, but modern symbols for the elements were introduced by JJ Berzelius in 1814.
- These are defined as a short hand representation of the name of an element.

Symbols of Some Elements

Elements	Symbol	Elements	Symbol
Hydrogen	H	Helium	He
Boron	B	Carbon	C
Nitrogen	N	Oxygen	O
Fluorine	F	Neon	Ne
Sodium	Na	Magnesium	Mg
Aluminium	Al	Phosphorus	P
Sulphur	S	Chlorine	Cl
Potassium	K	Calcium	Ca
Chromium	Cr	Iron	Fe
Cobalt	Co	Nickel	Ni
Copper	Cu	Zinc	Zn
Bromine	Br	Silver	Ag
Tin	Sn	Antimony	Sb
Barium	Ba	Tungsten	W
Platinum	Pt	Gold	Au
Mercury	Hg	Lead	Pb
Radium	Ra	Uranium	U
Hafnium	Hf		

Chemical Formula

A chemical formula identifies each constituent element by its chemical symbol and indicates the proportionate number of atom of each element. For example, chemical formula of alcohol is C_2H_5OH.

Rules for Writing Chemical Formula

- The valencies or charges on the ion must balance e.g.

	For Hydrogen Chloride		For Magnesium Chloride	
Symbol	H	Cl	Mg	Cl
Valency/Change	1	1	+2	−1

- The symbol of positive part (i.e. Metal or Hydrogen) is written first.
- The symbol of negative part (i.e. Non-metal or oxygen) is written in last.
  e.g. HCl (For hydrogen chloride)
  $MgCl_2$ (For magnesium chloride)
- In case of polyatomic ions the ion is enclosed in a bracket with its balanced number of $Al_2(SO_3)_2$ (for aluminium sulphate).
- In case of solids, water of crystallisation is added as $.nH_2O$. e.g. $CaSO_4.2H_2O$ (For calcium sulphate)

Industrial names of some important compounds

Industrial Name	Chemical Name and Formula
Alum	Potassium aluminium sulphate ($K_2SO_4 \cdot Al_2(SO_4)_3 \cdot 24\,H_2O$)
Alcohol	Ethyl alcohol (C_2H_5OH)
Baking powder	Sodium bicarbonate ($NaHCO_3$)
Blue vitriol	Copper sulphate ($CuSO_4 \cdot 5H_2O$)
Bleaching powder	Calcium hypochlorite ($CaOCl_2$)
Borax	Sodium tetraborate decahydrate ($Na_2B_4O_7 \cdot 10H_2O$)
Brine or salt	Sodium chloride (NaCl)
Calomel	Mercurous chloride (Hg_2Cl_2 or HgCl)
Caustic potash	Potassium hydroxide (KOH)

Industrial Name	Chemical Name and Formula
Caustic soda	Sodium hydroxide ($NaOH$)
Chloroform	Trichloromethane ($CHCl_3$)
Dry ice	Solid carbon dioxide (CO_2)
Epsum	Magnesium sulphate ($MgSO_4 \cdot 7H_2O$)
Gypsum	Calcium sulphate ($CaSO_4 \cdot 2H_2O$)
Laughing gas	Nitrous oxide (N_2O)
Lunar caustic	Silver nitrate ($AgNO_3$)
Magnesia	Magnesium oxide (MgO)
Marble or chalk or pearl	Calcium carbonate ($CaCO_3$)
Marsh gas	Methane (CH_4)
Pearl ash	Potassium carbonate (K_2CO_3)
Plaster of Paris	Calcium sulphate hemihydrate $\left(CaSO_4 \cdot \frac{1}{2} H_2O\right)$
Quicklime	Calcium oxide (CaO)
Red lead	Lead peroxide (Pb_3O_4)
Rock salt	Sodium chloride ($NaCl$)
Ruby or sapphire	Aluminium oxide, (Al_2O_3)
Sand	Silicon dioxide (SiO_2)
Spirit	Methyl alcohol (CH_3OH)
Soda ash	Sodium carbonate (Na_2CO_3)
Vinegar	Acetic acid (CH_3COOH)
Washing soda	Sodium carbonate decahydrate ($Na_2CO_3 \cdot 10H_2O$)
White vitriol	Zinc sulphate ($ZnSO_4 \cdot 7H_2O$)

Chemical Reactions

- A chemical reaction is a change in which one or more substance(s) or reactants react(s) to form new substance(s) with entirely different properties.
- Breaking of the old bonds and formation of the new bonds are responsible for the occurrence of a chemical reaction.

e.g. $$\underbrace{\underset{\text{Sodium}}{Na(s)} + \underset{\text{Water}}{H_2O(l)}}_{\text{Reactants}} \longrightarrow \underbrace{\underset{\text{Sodium hydroxide}}{NaOH(aq)} + \underset{\text{Hydrogen}}{H_2(g)\uparrow}}_{\text{Products}}$$

- In the above chemical reaction, sodium hydroxide and hydrogen are the **products** and sodium and water are the **reactants**.

Representation of Chemical Reactions : The Chemical Equation

- The short representation of a chemical reaction with the help of symbols of elements or formula of compounds is called chemical equation.
- The substances or compounds which take part in a reaction are called **reactants.** These are written on the left hand side (LHS) with a plus sign (+) in between them.
- The substances or compounds formed in the course of reaction are called **products.** These are written on the right hand side (RHS) with a plus sign (+) in between them.
- The arrow head (→) points toward the products which shows the direction of reaction. e.g. Zinc reacts with sulphuric acid to form zinc sulphate and hydrogen gas.

$$\underbrace{Zn + H_2SO_4}_{\text{(Reactants)}} \longrightarrow \underbrace{ZnSO_4 + H_2(g)}_{\text{(Product)}}$$

Rules for Writing a Balanced Chemical Equations

- The number of atoms of a particular element in reactants should be equal to the number of atom of similar element in products. e.g.

	Reactants		Products	
	Fe	H_2O	Fe_3O_4	H_2
No. of atoms	1	2 1	3 4	2

As per rule, the above equation is incorrect and can be correctly written as :

$$3Fe + 4H_2O \longrightarrow Fe_3O_4 + 4H_2$$

- The physical states of reactants and products should be mentioned along with their chemical formula in parenthesis.

The above equation can be written in accordance to rule as :

$$3Fe(s) + 4H_2O(g) \longrightarrow Fe_3O_4(s) + 4H_2(g)$$

(*s*) : solid, (*g*) : gas

Types of Chemical Reactions

Different types of chemical reactions are as follows

- **Combination Reaction** A reaction in which a single new product is formed from two or more reactants, is known as combination reaction.

  e.g. $\underset{\text{Carbon}}{C(s)} + \underset{\text{Oxygen}}{O_2(g)} \longrightarrow \underset{\text{Carbon dioxide}}{CO_2(g)}$

- **Decomposition Reaction** A reaction in which a single reactant breaks down to form two or more products, is known as decomposition reaction.

  e.g. $\underset{\text{Calcium carbonate}}{CaCO_3(s)} \longrightarrow \underset{\text{Calcium oxide}}{CaO(s)} + \underset{\text{Carbon dioxide}}{CO_2(g)}$

- **Displacement Reaction** A reaction in which more reactive element displaces less reactive element from its compound present in dissolved state, is known as displacement reaction. e.g.

  $\underset{\text{Zinc metel}}{Zn(s)} + \underset{\text{Copper sulphate solution}}{CuSO_4(aq)} \longrightarrow \underset{\text{Zinc sulphate solution}}{ZnSO_4(aq)} + \underset{\text{Copper metal}}{Cu(s)}$

- **Neutralisation Reaction** Acids and bases neutralise each other to form corresponding salts and water. This reaction is known as neutralisation reaction.

  e.g. $\underset{\text{Sodium hydroxide}}{2NaOH} + \underset{\text{Sulphuric acid}}{H_2SO_4} \longrightarrow \underset{\text{Sodium suphate}}{Na_2SO_4} + \underset{\text{Water}}{H_2O}$

- **Reversible and Irreversible Reaction**

  A chemical reaction which proceeds in both directions, is called a reversible reaction.

  – For example, formation of ammonia from nitrogen and hydrogen by Haber's process.

  $$N_2 + 3H_2 \xrightleftharpoons{\text{Fe,Mo}} 2NH_3$$

  – A chemical reaction which proceeds only in one direction, is called irreversible reaction. For example,

  $$2NaOH + H_2SO_4 \longrightarrow Na_2SO_4 + 2H_2O$$

Exothermic and Endothermic Reactions

Reactions occurring with the evolution of heat/energy are called **exothermic reactions**, e.g. respiration, decomposition, burning of natural gas, etc.

The reactions which occur by the absorption of heat/energy are called **endothermic reactions**, e.g. digestion of food, photosynthesis process.

$$A + B \longrightarrow C + \Delta E \quad \text{(exothermic)}$$

$$A + B \longrightarrow C - \Delta E \quad \text{(endothermic)}$$

Corrosion

- It is the process of oxidative deterioration of a metal surface by the action of substances present in environment to form unwanted corrosion products.
- In other words, it is the process of formation of oxide or other salts on the surface of a metal when it is exposed to the atmosphere.

  e.g. Conversion of iron into rust $[Fe_2O_3 \cdot xH_2O]$

  $$\underset{\text{Iron}}{2Fe(s)} + \underbrace{\frac{3}{2}O_2(g) + xH_2O(l)}_{\text{From moist air}} \rightarrow \underset{\text{Hydrated ferric oxide (Rust)}}{Fe_2O_3 \cdot xH_2O(s)}$$

- Corrosion of iron is called rusting.

Exam Pattern Questions

1 Who introduced the symbols for representing the elements?

(a) Bohr (b) Dalton
(c) Lavoiser (d) Proust

2 Symbol of antimony is

(a) Sb (b) Tb (c) An (d) W

3 Symbol of sodium is

(a) Ne (b) So (c) S (d) Na

4 Chemical formula of alcohol is

(a) C_2H_5OH (b) C_2H_5COOH
(c) KOH (d) CH_3

5 Chemical name of baking soda is

(a) sodium carbonate (b) sodium bicarbonate
(c) sodium hydroxide (d) calcium hydroxide

6 The chemical formula of soda ash is

(a) Na_2CO_3 (b) $NaHCO_3$
(c) NaOH (d) NaO

7 Sodium hydroxide is also known as
(a) caustic soda (b) hypo
(c) quicklime (d) slaked lime

8 The chemical formula of calcium hydrogen carbonate is
(a) $CaHCO_3$ (b) $Ca(HCO_3)_2$
(c) Ca_2HCO_3 (d) $Ca(HCO_3)_3$

9 Spirit is
(a) propyl alcohol (b) ethyl alcohol
(c) methyl alcohol (d) None of these

10 The chemical formula of chalk is
(a) $CaCO_3$ (b) $Ca(OH)_2$
(c) CaO (d) $CaHCO_3$

11 Marsh gas is
(a) CH_4 (b) CH_2OH
(c) HCHO (d) CH_3COOH

12 The chemical formula of ammonium chloride is
(a) NH_2Cl (b) NH_2Cl_2
(c) NH_4Cl (d) NH_3Cl

13 The reaction in which one or more substances react to form new substance(s) with entirely different process is called
(a) a biochemical reaction
(b) a nuclear reaction
(c) a physical reaction
(d) a chemical reaction

14 Chemical reaction can be identified by
(a) change in state (b) change in temperature
(c) evolution of gas (d) All of these

15 Formation of slaked lime by the reaction of calcium oxide with water is the
(a) decomposition reaction
(b) displacement reaction
(c) combination reaction
(d) exothermic reaction

16 Which of the following is a decomposition reaction?
(a) $CaO + H_2O \longrightarrow Ca(OH)_2 + \text{Heat}$
(b) $2FeSO_4(s) \xrightarrow{\Delta} Fe_2O_3(s) + SO_2(g) + SO_3(g)$
(c) $Na_2SO_4 + BaCl_2 \longrightarrow BaSO_4 + 2NaCl$
(d) $CuO + H_2 \longrightarrow Cu + H_2O$

17 $Fe_2O_3 + 2Al \longrightarrow Al_2O_3 + 2Fe$
The above reaction is an example of a
(a) combination reaction
(b) double displacement reaction
(c) decomposition reaction
(d) displacement reaction

18 Chemical reaction occurring in nature is generally
(a) reversible (b) irreversible
(c) oxidative (d) None of these

19 Burning of natural gas is an example of
(a) exothermic reaction
(b) endothermic reaction
(c) neutralisation reaction
(d) None of the above

20 The reaction which is accompained by the absorption of heat is known as
(a) combustion reaction (b) exothermic reaction
(c) endothermic reaction (d) All of these

21 A balanced chemical equation is in accordance with
(a) Avogadro's law
(b) law of multiple proportion
(c) law of conservation of mass
(d) law of gaseous volumes

22 In the following equation:
$Na_2CO_3 + xHCl \longrightarrow 2NaCl + CO_2 + H_2O$,
the value of x is
(a) 1 (b) 2 (c) 3 (d) 4

23 In the following reaction
$Be_2C + xH_2O \longrightarrow yBe(OH)_2 + CH_4$ the value of x and y is
(a) 4 and 2 (b) 2 and 4
(c) 3 and 4 (d) 4 and 4

24 Complete this equation
$BaSO_4 + NaCl \longrightarrow — + Na_2SO_4$
(a) BaCl (b) $BaCl_2$ (c) $NaCl_2$ (d) $2BaCl_2$

25 Corrosion is a
(a) slow oxidation (b) fast oxidation
(c) reduction (d) None of these

26 Corrosion of iron is called
(a) Rusting (b) reversible reaction
(c) oxidation (d) None of these

Answers

1 *(b)*	2 *(a)*	3 *(d)*	4 *(a)*	5 *(b)*	6 *(a)*	7 *(a)*	8 *(b)*	9 *(c)*	10 *(a)*
11 *(a)*	12 *(c)*	13 *(d)*	14 *(d)*	15 *(c)*	16 *(b)*	17 *(b)*	18 *(b)*	19 *(a)*	20 *(c)*
21 *(c)*	22 *(b)*	23 *(d)*	24 *(b)*	25 *(a)*	26 *(a)*				

Chapter 05 Laws of Chemical Combinations

Elements combined to form molecules in accordance to the following five basic laws, called the laws of chemical combinations.

1. Law of Conservation Mass
2. Law of Definite Proportions
3. Law of Multiple Proportions
4. Law of Reciprocal Proportions
5. Gay Lussac's Law of Gaseous Volumes

Law of Conservation of Mass

- This law was put forth by **Antoine Lavoisier** in 1789.
- According to this law, 'matter can neither be created nor destroyed but one form of matter can be converted into other.'
- This law is also known as **law of indestructibility of matter.**
- The other statement for this law is 'In all physical and chemical changes, the total mass of the reactants is equal to that of the products.'
  i.e. sum of masses of reactants
  = Sum of masses of products

Law of Definite Proportions

- This law was given by, a French chemist, Joseph Proust in 1799.
- According to this law, "a given compound always contains exactly the same proportion of elements by weight."
- It is sometimes also referred to as law of definite composition.

e.g. pure water obtained from any source (well, river, lake or sea) or any country will always be made up of only hydrogen and oxygen elements combined together in the same fixed ratio of 1 : 8 by mass.

Law of Multiple Proportions

- This law was proposed by Dalton in 1803.
- It states that "if two elements can combine to form more than one compound, the masses of one element that combine with a fixed mass of the other element, are in the ratio of small whole numbers".
- For example, two compounds, water and hydrogen peroxide are formed when hydrogen combines with oxygen.

$$\underset{2\text{ g}}{\text{Hydrogen}} + \underset{16\text{ g}}{\text{Oxygen}} \rightarrow \underset{18\text{ g}}{\text{Water}}$$

$$\underset{2\text{g}}{\text{Hydrogen}} + \underset{32\text{ g}}{\text{Oxygen}} \rightarrow \underset{34\text{ g}}{\text{Hydrogen peroxide}}$$

- Here, the masses of oxygen (i.e. 16 g and 32 g) that combine with a fixed mass of hydrogen (i.e. 2 g) bear a simple ratio, i.e. 16 : 32 or 1 : 2.

Law of Reciprocal Proportions

- This law was given by Richter in 1792.
- It states that, "the ratio of the masses of two elements A and B which combine separately with a fixed mass of the third element C is either the same or some simple multiple of the ratio of the masses in which A and B combine directly with each other".

Gay Lussac's Law of Gaseous Volumes

- As the name implies this law was given by Gay Lussac in 1808.
- He stated that "when gases combine or are produced in a chemical reaction they do so in a simple ratio by volume provided all the gases are at same temperature and pressure".
- For example, one volume of hydrogen and one volume of chlorine always combine to form two volumes of hydrogen chloride gas.

$$\underset{1\text{ vol}}{H_2} + \underset{1\text{ vol}}{Cl_2} \longrightarrow \underset{2\text{ vol}}{2\,HCl}$$

- The ratio between the volumes of the reactants and the product in this reaction is simple, i.e. 1 : 1 : 2

Hence, it illustrates the law of combining volumes.

Avogadro's Law

Avogadro put forward the hypothesis known as Avogadro's hypothesis or Avogadro's Law, which states that equal volumes of gases at the same temperature and pressure should contain equal number of molecules.

Exam Pattern Questions

1. Who put the law of conservation of mass
(a) Antonie Lavoisier
(b) Joseph proust
(c) Dalton
(d) P. V proust

2. Which law is known as law of indestructibility of matter ?
(a) Law of multiple proportion
(b) Law of definite proportion
(c) Law of conservation of mass
(d) Avogadro's law

3. If 6.3 g of $NaHCO_3$ are added to 15.0 g of CH_3COOH solution, the residue is found to weight 18.0 g. What is the mass of CO_2 released in the reaction ?
(a) 3.3 g (b) 3.31 kg
(c) 33 g (d) 3 g

4. Which law states that matter can neither be created nor destroyed?
(a) Law of definite proportions
(b) Law of conservation of mass
(c) Law of multiple proportions
(d) Avogadro's law

5. A chemical equation is balanced according to the law of
(a) multiple proportions
(b) constant proportions
(c) reciprocal proportions
(d) conservation of mass

6. Potassium combines with two isotopes of chlorine (^{35}Cl and ^{37}Cl) respectively to form two samples of KCl. Their formation follows the law of
(a) constant proportions
(b) multiple proportions
(c) reciprocal proportions
(d) low of conservation of mass

7. 4.88 g of $KClO_3$ when heated, produces 1.92 g of O_2 and 2.96 g of KCl. The result of the following experiment illustrates
(a) the law of conservation of mass
(b) the law of multiple proportion
(c) the law of constant proportion
(d) None of the above

8. Which law states that if two elements can combine to form more than one compound, the masses of one element that combine with a fixed mass of other element, are in the ratio of small whole numbers?
(a) Avogadro's law
(b) Law of definite composition
(c) Law of multiple proportions
(d) Gay Lussac's law of gaseous volumes

9. Three oxides of nitrogen contained 53.6%, 46.7% and 30.4% nitrogen respectively. Show that these figures illustrate the law of multiple proportions.
(a) 1 : 2 : 4 (b) 4 : 2 : 1
(c) 1 : 4 : 2 (d) 1 : 2

10. Who give the law of reciprocal proportion?
(a) Richter
(b) Gay-Lussac
(c) Dalton
(d) Bohr

11. One part of an element *A* combines with two parts of *B* (another element). Six parts of element *C* combine with four parts of element *B*. If *A* and *C* combine together, the ratio of their masses will be governed by
(a) law of definite proportions
(b) law of multiple proportions
(c) law of reciprocal proportions
(d) law of conservations of mass

12. In the reaction, $N_2 + 3H_2 \longrightarrow 2NH_3$, the ratio of volumes of nitrogen, hydrogen and ammonia is 1 : 3 : 2. These ratio illustrate the law of
(a) constant properties
(b) Gay-Lussac
(c) multiple proportions
(d) reciprocal proportions

13. Avogadro's found the smallest particle of a gas which can exist independently
(a) element
(b) molecule
(c) atom
(d) All of these

14. Copper oxide was prepared by the 1.75 g of the metal was dissolved in nitric acid and igniting the residual copper nitrate yielded 2.19 g of copper oxide.
(a) 89.91 (b) 79
(c) 79.91 (d) 70.91

15. Avogadro proposed that equal volumes of gases at the same *A* and *B* should contain equal number of molecules. *A* and *B* respectively are at same
(a) temperature and pressure
(b) density and mass
(c) molarity and normality
(d) Avogadro constant and Planck's constant

Answers

1 (a)	2 (c)	3 (a)	4 (b)	5 (d)	6 (d)	7 (a)	8 (c)	9 (b)	10 (a)
11 (c)	12 (b)	13 (b)	14 (c)	15 (a)					

Chapter 06 Oxidation and Reduction

Oxidation

- It is a process in which a substance loses electrons.
- According to classical concept oxidation is defined as a process that involves
  - (i) **Addition of oxygen**

    e.g. $2Mg(s) + O_2(g) \longrightarrow 2MgO(s)$

    All the combustion processes are examples of it, e.g. combustion of methane to produce CO_2 and water.

    $CH_4(g) + 2O_2(g) \longrightarrow CO_2(g) + 2H_2O(l)$
  - (ii) **Addition of an electronegative elements**

    $Mg(s) + \underset{\text{Electronegative element}}{Cl_2(g)} \longrightarrow MgCl_2(s)$
  - (iii) **Removal of hydrogen**

    $2H_2S(g) + O_2(g) \longrightarrow 2S(s)\ 2H_2O(l)$
  - (iv) **Removal of an electropositive elements**

    $2K_4[Fe(CN)_6](aq) + H_2O_2(aq) \longrightarrow 2K_3[Fe(CN)_6](aq) + 2KOH(aq)$

Reduction

- It is a process in which a substance gains electrons.
- According to classical concept, reduction is defined as a process that involves
  - (i) **Addition of hydrogen** e.g.

    $\underset{\text{Ethane}}{CH_2}\quad CH_2(g) + H_2(g) \longrightarrow \underset{\text{Ethane}}{CH_3{-}CH_3(g)}$
  - (ii) **Addition of an electropositive element**

    e.g. $HgCl_2 + Hg \longrightarrow Hg_2Cl_2$
  - (iii) **Removal of oxygen**

    e.g. $2HgO(s) \longrightarrow 2Hg(l) + O_2(g)$
  - (iv) **Removal of an electronegative element**

    e.g. $2FeCl_3(aq) + H_2(g) \longrightarrow 2FeCl_2(aq) + 2HCl(aq)$

Redox Reactions

- The reactions that involve oxidation and reduction as its two half reactions are called **redox reactions.**

Or

- In other words, redox reactions are the reactions in which oxidation and reduction processes occur simultaneously.
- For example, if we consider the following reaction

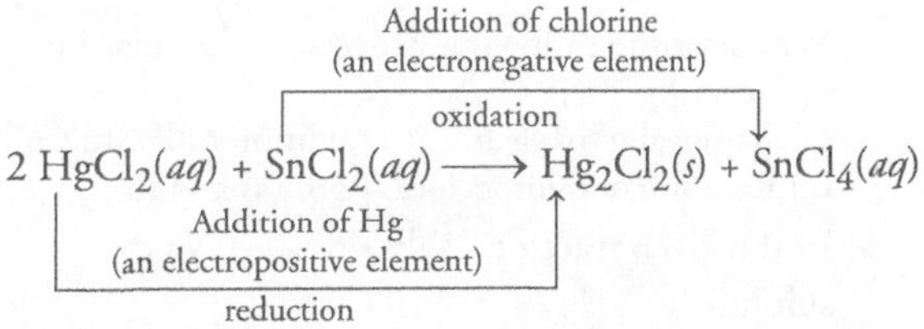

- Since, in the above reaction oxidation and reduction occur simultaneously, so it is an example of redox reaction.

Oxidising and Reducing Agents

- In a redox reaction, the substance which oxidises the other or which itself undergoes reduction is called the **oxidising agent.**
- The substance that reduces the other and itself undergoes oxidation is called the **reducing agent.**

Exam Pattern Questions

1 The process in which a substance losses electron
(a) oxidation (b) reduction
(c) combustion (d) reversible

2 Identify the species undergoing oxidation
$H_2S + Cl_2 \longrightarrow 2HCl + S$
(a) Cl_2 (b) H_2S
(c) HCl (d) H_2O

3 The process also named as de-electronation
(a) combustion (b) oxidation
(c) reduction (d) All of these

4 In oxidation process
(a) oxidation number decreases
(b) number of electrons decreases
(c) oxygen content decreases
(d) number of ions decreases

5 In the reaction,
$SO_2 + 2H_2S \longrightarrow 3S + 2H_2O$, the substance oxidised is
(a) H_2S (b) SO_2
(c) S (d) H_2O

6 Identify the substance that get reduced in this reaction
$Fe_2O_3 + 3CO \longrightarrow 2Fe + 3CO_2$
(a) Fe_2O_3 (b) FeO_3
(c) 2Fe (d) CO

7 Which of the following processes takes place in reduction?
(a) Removal of oxygen (b) Addition of hydrogen
(c) Removal of hydrogen (d) Both (a) and (b)

8 In the given reaction, $2Na + S \longrightarrow Na_2S$, sulphur is
(a) oxidised (b) reduced
(c) reducing agent (d) None of these

9 Reduced form of HNO_3 is
(a) NO_2 (b) H_2O
(c) $NO_2 + H_2O$ (d) NO

10 Oxidised form of H_2S is
(a) S (b) SO_2
(c) Both (a) and (b) (d) SO_3

11 The reaction that involve oxidation and reduction as its two half reactions are called
(a) reduction (b) oxidation
(c) combustion (d) redox reactions

12 Both oxidation and reduction takes place in
(a) $NaBr + HCl \longrightarrow NaCl + HBr$
(b) $HBr + AgNO_3 \longrightarrow AgBr + HNO_3$
(c) $H_2 + Br_2 \longrightarrow 2HBr$
(d) $CaO + H_2SO_4 \longrightarrow CaSO_4 + H_2O$

13 In the reaction,
$$2H_2O_2 \longrightarrow 2H_2O + O_2$$
oxygen is
(a) oxidised only
(b) reduced only
(c) neither oxidised nor reduced
(d) Both oxidised and reduced

14 Which of the following acts as an oxidising agent?
(a) HNO_3 (b) Cl_2
(c) $FeCl_3$ (d) All of these

15 Which of the following is the most powerful oxidising agent?
(a) F_2 (b) O_2
(c) Br_2 (d) I_2

16 Which one of the following cannot act as a reducing agent?
(a) CO_2 (b) SO_2
(c) NO_2 (d) ClO_2

17 An element which donates electrons is called as
(a) reducing agent
(b) oxidising agent
(c) complexing agent
(d) None of the above

Answers

1 (a)	2 (b)	3 (b)	4 (b)	5 (a)	6 (a)	7 (d)	8 (b)	9 (c)	10 (c)
11 (d)	12 (c)	13 (d)	14 (d)	15 (a)	16 (a)	17 (a)			

Chapter 07 Properties of Water and Air

Water (H_2O)

- It is a compound of hydrogen and oxygen, in which these are present in 1 : 8 by weight. Its formula is H_2O. It is very essential for existence of all form of life.
- Water is the most common, abundant and easily obtainable compound as compared to all other known compounds.
- It can exist in solid, (as ice, snow etc.), liquid (as lakes, river, sea etc.) or gaseous (as water, vapour) states.
- It constitutes a major part of all the living organism, e.g. it forms about 65% of human body and almost 95% of some plants.
- Its distribution over the earth's surface is not uniform.
- However, the fraction of water available for human use is oblique only 0.003% of the total global water availability.

Physical Properties of Water

The important physical properties of water are as follows :

- Pure water is a transparent, colourless, tasteless and odourless substance.
  - It takes the odour of the substance, which is dissolved in it. Thick layer of water appears as greenish blue.
- Its freezing point, boiling point, heat of vaporisation and heat of fusion is higher than the hydrides of other elements of group 16.
  - This is because of the presence of intermolecular hydrogen bonding in between water molecules.
- Water has a high specific heat, thermal conductivity, surface tension, dipole moment and dielectric constant than many other liquids and thus, plays a vital role in the biosphere.

Chemical Properties of Water

Water reacts with a wide range of compounds. Some of its important chemical reactions are described below :

Amphoteric Nature

- Water is amphoteric in nature, i.e. it behaves as a Bronsted acid as well as a Bronsted base.

$$\underset{\text{Acid}_1}{H_2O(l)} + \underset{\text{Base}_2}{NH_3(aq)} \longrightarrow \underset{\text{Acid}_2}{NH_4^+(aq)} + \underset{\text{Base}_1}{OH^-(aq)}$$

$$\underset{\text{Base}_1}{H_2O(l)} + \underset{\text{Acid}_2}{H_2S(aq)} \longrightarrow \underset{\text{Acid}_1}{H_3O^+(aq)} + \underset{\text{Base}_2}{HS^-(aq)}$$

Auto-protolysis or Self-ionisation

- When one water molecule behaves as an acid and the other behaves as a base, the water undergoes self-ionisation and the reaction is called auto-protolysis.
- Amphoteric nature of water is responsible for its auto-protolysis.

$$\underset{\substack{\text{Acid}_1\\\text{(acid)}}}{H_2O(l)} + \underset{\substack{\text{Base}_2\\\text{(base)}}}{NH_3(aq)} \longrightarrow \underset{\substack{\text{Acid}_2\\\text{(conjugate acid)}}}{NH_4^+(aq)} + \underset{\substack{\text{Base}_1\\\text{(conjugate base)}}}{OH^-(aq)}$$

Hydrolysis Reaction

- When H^+ and OH^- ions of water interact with the anion and cation of the salt respectively to give original acid and original base, the reaction is called hydrolysis.

e.g.

$$SiCl_4(l) + 2H_2O(l) \longrightarrow SiO_2(s) + 4HCl(aq)$$

or $N^{3-}(s) + 3H_2O(l) \longrightarrow NH_3(g) + 3OH^-(aq)$

$$\underset{\text{Aluminium nitride}}{AlN} + 3H_2O \longrightarrow Al(OH)_3 + \underset{\text{Ammonia}}{NH_3}$$

Hard and Soft Water

- Water that lathers with soap is called **soft water**; e.g; rain water, distilled water etc., and which does not lather is called **hard water**, e.g. sea water, well water etc.
- The hardness of water is because of the presence of bicarbonates (hydrogen carbonates), chlorides and sulphates of calcium and magnesium.

Air

- Air around us is a mixture of many gases and dust particles. It is the clear gas in which living things live and breathe.
- It has an indefinite shape and volume. It has no colour or smell.
- Air is a mixture of about 78% nitrogen, 21% oxygen, 0.9% argon, 0.03% carbon dioxide and 0.04% amounts of other gases.
- Our atmosphere is divided into five layers starting from the earth's surface.
- These are **troposphere, stratosphere, mesosphere, thermosphere** and **exosphere.**

Troposphere

- This layer is the most important layer of the atmosphere. Its average height is 13 km.
- The air we breathe exists here. Almost all the weather phenomena like rainfall, fog and hailstorm occur in this layer.

Stratosphere

- Above the troposphere lies the stratosphere. It extends up to a height of 50 km.
- This layer is almost free from clouds and associated weather phenomenon, making conditions most ideal for flying aeroplanes.
- One important feature of stratosphere is that it contains a layer of ozone gas.

Mesosphere

This is the third layer of the atmosphere. It lies above stratosphere. It extends up to the height of 85 km.

Thermosphere

- In thermosphere temperature rises very rapidly with increasing height. It extends upto 640 km. This layer helps in radio transmission.
- Mesosphere and thermosphere are collectively called ionosphere.

Exosphere

The upper most layer of the atmosphere is known as exosphere (500-1600 km.

Light gases like helium and hydrogen float into the space from here.

Exam Pattern Questions

1 In which ratio hydrogen and oxygen are present in water

(a) 1 : 8 (b) 8 : 1
(c) 2 : 4 (d) None of these

2 The fraction of water available for human use is oblique ...... of the total global water.

(a) 0.3% (b) 0.001%
(c) 0.003% (d) 3%

3 The percentage of water present in plants is

(a) 70 (b) 65 (c) 95 (d) 45

4 Water has high freezing and boiling point than the hydrides of other element of group 16 because it has

(a) intermolecular hydrogen bonding
(b) intramolecular hydrogen bonding
(c) hydrogen bonding
(d) All of the above

5 Water has high density at
(a) 277 K (b) 273 K
(c) 270 K (d) 0°C K

6 Atmospheric nature of water is responsible for its
(a) hydrolysis (b) auto-protolysis
(c) ionisation (d) All of these

7 Water that lathers with soap
(a) soft water (b) hard water
(c) mineral water (d) Both (a) and (b)

8 The hardness of water is because of the presence of
(a) bicarbonates (b) chlorides
(c) sulphates of calcium (d) All of these

9 How much nitrogen is present in air?
(a) 21% (b) 78%
(c) 0.9% (d) 70%

10 Atmospheric content of CO_2 is
(a) 0.0034% (b) 0.034%
(c) 0.34% (d) 3.4%

11 Our atmosphere is divided into ……… layers.
(a) five (b) four
(c) seven (d) None of these

12 The average height of troposphere layer
(a) 10 km (b) 12 km
(c) 13 km (d) 9 km

13 Which region of atmosphere has human beings alongwith organisms?
(a) Stratosphere (b) Trosphere
(c) Hydrosphere (d) Mesosphere

14 Which of the following atmospheric layer contains clouds, water vapour and air?
(a) Stratosphere (b) Troposphere
(c) Mesosphere (d) All of these

15 Stratosphere extends up to a height of
(a) 50 km (b) 40 km
(c) 45 km (d) 80 km

16 Which layer is consist of ozone layer?
(a) Mesophere
(b) Stratosphere
(c) Thermosphere
(d) None of the above

17 In which layer meteorites burn up on entering from the space
(a) thermosphere
(b) mesosphere
(c) troposphere
(d) stratosphere

18 Which of the following region is the coldest?
(a) Stratosphere
(b) Troposphere
(c) Mesosphere
(d) Thermosphere

19 Thermosphere extends up to
(a) 650 km (b) 400 km
(c) 80-200 km (d) 80 km

20 The uppermost layer of the atmosphere is known as
(a) exosphere (b) mesosphere
(c) stratosphere (d) thermosphere

Answers

1 (a)	2 (c)	3 (a)	4 (a)	5 (a)	6 (b)	7 (a)	8 (d)	9 (b)	10 (b)
11 (a)	12 (c)	13 (b)	14 (b)	15 (a)	16 (b)	17 (b)	18 (c)	19 (a)	20 (a)

Chapter 08

Preparation and Properties of Hydrogen, Oxygen, Nitrogen

Hydrogen (H_2)

Hydrogen is the most abundant molecule in the universe. It is the principal element in the solar atmosphere.

Preparation of Hydrogen

- In laboratory, it is prepared by the reaction of granulated zinc with dilute hydrochloric acid.
- Commercially, it is prepared by electrolysis of acidified water using platinum electrodes and by the reaction of steam on hydrocarbons or coke at high temperature in the presence of catalyst.
- It is also prepared by passing water vapours over red hot iron or by treating hydrolith or sodium with water.

Properties of Hydrogen

- It is a colourless, odourless, tasteless and combustible gas.
- It is lighter than air and insoluble in water.
- Its melting point is 13.96 K and boiling point is 20.39 K. Its density is $0.09\ gL^{-1}$.
- It reacts with oxygen (or air) at high temperature to form water. The reaction is highly exothermic.

$$2H_2(g) + O_2(g) \xrightarrow[\text{heating}]{\text{Catalyst or}} 2H_2O\ (l) + \text{Heat}$$

- It reacts with dinitrogen to form ammonia (Haber's process).

$$3H_2(g) + N_2(g) \xrightarrow[\text{Fe, Mo}]{\text{673 K, 200 atm}} 2NH_3\ (g) + \text{Heat}$$

Uses of Hydrogen

- The largest single use of dihydrogen is in the synthesis of ammonia by Haber's process, which is used in the manufacture of nitric acid and nitrogenous fertillizers.
- It is used in the manufacturing of vanaspati fat by the hydrogenation of poly unsaturated vegetable oils like soyabean, cotton seeds, etc.
- It is used in the manufacturing of bulk organic chemicals particularly methanol.
- It is widely used for the manufacturing of metal hydrides, hydrogen chloride, etc.

Oxygen (O_2)

- It was first discovered by Sweden scientist **Scheele** (1772) and the name oxygen was given by **AL Lavoisier** in 1977. Its atomic number is 8 and mass number is 16.
- It belongs to group-16 or VI A, 2nd period and *p*-block of the periodic table. Its electronic configuration is $1s^2, 2s^2 2p^4$.
- It exists in the following isotopic forms $^{16}_{8}O$, $^{17}_{8}O$ and $^{18}_{8}O$.

Preparation of Oxygen

- The main source of atmospheric oxygen is photosynthesis.
- In laboratory, it is prepared by heating (at 375°C) potassium chlorate ($KClO_3$) in the presence of a catalyst manganese dioxide (MnO_2).

$$2KClO_3 \xrightarrow[MnO_2]{\text{Heat}} 2KCl + 3O_2$$

- By thermal decomposition of the oxides of metals present at lower side in electrochemical series and higher oxide of some metals.

$$2Ag_2O(s) \longrightarrow 4Ag(s) + O_2(g)$$

- Industrially, it is obtained from air by fractional distillation.

Properties of Oxygen

- Dioxygen is colourless, odourless gas which gets converted into deep blue liquid on cooling.
- It is slightly heavier than air. It does not burn itself but is a supporter of combustion.
- Its solubility in water is just sufficient for the vital support of marine and aquatic life.
- It is paramagnetic in nature.
- It reacts with nearly all metals (except Au, Pt) and non-metals and some noble metals.

Uses of Oxygen

- It is used in oxyacetylene welding and in the manufacturing of many metals such as steel.
- Oxygen cylinders (which contain oxygen diluted with helium) are used in hospitals, high altitude flying and in mountaineering.
- Liquid oxygen is used in rocket fuel as an oxidiser.

Nitrogen (N_2)

- It was discovered by D Rutherford (1772). Its atomic number is 7 and mass number is 14.
- It belongs to group-15 or V A, 2nd period and *p*-block of the periodic table. Its electronic configuration is $1s^2, 2s^2 2p^3$.

Preparation of Nitrogen

- Industrially, it is prepared by the liquefaction and fractional distillation of air.
- In laboratory, it is prepared by treating an aqueous solution of ammonium chloride with sodium nitrite.

$$NH_4Cl + NaNO_2 \longrightarrow \underset{\text{Unstable}}{[NH_4NO_2]} + NaCl$$

$$[NH_4NO_2] \xrightarrow{\Delta} N_2 + 2H_2O$$

- Very pure nitrogen can be obtained by thermal decomposition of sodium or barium azide.

$$Ba(N_3)_2 \longrightarrow Ba + 3N_2$$

Properties of Nitrogen

- It is a colourless, odourless, tasteless, diatomic, non-polar and non-toxic gas.
- It is inert at room temperature. At high temperature, it reacts with oxygen and hydrogen to form oxides and hydrides respectively.
- It also reacts with metals (like Mg, Li, etc) to form nitrides (Mg_3N_2, Li_3N).

Uses of Nitrogen

- It is used in the manufacturing of ammonia and other industrial chemicals containing nitrogen (e.g. calcium cyanamide).
- It is used to produce inert atmosphere in iron and steel industry.
- liquid N_2 is used as a refrigerant to preserve biological materials, food items and sperm of bull and in cryosurgery, etc.
- It is used in electric bulb and thermometer of measuring high temperature.

Exam Pattern Questions

1 Hydrogen is much less abundant in the earth's atmosphere because of its
(a) low enthalpy of fusion
(b) low enthalpy of vaporisation
(c) light nature
(d) All of the above

2 How many neutrons are present in protium, deuterium and tritium respectively?
(a) 1, 0 and 2 (b) 0, 2 and 1
(c) 0, 1 and 2 (d) 2, 1 and 0

3 Which of the following metal and acid are used to prepare dihydrogen respectively?
(a) Crystalline zinc with dil. HCl
(b) Granulated zinc with dil. HCl
(c) Granulated zinc with conc. HCl
(d) Crystalline zinc with conc. HCl

4 Dihydrogen is not obtained when zinc reacts with
(a) cold water (b) hot NaOH solution
(c) dil. H_2SO_4 (d) dil. HCl

5 Which of the following gas is/are obtained by electrolysis of acidified water using platinum electrodes?
(a) H_2 (b) O_2 (c) N_2 (d) H_2 and O_2

6 The maximum percentage of the industrial dihydrogen is produced from
(a) petrochemicals
(b) coal
(c) electrolysis of aqueous solution of salts
(d) other sources except these

7 Very pure hydrogen (99.9%) can be made by which of the following processes?
(a) Reaction of methane with steam
(b) Mixing natural hydrocarbons of high molecular weight
(c) Electrolysis of water
(d) Reaction of salts like hydrides with water

8 Which of the following properties of dihydrogen is incorrect?
(a) It is colourless, odourless, tasteless
(b) It is combustible gas
(c) It is lighter than air
(d) It is soluble in water

9 Hydrogenation of vegetable oils using nickel as a catalyst gives edible fat which is
(a) coconut oil
(b) soyabean oil
(c) margarine and vanaspati ghee
(d) peanut oil

10 Electronic configuration of oxygen
(a) $1s^2 2p^4$ (b) $2s, 2s^2 2p$
(c) $1s^2, 2s^2, 2p^4$ (d) $1s, 2s^2, 2p^4$

11 Number of allotropic forms of oxygen is
(a) 3 (b) 4 (c) 2 (d) 5

12 Oxygen shows only negative oxidation state as −2 except in the case of
(a) OH_2 (b) OF_2
(c) OCl_2 (d) CO_2

13 Oxygen is
(a) coloured, odourless gas
(b) slightly havier than air
(c) reactive with Au
(d) a combustible gas

14 Ozone (O_3) is
(a) an allotropic form of oxygen
(b) too reactive to remain for long in the atmosphere at sea level
(c) formed from atmospheric oxygen in the presence of sunlight at a height of about 20 km
(d) All the above statements are correct

15 Which gas is used as an oxidise
(a) O_2 (b) H_2O
(c) H_2 (d) CO_2

16 Oxygen is used in
(a) oxyacetylene welding
(b) the manufacture of steel
(c) oxygen cylinders in hospitals, high altitude flying and mountain
(d) All of the above

17 The highest volume of gases in lower atmosphere is comprised of
(a) hydrogen (b) carbon dioxide
(c) oxygen (d) nitrogen

18 Which gas is inert at room temperature?
(a) Ne (b) O_2 (c) Li (d) N_2

19 Dinitrogen
(a) is a colourless, odourless, tasteless and non-toxic gas
(b) has a very low solubility in water
(c) is rather inert at room temperature
(d) All of the above

20 Ammonium chloride on treatment with sodium nitrile forms
(a) He (b) H_2
(c) O_2 (d) N_2

21 Extra pure N_2 can be obtained by heating
(a) NH_3 with CuO (b) NH_4NO_3
(c) $(NH_4)_2Cr_2O_7$ (d) $Ba(N_3)_2$

22 Which of the following liquid is used as refrigerant for cryo-preservation of items?
(a) Liquid sodium (b) Liquid nitrogen
(c) Liquid oxygen (d) Bromine

23 Which of the following gas is used in thermometer of measuring high temperature?
(a) N_2 (b) CO_2
(c) O_2 (d) H_2

Answers

1 (c)	2 (c)	3 (b)	4 (a)	5 (d)	6 (a)	7 (c)	8 (d)	9 (c)	10 (c)
11 (a)	12 (b)	13 (b)	14 (d)	15 (a)	16 (d)	17 (d)	18 (d)	19 (d)	20 (d)
21 (d)	22 (b)	23 (a)							

Chapter 09

Carbon and Its Forms

Carbon (C)

- Carbon is the seventeenth most abundant element by mass in earth's crust. Its atomic number is 6 and mass number is 12.
- It belongs to group-14 or IV A, 2nd period and *p*-block of the periodic table. Its electronic configuration is $1s^2, 2s^2, 2p^2$.

Allotropes of Carbon

- Carbon exhibits many allotropic forms; both crystalline as well as amorphous.
- Diamond, graphite and fullerene are crystalline forms of carbon. While, carbon black, coke, wood charcoal, coal, etc. are its amorphous forms.

Diamond

- It is a precious gem stone that occurs in nature in the form of kimberlite stone.
- Its purity is measured in terms of carat (1 carat = 200 mg). Different varities of diamond are known by the name cullinan (3107 carat), hope (45.52 carat), kohinoor (141 carat) etc.
- In diamond, each carbon atom is bonded to four other carbon atoms in tetrahedral fashion forming a rigid three-dimensional structure.
- It is very difficult to break extended covalent bonding and therefore, diamond is the hardest substance on earth.

Graphite

- In graphite, each carbon atom is bonded to three other carbon atoms in the same plane giving a hexagonal array.
- The fourth electron of each carbon is free and moves in entire crystal lattice making graphite a good conductor of electricity.

Fullerene

- It is made by heating graphite in an electric arc in the presence of inert gases such as helium or argon.
- These are cage, like molecules. C_{60} molecule has a shape like soccer ball and is called as **Buckminster fullerene.**

Charcoal

- It is the impure form of carbon because of its porous structure and large surface area.
- It has high capacity of absorbing gases.

Coke

- It is obtained by heating coal in the absence of air at high temperature, by this volatile components get removed from the coke. It contains 80-85% carbon.
- It is used as a fuel and as a reducing agent in metallurgy.

Coal

- About 90% coal is found in northern hemisphere. It is obtained by the process of carbonisation from vegetable substances and is considered as a unlimited source of energy.
- It is used as fuel, in the production of coal gas and synthetic petrol.

Compounds of Carbon

The different types of compounds of carbon are as follow.

Carbon Dioxide (CO_2)

- In our atmosphere, only 0.03%-0.05% (by volume) CO_2 is present.
- It comes to the atmosphere from animal breathing, decay of vegetable matter, burning of carbon and carbonaceous matter etc.

- However, green plants by the process of **photosynthesis** removes it from the atmosphere. Photosynthesis is the process in which green plant prepare their own food (and also for animals and human beings), i.e. carbohydrates from CO_2 in the presence of chlorophyll and sunlight.

$$6CO_2 + 12H_2O \xrightarrow[\text{Chlorophyll}]{h\nu} C_6H_{12}O_6 + 6O_2 + 6H_2O$$

- Unlike CO, CO_2 is non-poisonous. But, if the concentration of CO_2 in the atmosphere increases (by combustion of fossil fuel and decomposition of lime stone for manufacturing cement), the green house effect increases, which raises the temperature of the atmosphere, i.e. causes global warming; consequences of which might be very serious.

Methods of Preparation

Following methods can be used to prepare CO_2

- **General method** When carbon or carbon containing fuels are heated in excess of air, CO_2 is obtained.

$$C(s) + O_2(g) \xrightarrow{\Delta} CO_2(g)$$

$$CH_4(g) + 2O_2(g) \xrightarrow{\Delta} CO_2(g) + 2H_2O(g)$$

- **Laboratory method** In laboratory, it is obtained by treating calcium carbonate with dilute HCl.

$$CaCO_3(s)\ 2HCl(aq) \longrightarrow CaCl_2(aq) + CO_2(s) + H_2O(l)$$

- **Commercial method** On commercial scale, it is obtained by heating limestone.

$$\underset{\text{Limestone}}{CaCO_3(s)} \xrightarrow{\Delta} CaO(s) + CO_2(g)$$

Physical Properties

- It is a colourless and odourless gas, which is heavier than air (density $1.977 g\ L^{-1}$ at 273 K).
- It is less soluble in water and because of this property, it is biochemically and geochemically an important molecule.
- It is an acidic gas. So, it forms metal carbonates when treated with alkalies.
  e.g. $2NaOH + CO_2 \longrightarrow Na_2CO_3 + H_2O$

Chemical Properties

- It turns lime water milky which disappears, if CO_2 is passed for a long time due to the formation of soluble calcium bicarbonate.
- It reacts with liquid NH_3 at 473 K and 220 atm and gives ammonium carbonate which subsequently decomposes to give urea.
- When liquified CO_2 is allowed to expand rapidly, it gets converted in the form of solid CO_2, which is also called dry ice.
  - It is a soft white snow, like compound with specific gravity 1.53 and melting point $-56.6°C$ at 5.2 atm pressure.

Use of Carbon-dioxide

- It is used as a refrigerant for ice-cream and frozen food under the commercial name **drikold**.
- Gaseous CO_2 is used to carbonate soft drinks.
- In hospitals, it is used for surgical operations of sores.
- Carbogen (a mixture of 95% O_2 and 5% CO_2) is used for artificial respiration.
- Being heavier than air and non supporter of combustion, it is used to extinguish fires.
- In substantial quantities, it is used for making urea.

Hydrocarbons

These are compounds of only carbon and hydrogen. These are of three types, which are as follows :

Saturated Hydrocarbons

They contain only single bonds. These are also called **alkanes** or **paraffins** and have general formula C_nH_{2n+2}, where $n = 1,2,3$. Methane is the first member of this group.

Unsaturated Hydrocarbons

They have general formula C_nH_{2n} for alkene and C_nH_{2n-2} for alkynes. These have atleast one double (=) or triple (≡) bond and are called alkenes and alkynes respectively. e.g. Ethylene

Aromatic Hydrocarbons

They have ring structure with alternate double bonds and $(4n+2)\pi e^-$ (**Huckel's rule**), e.g. benzene, acetylene.

Exam Pattern Questions

1 The pure form of carbon is
(a) diamond (b) graphite
(c) charcoal (d) fullerene

2 Which allotrope of carbon is in rigid three-dimensional structure?
(a) Graphite (b) Fullerene
(c) Diamond (d) Carbon black

3 Hardest allotrope of carbon is
(a) diamond (b) graphite
(c) coke (d) lamp black

4 The material used in the manufacture of lead pencil is
(a) graphite (b) lead (c) carbon (d) mica

5 Which have high capacity of absorbing gas?
(a) Coal (b) Coke
(c) Charcoal (d) All of these

6 Which is used as reducing agent in metallurgy?
(a) Graphite (b) Coke (c) Coal (d) Fullerene

7 Which of the following is not a form of carbon?
(a) Soot (b) Haematite
(c) Graphite (d) Charcoal

8 Which gas is used as a fire extinguisher?
(a) Carbon dioxide (b) Carbon monoxide
(c) Carbon suboxide (d) Sulphur dioxide

9 CO_2 in water behaves as
(a) weak dibasic acid H_2CO_3
(b) weak monobasic acid HO—COOH
(c) weak diacid base $CO(OH)_2$
(d) weak monoacid base HO—COOH

10 CO_2 is a colourless, odourless gas and less soluble in water, but forms
(a) dibasic acid with water
(b) carbonic acid with water
(c) Both (a) and (b)
(d) None of the above

11 Which of the following statement(s) is/are incorrect regarding carbon dioxide?
(a) It is acidic in nature
(b) It combines with alkali to form metal carbonates
(c) It is present in atmosphere to the extent of 0.03% by volume
(d) None of the above

12 0.03% of carbon dioxide present in the atmosphere can be removed by
(a) conversion of CO_2 to glucose
(b) photosynthesis
(c) chemical change of CO_2 to carbohydrate
(d) All of the above

13 Which one among the following is responsible for the expansion of water in ocean?
(a) Carbon dioxide (b) Nitrogen dioxide
(c) Carbon monoxide (d) Sulphur dioxide

14 General formula of alkane
(a) C_nH_{2n+2} (b) C_nH_{2n}
(c) $C_{2n}H_{2n+2}$ (d) None of these

15 Paraffin are called
(a) Unsaturated hydrocarbon
(b) Saturated hydrocarbon
(c) Aromatic hydrocarbon
(d) None of the above

16 The first stable member of alkane series is known as
(a) ethane (b) methane
(c) propane (d) None of these

17 What is the nature of hydrocarbon that contains at least one double bond?
(a) Saturated (b) Unsaturated
(c) Aromatic (d) Cyclic

18 General formula of alkenes is
(a) C_nH_{2n-2} (b) C_nH_{2n+2}
(c) C_nH_{2n} (d) C_nH_{2n-1}

19 The general formula for alkynes is
(a) C_nH_{2n-2} (b) C_nH_{2n-4}
(c) C_nH_{2n+2} (d) C_nH_{2n-1}

20 Aromatic compounds are
(a) cyclic compounds
(b) aliphatic compounds
(c) saturated compounds
(d) All of the above

Answers

1 *(a)*	2 *(c)*	3 *(a)*	4 *(a)*	5 *(c)*	6 *(b)*	7 *(b)*	8 *(a)*	9 *(a)*	10 *(c)*
11 *(d)*	12 *(d)*	13 *(a)*	14 *(a)*	15 *(b)*	16 *(b)*	17 *(b)*	18 *(c)*	19 *(a)*	20 *(a)*

Chapter 10 Acids, Bases and Salts

Acids

- Substances, which are sour in taste and turns blue litmus to red are called acids.
- Some common fruits such as unripe mango, lemon, orange, tamarind etc., are sour in taste. This suggests that these fruits contain acids.
- Acids are also defined as those substances which furnish hydrogen ions (H^+) or hydronium ions (H_3O^+) on dissociation or ionisation in an aqueous solution.

Chemical Properties of Acids

- Acids form salts on reacting with most of the metals with the evolution of hydrogen gas.
  e.g. $Zn + H_2SO_4 \longrightarrow ZnSO_4 + H_2 \uparrow$
- Acids reacts with metal carbonates and metal hydrogen carbonates to produce salt, carbon dioxide gas and water.
  e.g. $CaCO_3 + 2HCl \longrightarrow CaCl_2 + H_2O + CO_2 \uparrow$
- Acids give salt and water on reaction with metallic (basic) oxides.
  e.g. $CuO + 2HCl \longrightarrow CuCl_2 + H_2O$

  Some naturally occurring acids are :

Natural source	Acid
Vinegar	Acetic acid
Orange and Lemon	Citric acid
Tamarind	Tartaric acid
Tomato	Oxalic acid
Curd	Lactic acid
Ant sting and Nettle sting	Methanoic acid

Bases or Alkalies

- Substances that furnish hydroxide ions (OH^-) on dissociation or ionisation in an aqueous solution are called bases.
- They are bitter in taste and soapy to touch and turn red litmus solution to blue.
- Bases, which are soluble in water are called alkalies. Thus all alkalies are basis, but all bases are not alkalies

Chemical Properties of Bases

- Strong bases react with active metals to form salt and produce hydrogen gas.
  e.g. $Zn + 2NaOH \longrightarrow Na_2ZnO_2 + H_2 \uparrow$
- Oxides of non-metal (acidic) on reaction with base give salt and water.
  e.g. $CO_2 + Ca(OH)_2 \longrightarrow CaCO_3 + H_2O$
- Strong bases (like NaOH, KOH, $Ca(OH)_2$, etc.) are completely dissociated or ionised in water, whereas weak bases (like NH_4OH, $Al(OH)_3$ etc.) ionises only partially.

Now, we will study about sodium hydroxides which is a strong base.

Caustic Soda (NaOH)

Chemical Name Sodium hydroxide
Common Name Caustic soda

Uses

- It is used as a reagent in laboratory. It is used in de-greasing metals.
- It is used to manufacture the soap, paper, rayon, dyes, pure fat and oils.
- It is used in purification of bauxite and in petroleum refining.

Reaction Between Acids and Bases

- Acids react with bases to produce salt and water.
- In this reaction, an acid neutralises a base, i.e. acid nullifies or reduces the effect of a base or *vice-versa*, thus reaction is known as **neutralisation reaction.**

$$\text{Base} + \text{Acid} \longrightarrow \text{Salt} + \text{Water}$$

$$HX + MOH \longrightarrow MX + HOH,$$
[where, M = metal]

$$H^+ + OH^- \longrightarrow H_2O(l)$$

- Mixing of an acid or base with water is called **dilution.** It results in decrease in the concentration of ions (H_3O^+ / OH^-) per unit volume.
- Dissolving an acid or base in water is highly exothermic (heat generating) reaction. So, care must be taken while doing it.

pH Scale

- It is a scale used for measuring hydrogen ion concentration. It has values ranging from 0 (very acidic) to 14 (very alkaline). Thus, pH is a number, which indicates the acidic or basic nature of a solution. $pH = -\log[H^+]$
  - If $pH > 7$, solution is basic.
  - If $pH < 7$, solution is acidic.
  - If $pH = 7$, solution is neutral.

Salts

- Salts are produced by the neutralisation reaction between acid and base.
- Salts of a strong acid and a strong base are neutral with pH value of 7.
- Salts of a strong acid and weak base are acidic with pH value less than 7.
- Salts of strong base and weak acid are basic in nature with pH value more than 7. Now, we will study about some salts and their uses.

Common Salt (NaCl)

Chemical Name Sodium chloride

Uses

- It is used in cooking as well as in cooking gas.
- It is commonly used as condiment and food preservative.
- It is used in many industrial processes.
- It is an important rawmaterial for various materials of daily use, like baking powder, bleaching powder etc.

Bleaching Powder $Ca(OCl)Cl$ or $CaOCl_2$

Chemical Name Calcium hypochlorite or calcium oxychloride or chlorite of lime or chlorinated lime.

Uses

- It is used as bleaching agent for cotton, linen and wood pulp.
- It is used as a disinfectant and germicide especially in the sterilisation of drinking water.
- It is used for manufacturing of chloroform.
- It is used as an oxidising agent in many chemical industries.
- It is used as cleaning process of sugar.

Baking Soda ($NaHCO_3$)

Chemical Name Sodium hydrogen carbonate or sodium bicarbonate.

Uses

- It is used as baking powder which is a mixture of baking soda (sodium hydrogen carbonate) and mild edible acid (such as tartaric acid).
- It is used as foamy drinking substances.
- It is used in medicines. It is also present as an ingredient in antacids. Being alkaline, it neutralises excess acid in the stomach.
  $$NaHCO_3(s) + HCl(l) \longrightarrow NaCl(aq) + H_2O(l) + CO_2(g)$$
- It is also used in fire extinguishers.

Washing Soda ($Na_2CO_3 \cdot 10H_2O$)

Chemical Name Sodium carbonate

Uses

- It is used for washing purposes, for removing the hardness of water, in manufacturing of glass, paper, caustic soda, detergent, etc.
- It is used in the form of laboratory reagent.
- It is used as medicine of eye and in the form of anti-bacterial agent.

Plaster of Paris $\left(CaSO_4 \cdot \frac{1}{2} H_2O\right)$

Chemical Name Calcium sulphate hemihydrate

Uses

- It is used as plaster to joint the broken bones.
- It is used to form scalpture's and toy's.
- It is used in dental treatment to smooth the walls and to decorate them.
- It is used as fire resistance substance.

Exam Pattern Questions

1 Which is present more in aqueous solution of a strong acid?
(a) H^+ ions (b) OH^- ions
(c) Cl^- ions (d) Na^+ ions

2 Which of the following is a strong base?
(a) $Ca(OH)_2$ (b) KOH
(c) $Mg(OH)_2$ (d) NH_4OH

3 Acetic acid is a weak acid because
(a) quantity of water is greater
(b) its ionisation is small
(c) it is an organic acid
(d) it is an inorganic acid

4 Number of acidic hydrogen atoms present in sulphuric acid are
(a) 2 (b) 1 (c) 3 (d) zero

5 Citric acid is present in free form in
(a) tamarird (b) milk (c) apple (d) lemon

6 Substances that furnish (OH^-) on dissociation or ionisation in a aqueous solution are called
(a) acids (b) bases
(c) salts (d) All of these

7 Which one among the following statements about the bases is correct?
(a) All bases are alkalies
(b) None of the bases is alkali
(c) $SnCl_2$ is an alkali
(d) All alkalies are bases, but all bases are not alkalies

8 Mixing of acids or bases in water are called
(a) neutralisation (b) dilution
(c) decomposition (d) dissociation

9 Which of the following statement is correct about a neutral solution?
(a) pH value is greater than 7
(b) pH value is smaller than 7
(c) pH value is zero
(d) pH value is 7

10 pH value of acidic solution is
(a) 7 (b) less than 7
(c) more than 7 (d) zero

11 pH value of pure water is
(a) 0 (b) 1 (c) 7 (d) 14

12 Which of the following is an acidic salt?
(a) NaCl (b) $NaHSO_4$
(c) Na_2SO_4 (d) KCN

13 The aqueous solution of sodium carbonate is
(a) weakly acidic (b) strongly acidic
(c) basic (d) neutral

14 The combination of hydrochloric acid and sodium hydroxide solution forms
(a) common salt (b) caustic soda
(c) bleaching powder (d) baking soda

15 The chemical name of caustic soda is
(a) sodium hydroxide (b) sodium chloride
(c) sodium bicarbonate (d) calcium sulphate

16 The compound used for disinfecting water is
(a) washing soda (b) baking soda
(c) caustic soda (d) bleaching powder

17 The chemical formula of baking soda is
(a) Na_2CO_3 (b) $NaHCO_3$
(c) NaCl (d) NH_4Cl

18 Chemical name of washing soda is
(a) sodium bicarbonate (b) sodium hydroxide
(c) sodium carbonate (d) sodium oxide

19 Formula of plaster of Paris
(a) $CaSO_4 \cdot \frac{1}{2}H_2O$ (b) $Ca_2SO_3 \cdot \frac{1}{2}H_2O$
(c) $Ca_2 \cdot \frac{1}{2}H_2O$ (d) $CaSO_4 \cdot H_2O$

20 Common salt is not used as
(a) codiment (b) food preservative
(c) germicide (d) raw material

21 Bleaching powder can be used as
(a) baking soda (b) medicine
(c) germicide (d) antacid ingredient

22 A salt which can be used as anti bacterial agent for eye is
(a) common salt (b) baking soda
(c) $CaOCl_2$ (d) washing soda

Answers

1 *(a)*	2 *(b)*	3 *(b)*	4 *(a)*	5 *(d)*	6 *(b)*	7 *(d)*	8 *(b)*	9 *(d)*	10 *(b)*
11 *(c)*	12 *(c)*	13 *(b)*	14 *(c)*	15 *(a)*	16 *(a)*	17 *(d)*	18 *(b)*	19 *(c)*	20 *(c)*
21 *(c)*	22 *(d)*								

Chapter 11

Natural and Artificial Fertilisers

Natural Fertiliser

- Natural fertiliser or organic fertilisers are derived from animal matter, animal excreta, human excreta and vegetable matter.
- Naturally occurring organic fertilisers include animal wastes from meat processing, peat, manure slurry and guano.

Manure

- It is well decomposed refuse from the stable and barn yards including both animal excreta and straw or other litter.
- The term 'manure' implies to any material with the exception of water which when added to the soil makes it productive and promotes plant growth.
- Natural or organic manures which are bulky in nature and supply nutrients in small quantities and organic matter in large quantities.

Green Manuring

- It is a practice of ploughing in the green plant tissues in the field or adding green plants with tender twigs or leaves from outside and incorporating them into the soil for improving the physical structure as well as fertility of the soil.

Compost

The process of decomposing organic wastes is called composting and the decomposed material is called compost.

Vermicompost

- Vermicompost can be prepared in the field pit.
- In the lack of space in the garden, it can be started in containers like earthen pot, metal container, plastic tub, domestic waste and crop residues are to be stored in pit/container.
- Cowdung and red earthworms are added into the collected waste.

Artificial Fertilisers

- Fertilisers are inorganic substances that contain one or more ingredients of plant food in large proportions.
- Fertilisers which contain only one plant nutrient, called straight fertilisers. Such fertilisers are called nitrogenous or phosphatic or potassic fertilisers e.g. urea.
- Fertilisers which contain two or more nutrients, in one compound is known as complex or compound fertilisers.
- Complex fertilisers are granular and easy to apply, e.g. DAP, ammonium phosphate sulphate.

Nitrogenous Fertilisers

The nitrogenous fertilisers are broadly classified into four groups

- **Nitrate Fertilisers** Nitrate group of fertilisers are soluble in water and hygroscopic in nature.
  - These are alkaline in nature and contains less percentage of nitrogen than other groups.
  - The nitrate is not absorbed by the soil. They are applied in small doses.

- Examples of nitrate fertilisers are sodium nitrate (16%N), calcium nitrate (15.0% N), potassium nitrate (13% N).

- **Ammonium Fertilisers** This group of fertilisers are widely used, particularly ammonium sulphate.
- It is soluble in water but not hygroscopic.
  - They are acidic in nature.
  - Rice is the merely crop which can utilise the ammonical nitrogen.
  - This group of fertilisers may be used in basal application and top dressing.
- **Nitrate and Ammonium Fertilisers** These group of fertilisers are soluble in water but moderately hygroscopic like ammonium nitrate, ammonium sulphate, etc., in this group of fertilisers both ammonium and nitrate are present.
  - It is acidic in nature and used in top dressing and basal application.
- **Amide Fertilisers** It is soluble in water and hygroscopic in nature.
  - These fertilisers are converted to ammonium carbonate and then to nitrates due to action of microorganism.
  - The conversion of amides into ammonical and nitrate form takes about 6-7 days.
  - Amide fertilisers like– urea, calcium cynamide.

Phosphatic Fertilisers

- Those fertilisers, which contain and supply only the phosphorus content are phosphatic fertilisers they are expressed in oxidised form, P_2O_5,while its content in soil and plant is expressed in elemental form as 'P'.
- Phosphorus fertilisers are classified into three groups
  - (i) **Water soluble** SSP, DSP, TSP, etc.
  - (ii) **Citrate soluble** Basic slag, Di-calcium phosphate.
  - (iii) **Insoluble** Rock phosphate, raw bone meal, etc.

Some of there important examples are as follows:

- **Single super phosphate** $[Ca(H_2PO_4)_2]$ contain 16-20% P_2O_5.
- **Diammonium phosphate** $(NH_4)_2HPO_4$ contain 54% P_2O_5 and 21% nitrogen. It is acidic in nature.
- **Triple super phosphate** $[3Ca(H_2PO_4)_2]$ contain 40-48% P_2O_5.
- **Super phosphate** In rock phosphate is converted into a soluble form by treating with sulphuric acid and the resulting product is called super phosphate (ordinary).
- **Basic slag** It is much effective in high rainfall area and that are neutral to acidic in soil reaction. It contain 3-5% P_2O_5. It is alkaline in nature.
- **Rock phosphate** $[Ca_3(PO_4)_2]$ contain P_2O_5 20-30%. It is insoluble fertilisers.

Potassic Fertilisers

- **Potassium fertilisers** These are water soluble, but not hygroscopic in nature. There are no leachy loss.
- **Potassium chloride** Its use is found effective in acidic and heavy soils.
- **Chemical form** It is KCl.
- **Potassium chloride** It contains 60% K_2O.

NPK Fertilisers

These fertilisers supply N, P and K to the soil. They are also known as mixed fertilisers.

Exam Pattern Questions

1 The major nutrients are
(a) Fe, Zn, Mn (b) N, P, K
(c) Cu, Mo, B (d) None of these

2 Richest source of nitrogen is
(a) dried blood (b) raw bone meal
(c) fish manure (d) dry activated sludge

3 The most widely used source of nitrogen in agriculture in India is
(a) urea (b) FYM
(c) DAP (d) CAN

4 Which of the following is a biofertilizer?
(a) Green algae
(b) FYM
(c) Compost
(d) All of the above

5 A complex mixture of brown or dark brown amorphous and colloidal substances modified from the original tissues or synthesised by various soil organisms is referred as
(a) compost (b) FYM
(c) peat (d) humus

6 The presence of VAM enhances uptake of nutrients in general but particularly of
(a) Ca (b) Mg (c) Mo (d) P

7 Nitrogen is a major nutrient because
(a) it is available in soil more
(b) it is available in soil less
(c) it is required by plants more
(d) it is available in atmosphere more

8 Urea hydrolysis in the soil produces
(a) uric acid (b) amides
(c) ammonium carbonate (d) None of these

9 A straight fertiliser is one which
(a) comes straight from the factory
(b) has one major nutrient
(c) dissolves quickly
(d) None of the above

10 Complex fertilisers contain more than one major nutrient in a
(a) mixture
(b) combined form
(c) complicated combination
(d) None of the above

11 Fertilisers are added to increase a soils
(a) volume (b) fertility
(c) depth (d) life

12 AS is better than urea on S-deficient soils, because it has
(a) sulphur (b) ammonium
(c) sulphuric acid (d) water

13 Ammonium produced by urea can be absorbed by roots or it can
(a) change to nitrate
(b) go back to urea
(c) form complexes
(d) None of the above

14 Fertilisers SSP dissolve in soil to furnish phosphate, calcium and
(a) acid (b) chalk
(c) sulphur (d) boron

15 Plants absorb nutrients mostly through
(a) leaves (b) stem
(c) roots (d) seeds

16 Fertilizers contain one or more
(a) minerals (b) plant nutrients
(c) elements (d) atoms

17 In tree crops fertiliser is not added near the trunk because of
(a) less roots there (b) termites
(c) shade (d) All of these

18 The N in all fertilisers comes from
(a) naptha (b) gas
(c) air (d) water

19 The most common phosphate fertiliser in India
(a) SSP (b) 12-32-16
(c) DAP (d) Rock-P

20 The use of balanced fertiliser use is most desirable because it
(a) adds all nutrients (b) corrects all deficiencies
(c) adds NPK (d) None of these

21 The optimum fertiliser dose is one which maximises
(a) yield (b) soil fertility
(c) profits (d) water use

22 If fertiliser prices go up the optimum close should
(a) come down (b) stay unchanged
(c) also go up (d) None of these

23 Most common zinc fertiliser is
(a) zinc-chelate (b) zinc-oxide
(c) zinc-sulphate (d) zinc ash

24 India's rank in fertilisers consumption in the world is
(a) 6 (b) 10
(c) 21 (d) 3

25 The least hygroscopic fertiliser is
(a) SOP (b) CAN
(c) SSP (d) NPK Complex

26 A fertiliser not listed in the FCO cannot be labelled an sold as fertiliser because it is
(a) not recognised as fertiliser
(b) adulterated
(c) harmful
(d) None of the above

27 The central fertiliser quality control institute is located at
(a) Krishi Bhawan (b) Hyderabad
(c) Pune (d) Faridabad

28 Efficient fertilisers use results in
(a) more crop per kg fertiliser
(b) hold grains
(c) early maturity
(d) None of the above

29 Fertiliser needed to make 300 L of 1% solution is
(a) 3 kg (b) 1 kg
(c) 30 kg (d) 300 kg

30 Green manures are mostly used as a source of
(a) zinc (b) carbon
(c) chlorophyll (d) nitrogen

31 Greatest damage to fertiliser is caused by
(a) railways (b) free acid
(c) hooks (d) delays

32 Fertilisers containing free acid should be packed in
(a) HDEP bags (b) air tight bags
(c) jute bags (d) Both (a) and (b)

33 Which of the following is nitrogenous fertiliser for amide group?
(a) Ammonium sulphate
(b) Urea
(c) CAN
(d) Sodium nitrate

34 Potassic fertiliser containing maximum quantity of potash is
(a) muriate of potash
(b) potassium nitrate
(c) sulphate of potash
(d) None of the above

35 The P_2O_5 in all fertilisers comes from
(a) DAP (b) sulphur
(c) phosphate rock (d) electricity

Answers

1 (b)	2 (b)	3 (a)	4 (a)	5 (d)	6 (d)	7 (c)	8 (c)	9 (b)	10 (b)
11 (b)	12 (c)	13 (a)	14 (c)	15 (c)	16 (b)	17 (a)	18 (c)	19 (c)	20 (b)
21 (c)	22 (a)	23 (c)	24 (d)	25 (c)	26 (a)	27 (d)	28 (a)	29 (a)	30 (d)
31 (c)	32 (a)	33 (b)	34 (a)	35 (c)					

PRACTICE SETS
(1-2)

Indian Army

Nursing Assistant

Practice Set 1

1. The first Indian to get Nobel Prize
(a) Dr. C.V. Raman
(b) Rabindranath Tagore
(c) Amartya Sen
(d) Mahatma Gandhi

2. Which of the sites of Indus valley civilisation is found near Sutlej river?
(a) Ropar (b) Lothal
(c) Rakhigarhi (d) Banawali

3. The currency of Myanmar is known as
(a) Rufiyaa (b) Kyat
(c) Peso (d) Rupiah

4. On which date Vernal Equinox is observed?
(a) 21st March (b) 21st June
(c) 23rd September (d) 22nd December

5. What is the full form of UGC?
(a) University Grants Commission
(b) Union Goods Class
(c) United Grants Commission
(d) University Great Council

6. Under which articles of the Constitution are the cultural and educational rights granted?
(a) Article 29 and 30 (b) Article 25 and 26
(c) Article 31 and 32 (d) Article 23 and 24

7. The first Asian Games were held in
(a) Tokyo (b) Shanghai
(c) New Delhi (d) Mumbai

8. Find the 11th letter to the left of 20th letter from left in the English alphabet.
(a) D (b) J
(c) K (d) I

9. Pointing to a man Deepak said, "His only brother is the father of my daughter's father". How is the man related to Deepak?
(a) Grandfather (b) Father
(c) Uncle (d) Brother-in-law

10. If EARN is written as GCTP, how NEAR can be written in that code?
(a) CTGP (b) GPTC
(c) PGCT (d) PCGT

11. Which one is an irrational number?
(a) 22/7 (b) π
(c) 1.333 (d) 3.14

12. What is the least number by which 1470 must be divided to get a number which is a perfect square?
(a) 7 (b) 5
(c) 30 (d) 35

13. In how many year will a sum of ₹3000 yield a simple interest of ₹1080 at 12% per annum?
(a) 3 yr (b) $2\frac{1}{2}$ yr
(c) 2 yr (d) $3\frac{1}{2}$ yr

14. Cost price of an object is ₹1000. On selling it, the loss of 7% is incurred. Find the SP of that object.
(a) ₹ 980 (b) ₹ 930 (c) ₹ 940 (d) ₹ 950

15. The value of y in the solution of the equation $2^{x+y} = 2^{x-y} = \sqrt{8}$ is
(a) 0 (b) $\frac{1}{4}$ (c) $\frac{1}{2}$ (d) $\frac{3}{7}$

16. Which among the following is the fundamental quantity?
(a) Mass (b) Volume
(c) Velocity (d) Force

17. Which of the following is a scalar quantity?
(a) Velocity (b) Acceleration
(c) Force (d) Distance

18. Who defined the law of gravitation?
(a) Newton (b) Archimedes'
(c) Galileo (d) Faraday

19. The earth moving around the sun in a circular orbit is acted upon by a force and hence work done on the earth by the force is
(a) zero (b) positive
(c) negative (d) None of these

20. Out of solid, liquid and gas which has maximum elasticity?
(a) Solid (b) Gas
(c) Liquid (d) Cannot be compared

21. In which one of the following animals, skin is a respiratory organ?
(a) Cockroach (b) Frog
(c) Shark (d) Whale

22. Which of the following pairs has open type of circulatory system?
(a) Earthworm and leech (b) Man and whale
(c) Cockroach and silverfish (d) Tadpole larva and fish

23. Which of the following animals does not have nervous system?
(a) Leech (b) Tapeworm
(c) *Amoeba* (d) Snail

24. Cockroach cannot survive in the water because its respiratory organ is
(a) gill (b) trachea
(c) book lung (d) pulmonary sac

25. Types of vertebrate animals which creep and crawl are called
(a) mammalians
(b) amphibians
(c) molluscs
(d) reptilians

26. Which one of the following set belongs to the class Mammalia?
(a) Lion, hippopotamus, penguin, bat
(b) Lion, bat, whale, ostrich
(c) Hippopotamus, penguin, whale, kangaroo
(d) Whale, bat, kangaroo, hippopotamus

27. In coriander, the useful parts are
(a) roots and leaves
(b) leaves and flowers
(c) leaves and dried fruits
(d) flowers and dried fruits

28. Bryophytes resemble algae due to the feature
(a) no photosynthesis
(b) have photosynthetic activity but no vascular tissue
(c) have photosynthetic activity and vascular tissue both
(d) None of the the above

29. Amphibians are those animals that
(a) live on land (b) live under land
(c) live on land and water (d) live under water

30. Panda belongs to the same family as that of
(a) whale (b) bear
(c) kangaroo (d) porcupine

31. The type of tail found in shark is
(a) homocercal (b) heterocercal
(c) diphycercal (d) porcupine

32. Clitellum is found in
(a) leech (b) snail
(c) nereis (d) earthworm

33. The scavengers of earth are
(a) bacteria (b) viruses
(c) algae (d) fungi

34. Five-Kingdom, classification was given by
(a) Whittaker (b) Haeckel
(c) Linneus (d) Copeland

35. Animals with chitinous exoskeleton are
(a) insects (b) sponges
(c) sea-urchin (d) snails

36. Which of the following is the latest discovered state of matter?
(a) Solid (b) Gas
(c) Plasma (d) BEC

37. Atomic theory of matter was given by
(a) Avogadro(b) Dalton (c) Newton (d) Pascal

38. How many elements are found naturally?
(a) 18 (b) 98 (c) 108 (d) 118

39. Who introduced the symbols for representing the elements?
(a) Bohr (b) Dalton
(c) Lavoiser (d) Proust

40. Who put the law of conservation of mass
(a) Antonie Lavoisier (b) Joseph proust
(c) Dalton (d) P. V Proust

41. The process in which a substance losses electron
(a) oxidation (b) reduction
(c) combustion (d) reversible

42. In which ratio hydrogen and oxygen are present in water
(a) 1 : 8 (b) 8 : 1
(c) 2 : 4 (d) None of these

43. Hydrogen is much less abundant in the earth's atmosphere because of its
(a) low enthalpy of fusion
(b) low enthalpy of vaporisation
(c) light nature
(d) All of the above

44. The pure form of carbon is
(a) diamond (b) graphite
(c) charcoal (d) fullerene

45. Which is present more in aqueous solution of a strong acid?
(a) H^+ ions (b) OH^- ions
(c) Cl^- ions (d) Na^+ ions

46. The process also named as de-electronation
(a) combustion
(b) oxidation
(c) reduction
(d) All of the above

47. Which of the following metal and acid are used to prepare dihydrogen respectively?
(a) Crystalline zinc with dil. HCl
(b) Granulated zinc with dil. HCl
(c) Granulated zinc with conc. HCl
(d) Crystalline zinc with conc. HCl

48. Hardest allotrope of carbon is
(a) diamond (b) graphite
(c) coke (d) lamp black

49. Acetic acid is a weak acid because
(a) quantity of water is greater
(b) its ionisation is small
(c) it is an organic acid
(d) it is an inorganic acid

50. The most widely used source of nitrogen in agriculture in India is
(a) urea (b) FYM
(c) DAP (d) CAN

Answers

1 (b)	2 (a)	3 (b)	4 (a)	5 (a)	6 (a)	7 (c)	8 (d)	9 (c)	10 (c)
11 (b)	12 (c)	13 (a)	14 (b)	15 (a)	16 (a)	17 (d)	18 (a)	19 (a)	20 (a)
21 (b)	22 (c)	23 (c)	24 (b)	25 (d)	26 (d)	27 (c)	28 (b)	29 (c)	30 (b)
31 (b)	32 (d)	33 (a)	34 (a)	35 (d)	36 (b)	37 (b)	38 (b)	39 (b)	40 (a)
41 (a)	42 (a)	43 (c)	44 (a)	45 (a)	46 (b)	47 (b)	48 (a)	49 (b)	50 (a)

Indian Army

Nursing Assistant

Practice Set 2

1. Who was the first person to receive Jnanpith Award?
(a) G. Shankar Kurup (b) Rabindranath Tagore
(c) Munsi Premchand (d) Ashapoorna Devi

2. Which metal was not known to Indus valley people?
(a) Gold (b) Silver
(c) Bronze (d) Iron

3. Which is the deepest ocean in the world?
(a) Indian ocean (b) Atlantic ocean
(c) Pacific ocean (d) Arabian sea

4. On which date, National Science Day is celebrated?
(a) 30th January (b) 28th February
(c) 31st May (d) 5th June

5. How many parts are in Indian Constitution?
(a) 18 (b) 32
(c) 42 (d) 52

6. Currency of Saudi Arabia is
(a) Dinar (b) Lira
(c) Riyal (d) None of these

7. Santosh trophy is related with
(a) Cricket (b) Football
(c) Golf (d) Hockey

8. Find the next number in the series.
2, 15, 41, 80, ?
(a) 111 (b) 120
(c) 121 (d) 132

9. Pitch is related to Cricket, in the same way as Arena is related to ……
(a) Tennis (b) Gymnastic
(c) Badminton (d) Wrestling

10. Complete the second pair in the same way as first pair.
EGIK : LJHF : : SUWY : ?
(a) ZXVT (b) TVXZ
(b) LNPR (d) MOQS

11. The smallest odd prime number is
(a) 0 (b)1 (c) 2 (d) 3

12. Find the duplicate ratio of 7:9.
(a) 7:9 (b) $\sqrt{7}$:3 (c) 49:81 (d) 81:49

13. LCM of 15, 18, 36 and 144 is
(a) 144 (b) 360
(c) 1440 (d) 720

14. The degree of polynomial $336x^2 + 210x + 42$ is
(a) 3 (b) 4 (c) 42 (d) 2

15. If α and β are the roots of the equation $x^2 - 8x + p = 0$ and $\alpha^2 + \beta^2 = 40$, then p is equal to
(a) 12 (b) 10 (c) 9 (d) 11

16. Which of the following is not a vector quantity?
(a) Speed (b) Torque
(c) Momentum (d) Displacement

17. What is called 'change in position in a particular direction of an object'?
(a) Velocity (b) Acceleration
(c) Displacement (d) None of these

18. For the relation $F = \frac{GMm}{r^2}$, the quantity G
(a) depends on the value of g at the place of observation
(b) is used only when the earth is one of the two masses
(c) is greatest at the surface of the earth
(d) is universal constant of nature

19. If F force is applied on a body and body get displaced by s displacement, then work done on the body will be
(a) work = force/displacement
(b) work = displacement/force
(c) work = force × displacement
(d) None of the above

20. A body floats in a liquid, if the buoyant force is
(a) zero (b) greater than its weight
(c) less than its weight (d) equal to its weight

21. Which of the following is a tapeworm?
(a) Fasciola (b) Schistosoma
(c) Taenia (d) Enterobius

22. The medicine for epilepsis formed with the help of
(a) fungi (b) Lichen
(c) bacteria (d) algae

23. Which one of the following is incorrect?
(a) Leeuwenhoek–Microscope
(b) Robert Brown–Cell Theory
(c) Protoplasm–Purkinje
(d) Robert Hooke–Cell

24. Cellular totipotency is
(a) Capability of plant cells to form complete plant
(b) Formation of a new species
(c) Formation of a new plant
(d) Synthesis of new cell

25. Which of the pair is incorrect?
(a) Chlorophyll–green (b) Chromoplast–yellow
(c) Leucoplast–colourless (d) Elaioplast–red

26. Which organelle is also called director of the cell?
(a) Mitochondria (b) Nucleus
(c) Chloroplast (d) Ribosomes

27. In which phase of meiosis, centromere divides?
(a) Metaphase–I (b) Anaphase–II
(c) Anaphase–I (d) Metaphase–II

28. In the region of kinetochores, what attaches to the chromosomes?
(a) Centrosome (b) Spindle fibres
(c) Nucleus (d) Chromatids

29. Which one of the following corresponds for the start of M-phase?
(a) Cytokinesis
(b) G_1-phase
(c) Karyokinesis
(d) Karyogenesis

30. Nuclear envelope and nucleolus disappearance occur at the end of
(a) prophase (b) interphase
(c) metaphase (d) telophase

31. DNA or chromosome replication occurs during which phase?
(a) Prophase (b) Telophase
(c) Metaphase (d) Interphase

32. Which one among the following animal tissue transport hormones, heat and maintains water balance?
(a) Connective tissue (b) Blood
(c) Muscular tissue (d) Nervous tissue

33. Respiratory tract has
(a) compound epithelia
(b) pseudostratified epithelium
(c) stratified columnar epithelium
(d) stratified ciliated columnar epithelium

34. Shock resistive layer in human body is made up of
(a) proteins (b) fats
(c) carbohydrates (d) vitamins

35. Through 'photosynthesis' green plants generate
(a) inorganic materials
(b) minerals
(c) organic materials
(d) nutrients

36. Which of the following is/are in the plasma state?
(a) Mars (b) Jupiter
(c) Sun (d) All of these

37. What particles move around the nucleus of an atom and are negatively charged?
(a) Electrons (b) Protons
(c) Positrons (d) Neutrons

38. The heaviest naturally occurring element is
(a) osmium (b) uranium
(c) mercury (d) polonium

39. Symbol of antimony is
(a) Sb (b) Tb
(c) An (d) W

40. Which law is known as law of indestructibility of matter ?
(a) Law of multiple proportion
(b) Law of definite proportion
(c) Law of conservation of mass
(d) Avogadro's law

41. Identify the species undergoing oxidation

$$H_2S + Cl_2 \longrightarrow 2HCl + S$$

(a) Cl_2 (b) H_2S
(c) HCl (d) H_2O

42. The fraction of water available for human use is oblique ...... of the total global water.
(a) 0.3% (b) 0.001%
(c) 0.003% (d) 3%

43. How many neutrons are present in protium, deuterium and tritium respectively?
(a) 1, 0 and 2 (b) 0, 2 and 1
(c) 0, 1 and 2 (d) 2, 1 and 0

44. Which of the following is a strong base?
(a) $Ca(OH)_2$ (b) KOH
(c) $Mg(OH)_2$ (d) NH_4OH

45. Richest source of nitrogen is
(a) dried blood
(b) raw bone meal
(c) fish manure
(d) dry activated sludge

46. Which of the following consists of ionised gas?
(a) Plasma (b) BEC
(c) Carbon monoxide (d) Oxygen

47. The three basic components of an atom are
(a) protons, neutrons and ions
(b) protons, neutrons and electrons
(c) protium, deuterium and tritium
(d) protons, electrons and ions

48. Who classified elements into triads on the basis of their atomic weights?
(a) Mendeleev (b) Newlands
(c) Mosley (d) Dobereiner

49. Symbol of sodium is
(a) Ne (b) So (c) S (d) Na

50. If 6.3 g of $NaHCO_3$ are added to 15.0 g of CH_3COOH solution, the residue is found to weight 18.0 g. What is the mass of CO_2 released in the reaction ?
(a) 3.3 g (b) 3.31 kg
(c) 33 g (d) 3 g

Answers

1 (a)	2 (d)	3 (c)	4 (b)	5 (a)	6 (c)	7 (b)	8 (d)	9 (d)	10 (a)
11 (d)	12 (c)	13 (d)	14 (d)	15 (a)	16 (a)	17 (c)	18 (d)	19 (c)	20 (d)
21 (c)	22 (b)	23 (b)	24 (a)	25 (d)	26 (b)	27 (b)	28 (b)	29 (c)	30 (a)
31 (d)	32 (b)	33 (b)	34 (b)	35 (c)	36 (c)	37 (a)	38 (a)	39 (a)	40 (c)
41 (b)	42 (c)	43 (c)	44 (b)	45 (b)	46 (a)	47 (b)	48 (d)	49 (d)	50 (a)

CURRENT AFFAIRS

IMPORTANT CURRENT EVENTS

National

India Gets First Rafale Aircraft, Chinook & Apache Helicopters

- India has signed a €7.87 billion deal with France in Sept, 2016 to purchase 36 Rafale fighter jets out of which India has received first aircraft on October 8, 2019.
- Eight United States-made Apache AH-64E attack helicopters and four CH47 Chinook heavy-lift choppers inducted into Indian Air Force.

Mega Mergers of Public Sector Banks

- Finance Minister Niramala Sitharaman announced amalgamation of 10 public sector banks into four big banks and with this the number of public sector banks reduced from 27 to 12.
- Oriental Bank of Commerce and United Bank to be amalgamated with Punjab National Bank; Syndicate Bank to be merged with Canara Bank; Union Bank will subsume Andhra Bank and Corporation Bank; and Allahabad Bank will be merged with Indian Bank.

Article 370 Revoked

The Centre on August 5, 2019 scrapped the Article 370 of the Constitution which provided Special Status to the state of Jammu & Kashmir, thus converting the state into 2 union territories viz., UT of Jammu & Kashmir with a legislature and UT of Ladakh without a legislature.

National People's Party Designated as National Party

- The ruling NPP, in Meghalaya, was granted recognition as a National Party by the Election Commission of India.
- The NPP becomes the first party from the North-East to get the national party status.

Chandrayan-2 Launched

India has successfully launched its second lunar mission Chandrayan-2, aboard a GSLV Mk-III rocket from Satish Dhawan Space Centre, Sriharikota on July 22, 2019; consisting of an orbiter, a lander named Vikram and a rover dubbed Pragyaan to study the lunar surface.

First Lokpal Appointed

Former Supreme Court Judge Justice Pinaki Chandra Ghose was appointed as the India's first Lokpal by the President Ram Nath Kovind on March 20, 2019.

47th Chief Justice of India Appointed

President Ram Nath Kovind appointed Justice Sharad Arvind Bobde as the 47th Chief Justice of India, he succeeded Ranjan Gogoi.

Pradhan Mantri Kisan Maan Dhan Yojana Launched

Prime Minister Narendra Modi launched the Kisan Maan Dhan Yojana on September 12, 2019 at Ranchi, Jharkhand to improve the lives of 5 Crore small and marginal farmers of the country.

India's Tallest ATC Tower

India's tallest Air Traffic Control (ATC) tower built at Delhi's Indira Gandhi International Airport with 102-meter height.

India's Longest Electrified Train Tunnel Inaugurated

Vice President M. Venkaiah Naidu inaugurated the India's longest electrified rail tunnel between Cherlopalli and Rapuru and the electrified railway line between Venkatachalam and Obulavaripalli.

Ocean Energy Got Renewable Energy Status

- The Ministry of New and Renewable Energy has declared Ocean Energy as renewable energy.
- Energy produced using various forms of ocean energy such as tidal, wave, ocean thermal energy conversion among others shall be considered as renewable energy.

PM Narendra Modi Announced Appointment of CDS

In his Independence Day speech, PM Narendra Modi announced the appointment of a Chief of Defence Staff (CDS) who will be above the three Service Chiefs. A CDS is a high-ranking officer of the Army, Navy or Air Force and the single point of contact between the armed forces and the Prime Minister.

Standing Wheelchair Launched

IIT Madras has launched India's first indigenously-designed Standing Wheelchair – 'Arise'; for assisting the specially-abled person in day-to-day activities.

Government Granted 'Maharatna' Status to Hindustan Petroleum and Power Grid

The government accorded 'Maharatna'; status to state owned Public Sector Undertaking's (PSU's) Hindustan Petroleum and Power Grid Corporation.

International

First All Women Spacewalk

Two NASA astronauts namely Christina Koch and Jessica Meir made space history as they completed the first-ever spacewalk by an all-woman team on October 18, 2019.

New Definition of Kilogram

The kilogram had been given a new definition based on the most precise measurement ever made of the Planck constant, which can be expressed in terms of the SI units kilogram, meter and second.

NASA Discovered First Super Earth

NASA's Transiting Exoplanet Survey Satellite (TESS) mission, in July 2019, had discovered GJ 357d, a Super-Earth located 31 light years away from our Solar System.

Global Hunger Index 2019

Global Hunger Index 2019 is topped by Belarus, followed by Bosnia & Herzegovina and Bulgaria at the second and third place, respectively. While India ranked 102nd with a score of 30.3 out of 117 countries.

World's First Floating Nuclear Reactor

Russia has launched world's first floating nuclear reactor called Akademik Lomonosov; loaded with nuclear fuel from Arctic port of Murmansk for its 5,000 kilometre voyage to Pevek in North-Eastern Siberia.

Awards and Prizes

National

28th Vyas Samman 2019

Noted Hindi writer Nasira Sharma was conferred the 2019 Vyas Samman for her novel 'Kagaz Ki Naav'.

Dada Saheb Phalke Award 2019

Legendary actor Amitabh Bachchan has been selected for the 66th Dada Saheb Phalke award for the year 2018.

Rajiv Gandhi Khel Ratna Award 2019

Rajiv Gandhi Khel Ratna award 2019 was awarded to Paralympic silver-medallist Deepa Malik and wrestler Bajrang Punia.